Evidence-Based Infectious Diseases

Evidence-Based Infectious Diseases

Third Edition

Edited by

Dominik Mertz
Associate Professor, Division of Infectious Diseases
McMaster University
Hamilton, Ontario, Canada

Fiona Smaill
Professor, Department of Pathology and Molecular Medicine
McMaster University
Hamilton, Ontario, Canada

Nick Daneman
Clinician-Scientist, Division of Infectious Diseases
Sunnybrook Health Sciences Centre
University of Toronto
Toronto, Ontario, Canada

WILEY Blackwell

Registered Office(s)
John Wiley & Sons, Inc., 111 River Street, Hoboken, NJ 07030, USA
John Wiley & Sons Ltd, The Atrium, Southern Gate, Chichester, West Sussex, PO19 8SQ, UK

Editorial Office
9600 Garsington Road, Oxford, OX4 2DQ, UK

For details of our global editorial offices, customer services, and more information about Wiley products visit us at www.wiley.com.

Wiley also publishes its books in a variety of electronic formats and by print-on-demand. Some content that appears in standard print versions of this book may not be available in other formats.

Library of Congress Cataloging-in-Publication Data

Names: Mertz, Dominik, editor. | Smaill, Fiona, editor. | Daneman, Nick, editor.
Title: Evidence-based infectious diseases / edited by Dominik Mertz, Fiona Smaill, Nick Daneman.
Description: Third edition. | Hoboken, NJ : Wiley, 2018. | Includes bibliographical references and index. |
Identifiers: LCCN 2018010575 (print) | LCCN 2018011367 (ebook) | ISBN 9781119260332 (pdf) |
    ISBN 9781119260356 (epub) | ISBN 9781119260318 (paperback)
Subjects: | MESH: Communicable Diseases–diagnosis | Communicable Diseases–therapy |
    Evidence-Based Medicine
Classification: LCC RC112 (ebook) | LCC RC112 (print) | NLM WC 100 | DDC 616.9–dc23
LC record available at https://lccn.loc.gov/2018010575

Cover Design: Wiley
Cover Image: © Raycat/Gettyimages

Set in 10/12pt Warnock by SPi Global, Pondicherry, India

10 9 8 7 6 5 4 3 2 1

Contents

List of Contributors

Ali Amini, MA, MB, BChir, MRCP, DTM&H
Infectious Diseases
University of Oxford
Oxford, UK

Monique Andersson, MBBS, MD, MRCP, FRCPath, DTM&H
Department of Medical Virology
University of Stellenbosch
Cape Town, South Africa
and
Department of Infectious Diseases
and Microbiology
Oxford University Hospitals NHS
Foundation Trust
Oxford, UK

Brian Angus, BSc, MBChB, DTM&H, MD, FRCP, FFTM
Nuffield Department of Medicine
Oxford University
Oxford, UK

Douglas Austgarden, BSc, MD, FRCPC
Department of Critical Care
Royal Victoria Regional Health Centre
Barrie, Ontario, Canada

Lise Bondy, MD, FRCP
Division of Infectious Diseases
Western University
London, Ontario, Canada

Eric J. Bow, MD, MSc, D Bacteriol, FRCPC
Departments of Medical Microbiology and
Infectious Diseases, and Internal Medicine
Sections of Infectious Diseases and
Haematology/Oncology
Max Rady College of Medicine
The University of Manitoba
Winnipeg, Manitoba, Canada

Peter Daley, MD, MSc, FRCPC, DTM&H
Disciplines of Medicine and Laboratory
Medicine
Memorial University
Eastern Health
St. John's, Newfoundland, Canada

Guilio DiDiodato, MD, FRCPC, MPH
Department of Medicine
University of Toronto
Antimicrobial Stewardship Program
Royal Victoria Regional Health Centre
Barrie, Ontario, Canada

Mark Downing, MD
Division of Infectious Diseases
Saint Joseph's Health Centre
Toronto, Ontario, Canada

Thomas Fekete, MD
Temple University School of Medicine
Philadelphia, PA, USA

Bahareh Ghadaki, BSc, MD, FRCPC
Division of Infectious Disease
Department of Medicine
Niagara Health
St. Catharines, Ontario, Canada

Wayne L. Gold, MD, FRCPC
Department of Medicine
University Health Network
University of Toronto
Toronto, Ontario, Canada

Ravindra Gupta, MA, BMBCh, MPH, PhD, FRCP, FRCPath
Division of Infection and Immunity
University College London
London, UK

Alainna J. Jamal, Hon BSc
Faculty of Medicine
University of Toronto
Toronto, Ontario, Canada

Jennie Johnstone, MD, PhD
St. Joseph's Health Center
Public Health Ontario
and
Dalla Lana School of Public Health
University of Toronto
Toronto, Ontario, Canada

Christopher E. Kandel, MD, FRCPC
University Health Network
University of Toronto
Toronto, Ontario, Canada

Joanne M. Langley, MD, MSc
Community Health and Epidemiology
Dalhousie University
Halifax, Nova Scotia, Canada

Christine H. Lee, MD, FRCPC
Department of Pathology and Molecular Medicine
McMaster University
Hamilton, Ontario
and
Department of Pathology and Laboratory Medicine
University of British Columbia
Vancouver, British Columbia, Canada

Paul A. Moroz, BSc
University of British Columbia
Vancouver, British Columbia, Canada

Andrew M. Morris, MD, SM (Epi)
Department of Medicine
Sinai Health System
University Health Network
and
University of Toronto
Toronto, Ontario, Canada

Eli N. Perencevich, MD, MSc
Internal Medicine and Epidemiology
University of Iowa
Carver College of Medicine
Iowa City, IA, USA

Nora Renz, MD
Attending Internal Medicine Physician
Septic Surgery Unit
Center for Musculoskeletal Surgery
Charité - Universitätsmedizin Berlin
Berlin, Germany

Ashley Roberts, MD, MEd, FRCPC
Division of Pediatric Infectious Diseases
British Columbia Children's Hospital/
University of British Columbia
Vancouver, British Columbia, Canada

Bram Rochwerg, MD, MSc
Department of Medicine (Critical Care)
McMaster University
Department of Health Research Methods, Evidence and Impact
McMaster University
Hamilton, Ontario, Canada

Gregory W. Rose, MD, MSc (Epi), FRCPC
Infection Prevention and Control
Infectious Diseases consultant
Queensway Carleton Hospital
Ottawa, Ontario, Canada

Michael S. Silverman, MD, FRCP, FACP
Division of Infectious Diseases
Western University
London, Ontario, Canada

Marek Smieja, MD, PhD, FRCPC
Pathology and Molecular Medicine
McMaster University
Hamilton, Ontario, Canada

Graham M. Snyder, MD, SM
Division of Infectious Diseases
Beth Israel Deaconess Medical Center
Boston, MA, USA

Jocelyn A. Srigley, MD, MSc
Infection Prevention and Control
Provincial Health Services Authority
and
Department of Pathology & Laboratory
Medicine
BC Children's & Women's Hospitals
and
Department of Pathology & Laboratory
Medicine
University of British Columbia
Vancouver, British Columbia, Canada

**Kaede Sullivan, MD, MSc, FRCPC, FAAP, FCCM,
D(ABMM)**
Department of Pathology and Laboratory
Medicine
Lewis Katz School of Medicine
Temple University
Philadelphia, PA, USA

Darrell H. S. Tan, MD, FRCPC, PhD
Division of Infectious Diseases
University of Toronto
Toronto, Ontario, Canada

Courtney A. Thompson, MD, FRCPC
Division of Infectious Diseases
University Health Network
Toronto, Ontario, Canada

Andrej Trampuz, MD
Center for Musculoskeletal Surgery
Charité - Universitätsmedizin Berlin
Berlin, Germany

Louis Valiquette, MD
Department of Microbiology and Infectious
Diseases
Faculté de Médecine et des Sciences de la Santé
Université de Sherbrooke
Sherbrooke, Québec, Canada

Deborah Yamamura, BSc, MD, FRCPC
Hamilton Health Sciences
Hamilton General Site
and
Associate Professor
Department of Pathology and
Molecular Medicine
McMaster University
Hamilton, Ontario, Canada

Preface

Following the success of our original edition in 2004 and the second edition in 2009, we are privileged to have this opportunity to edit an updated version of *Evidence-Based Infectious Diseases*. We have targeted this book to general internists and to trainees and staff physicians in infectious diseases and hospital epidemiology, as feedback from the previous editions indicated that our textbook was particularly helpful to these groups.

We hope that this new edition will bring added value, while continuing to serve as an evidence-based resource for physicians who manage patients with infections. Major updates in the current edition include: a) introducing wording that reflects the level of evidence supporting the recommendations made, b) adding new chapters on health-care associated pneumonia, *Clostridium difficile* infection, and antimicrobial stewardship, and c) in order to fit these chapters into the book, we needed to cut the other chapters which resulted in more concise and condensed text.

We are grateful to the chapter authors for all of their hard work. We hope that you will find this edition informative and we welcome any feedback.

Chapter 1

Introduction to Evidence-based Infectious Diseases

Dominik Mertz, Nick Daneman, and Fiona Smaill

The purposes of this first chapter are to provide brief overviews of the scope of the third edition of this book as well as evidence-based infectious diseases (EBID) practice, and to introduce the approach we implemented to reflect the level of evidence supporting recommendations made in this book.

1.1 What is Evidence-based Medicine?

Evidence-based medicine was born in the 1980s of the last century [1,2]. David Sackett, the founding chair of the Department of Clinical Epidemiology and Biostatistics at McMaster University, defined *evidence-based medicine* as "the conscientious, explicit and judicious use of current best evidence in making decisions about the care of patients" [3]. One of the key aspects of evidence-based medicine is a focus on randomized clinical trials (RCTs) for assessing treatment, which now is a standard requirement for the licensing of new therapies.

1.2 Evidence-based Infectious Diseases (EBID)

The field of infectious diseases, or more accurately the importance of illness due to infections, played a major role in the development of epidemiological research in the 19th and early 20th centuries. Classical observational epidemiology was derived from studies of epidemics—infectious diseases such as cholera, smallpox, and tuberculosis. Classical epidemiology was nevertheless action-oriented. For example, John Snow's observations regarding cholera led to his removal of the Broad Street pump handle in an attempt to reduce the incidence of cholera. Pasteur, on developing an animal vaccine for anthrax, vaccinated a number of animals with members of the media in attendance [4]. When unvaccinated animals subsequently died, while vaccinated animals did not, the results were immediately reported throughout European newspapers.

In the era of clinical epidemiology, it is notable that the first true RCT is widely attributed to Sir Austin Bradford Hill's 1947 study of streptomycin for tuberculosis [5]. In subsequent years, and long before the "large simple trial" was rediscovered by the cardiology community, large-scale trials were carried out for polio prevention as well as tuberculosis prevention and treatment.

Infectious diseases were at the frontiers of both classical and clinical epidemiology, but is current infectious diseases practice evidence-based? We believe the answer is "somewhat." We have excellent evidence for the efficacy and side effects of many modern vaccines and antiviral drugs for treatment of HIV and Hepatitis C. Furthermore, non-inferiority

Evidence-Based Infectious Diseases, Third Edition. Edited by Dominik Mertz, Fiona Smaill, and Nick Daneman.
© 2018 John Wiley & Sons Ltd. Published 2018 by John Wiley & Sons Ltd.

trials are mandatory for new antibiotics to receive approval from the FDA and other regulatory authorities for specific indications. This being said, the current use of many anti-infectives are not supported by high-level RCT data, and head-to-head comparisons of different anti-infectives and/or durations of treatment are largely missing. Thus, the acceptance of before-and-after data to prove the efficacy of antibiotics for syndromes such as bacterial meningitis is ethically appropriate and recommended in guidelines despite the fact that no RCT data exists. Therefore, it is not surprising that recommendations in Infectious Diseases Society of America (IDSA) guidelines are primarily based on low-quality evidence derived from non-randomized studies or expert opinion [6].

Furthermore, in treating many common infectious syndromes—from sinusitis and cellulitis to pneumonia—we have many very basic diagnostic and therapeutic questions that have not been optimally answered. How do we reliably diagnose pneumonia? Which antibiotic is most effective and cost-effective? Can we improve on the impaired quality of life that often follows such infections as pneumonia? Furthermore, there may not be a single "best" antibiotic for pneumonia, in contrast to treatment algorithms for myocardial infarction that apply uniformly to the majority of patients. Much of the "evidence" that guides therapy in infectious diseases, particularly for bacterial diseases, may not be clinical, but exists in the form of a sound biologic rationale, the activity of the antimicrobial against the offending pathogen, and the penetration at the site of infection (pharmacodynamics and pharmacokinetics). Still, despite having a sound biologic basis for choice of therapy, there are many situations where better RCTs need to be conducted and where clinically important outcomes, such as symptom improvement and health-related quality, are measured.

How, then, can we define *EBID*? Paraphrasing David Sackett, *EBID* may be defined as "the explicit, judicious and conscientious use of current best evidence from infectious diseases research in making decisions about the prevention and treatment of infection of individuals and populations." It is an attempt to bridge the gap between research evidence and the clinical practice of infectious diseases. Such an "evidence-based approach" may include critically appraising evidence for the efficacy and safety of a treatment option. However, it may also involve finding the best evidence to support (or refute) use of a diagnostic test to detect a potential pathogen. Additionally, EBID refers to the use of the best evidence to estimate prognosis of an infection or risk factors for the development of infection. EBID therefore represents the application of research findings to help answer a specific clinical question. In so doing, it is a form of knowledge transfer, from the researcher to the clinician. It is important to remember that use of research evidence is only one component of good clinical decision-making. Experience, clinical skills, and a patient-centered approach are all essential components. EBID serves to inform the decision-making process. For the field of infectious diseases, a sound knowledge of antimicrobials and microbiologic principles are also needed.

1.3 Posing a Clinical Question and Finding an Answer

The first step in practicing EBID is posing a clinically driven and clinically relevant question. To answer a question about diagnosis, therapy, prognosis, or causation, we can begin by framing the question [2]. The question usually includes a brief description of the patients, the intervention or exposure, the comparison, and the outcome (PICO). For example, if asking about the efficacy of antimicrobial-impregnated catheters in intensive care units [7], the question can be framed as follows: "In critically ill patients, does the use of antibiotic-impregnated catheters, compared with regular vascular catheters, reduce central line associated infections?" After framing the question, the second step is to search the literature. The most time-efficient approach is to search for evidence-based synopses and systematic reviews in a first step. Systematic reviews can be considered as concise summaries of the best available evidence that address sharply defined clinical questions. If there are no synopses or systematic reviews that can answer the clinical question, the next step is to search the primary literature itself, which, of course, is much more time-consuming. After finding the evidence the next step is to critically appraise it.

1.4 Evidence-based Diagnosis

Let us consider the use of a rapid antigen detection test for group A streptococcal infection in throat swabs. The first question to ask is whether there was a blinded comparison against an accepted reference standard. By *blinded*, we mean that the measurements with the new test were done without knowledge of the results of the reference standard.

Next, we would assess the results. Traditionally, we are interested in the sensitivity (proportion of reference-standard positives correctly identified as positive by the new test) and specificity (the proportion of reference-standard negatives correctly identified as negative by the new test).

Ideally, we would also like to have a measure of the precision of this estimate, such as a 95% confidence interval on the sensitivity and specificity, although such measures are unfortunately rarely reported in the infectious diseases literature.

Note, however, that while the sensitivity and specificity may help a laboratory to choose the best test to offer for routine testing, they do not necessarily help the clinician manage the patient. Thus, faced with a positive test with known 95% sensitivity and specificity, we cannot infer that our patient with a positive test for group A streptococcal infection has a 95% likelihood of being

infected. For this, we need a positive predictive value, which is calculated as the percentage of true positives among all those who test positive. If the positive predictive value is 90%, then a positive test would suggest a 90% likelihood that the person is truly infected. Similarly, the negative predictive value is the percentage of true negatives among all those who test negative. Both positive and negative predictive value change with the underlying prevalence of the disease, hence such numbers cannot be generalized to other settings.

A more sophisticated way to summarize diagnostic accuracy, which combines the advantages of positive and negative predictive values while solving the problem of varying prevalence, is to quantify the results using likelihood ratios. Like sensitivity and specificity, likelihood ratios are a constant characteristic of a diagnostic test and independent of prevalence. However, to estimate the probability of a disease using likelihood ratios, we additionally need to estimate the probability of the target condition (based on prevalence or clinical signs). Diagnostic tests then help us to shift our suspicion (pretest probability) about a condition depending on the result. Likelihood ratios tell us how much we should increase the probability of a condition for a positive test (positive likelihood ratio) or reduce the probability for a negative test (negative likelihood ratio). More formally, likelihood ratio positive (LR+) and negative (LR−) are defined as:

$$LR+ = \frac{\text{odds of a positive test in an individual with the condition}}{\text{odds of a positive test in an individual without the condition}}. \quad (1.1)$$

$$LR- = \frac{\text{odds of a negative test in an individual with the condition}}{\text{odds of a negative test in an individual without the condition}}. \quad (1.2)$$

A positive likelihood ratio is also defined as sensitivity/(1 – specificity), and the negative likelihood ratio as (1 – sensitivity)/specificity.

Having found that the results of the diagnostic test appear favorable for both diagnosing or ruling out disease, we ask whether the results of a study can be generalized to our patients. We might also call this "external validity" or "generalizability" of the study. Here, we are asking the question: "Am I likely to get the same results as in this study in my own patients?" This includes such factors as the severity and spectrum of patients studied, technical issues in how the test is performed outside the research setting, but also the epidemiology of pathogens in your area that affects pre-test probabilities—a unique additional challenge we face in infectious diseases.

Important caveats, however, are that (a) there may be no appropriate reference standard, and (b) the spectrum of illness may dramatically change the test characteristics, as may other co-interventions such as antibiotics. For example, let us assume that we are interested in estimating the diagnostic accuracy of a new commercially available polymerase chain reaction (PCR) test for the rapid detection of *Neisseria meningitidis* (*N. meningitidis*) in spinal fluid. The reference standard of culture may not be completely sensitive. Therefore, use of an expanded reference ("gold") standard might be used. For example, the reference standard may be growth of *N. meningitidis* from the spinal fluid, demonstration of an elevated white blood cell count in the spinal fluid along with gram-negative bacilli with typical morphology on Gram stain, or elevated white blood cell count along with isolation of *N. meningitidis* in the blood. It is also important to know in what type of patients the test was evaluated, such as the inclusion and exclusion criteria, as well as the spectrum of illness. Given that growth of microorganisms is usually progressive, test characteristics in infectious diseases can change depending when the tests are conducted. For example,

PCR conducted in patients who are early in their course of meningitis may not be sensitive as compared to patients who presented with late-stage disease.

1.5 Evidence-based Treatment

The term *evidence-based medicine* has become largely synonymous with the dictum that only double-blinded RCTs give reliable estimates of the true efficacy of a treatment. For the purposes of guidelines, "levels of evidence" have been proposed, with a hierarchy from large to small RCTs, prospective cohort studies, case-control studies, and case series. In newer iterations of these "levels of evidence," a meta-analysis of RCTs (without statistical heterogeneity, indicating that the trials appear to be estimating the same treatment effect), are touted as the highest level of evidence for a therapy.

In general, clinical questions about therapy or prevention are best addressed through RCTs. In observational studies, the choice of treatment may have been influenced by extraneous factors that influence prognosis (so-called "confounding factors"). One of the most important confounding factors when comparing treatment options in an observational study is confounding by indication, that is, the treatment decision is made based on how the patient presents. For example, patients who appear more severely sick may receive predominantly treatment A as the treating physicians believe that treatment A is better than treatment option B. Given the inferior prognosis of patients receiving predominantly treatment A, this treatment option may appear inferior to treatment B, which was mostly given to less severely ill patients. Statistical methods exist to "adjust" for identified potentially confounding variables, and we can use propensity scores to adjust for confounding by indication. However, not all such factors are known or accurately measured.

An RCT, if large enough, deals with such extraneous prognostic variables by equally apportioning them to the two or more study arms by randomization. Thus, both known and unknown confounders are distributed roughly evenly between the study arms. For example, a RCT would be the appropriate design to assess whether dexamethasone administered prior to antibiotics reduces mortality in adults who have bacterial meningitis [8]. We would evaluate the following characteristics of such a study: who was studied, was there true random assignment, were interventions and assessments blinded, what was the outcome, and can we generalize to our own patients?

When evaluating clinical trials, it is important to ensure that assignment of treatment was truly randomized. Studies should describe exactly how the patients were randomized, and how the allocation was concealed. It is especially important here to distinguish allocation concealment from blinding. Allocation of an intervention can always be concealed even though blinding of investigators, participants, or outcome assessors may be impossible. Consider an RCT of antibiotics versus surgery for appendicitis. Blinding participants and investigators after patients have been randomized would be difficult as sham operations are ethically problematic. However, allocation concealment occurs before randomization. It is an attempt to prevent selection bias by making certain that the investigator has no idea to what arm (antibiotics versus surgery) the next patient enrolled will be randomized. In many trials, this is done through a centralized randomized process whereby the study investigator is given the assignment after the patient has been enrolled. In some trials, the assignment is kept in envelopes. The problem with this is that, if the site investigator (or another clinician) has a preference for one particular intervention over another, the possibility for tampering exists.

The degree of blinding in a study should also be considered. It is important to recognize that blinding can occur at multiple levels such as the investigators, other health care providers, the patients, the outcome assessors, the data monitoring committee, the data analysts, and even the manuscript writers [9]. Describing a clinical trial as "double-blinded" is vague if, in fact, blinding can occur at so many different levels. It is better to describe who was blinded than using generic terms.

Similarity of groups at baseline should also be considered to assess whether differences in prognostic factors at baseline may have had an impact on the result. A careful consideration of the intervention is also important. We can ask what actually constitutes the intervention—was there a co-intervention that really may have been the "active ingredient"?

Follow-up is another important issue. It is important to assess whether all participants who were actually randomized are accounted for in the results. The expectation nowadays is that the analysis is based on the intention-to-treat population, which is the most conservative approach. That is, all patients randomized are accounted for and are analyzed with respect to the group to which they were originally allocated. For example, an individual in our hypothetical appendicitis trial who was initially randomized to antibiotics but later received surgery would be considered in the analysis to have received antibiotics.

In a next step, we examine the results of the RCT. Consider a randomized controlled trial of two antibiotics A and B for community-acquired pneumonia. If the mortality rate with antibiotic A is 2% and that with B is 4%, the absolute risk reduction is the difference between the two rates ($4 - 2 = 2\%$), the relative risk of A versus B is 0.5, and the relative risk reduction is 50% ($2/4 \times 100 = 50\%$). In studies with time-to-event data, the hazard ratio is measured rather than the relative risk, and can be thought of as an averaged relative risk over the duration of the study. These risk estimates are all commonly reported with a 95% confidence interval (CI) as a measure of precision. A 95% CI that does not cross 1.0 (for a relative risk or hazard ratio) or 0 (for the absolute risk reduction) has the same interpretation as a p value of <0.05, and we would declare these results as "statistically significant." Unlike the p value, the 95% CI gives us more information regarding the size of the treatment effect. Importantly, the lack of a statistically significant difference between two treatment options does not imply equal efficacy: The 95% CI presents a range of plausible treatment effects. As this plausible effect can be either superior or inferior to the comparison group, the study must be considered indeterminate rather than assuming non-inferiority. It is also important to be aware that statistical significance and clinical importance are not synonymous. A small study may miss an important clinical effect, whereas a very large study may reveal a small but statistically significant difference of no clinical importance. In well-designed studies, researchers pre-specify the size of a postulated "minimum clinically important difference" and power the study accordingly rather than solely relying on statistical significance.

A more practical way of determining the size of a treatment effect is to translate the absolute risk reduction into its reciprocal, the number needed to treat (NNT). In this example, the number needed to treat is the number of patients who need to be treated to prevent one death. It is the inverse of the absolute risk reduction (1/0.02), which is 50. Therefore, if 50 patients are treated with antibiotic B instead of A, one death would be prevented. A 95% CI can be calculated on the NNT, although this should only be done if the 95% CI of the absolute risk reduction is not crossing 0.

It is important to determine if all patient-important outcomes were considered in the RCT. For example, a RCT of a novel immunomodulating agent for patients with severe West Nile virus disease would need not only to consider neurologic signs and symptoms, but also to assess functional status and health-related quality of life. When deciding whether the results of a RCT can be applied to your patients, the similarity in the setting and patient population needs to be considered. Finally, you must consider whether the potential benefits of the therapy outweigh the potential risks.

Rather than relying on individual RCTs, it is generally preferable to try to identify systematic reviews on the topic. Systematic reviews, however, also need to be critically evaluated. First, you must ensure that the stated question of the review addresses the clinical question that you are asking. Similar to critical appraisal of RCTs, you should assess the validity of the systematic review itself, in particular, the comprehensiveness of the search strategy, how rigorously the search of titles, abstracts, and full texts were conducted–optimally by at least two investigators independently–and whether the statistical analysis were appropriate. Furthermore, it is an expectation that the authors of the systematic review have critically appraised the studies included in their review, preferably by using the Cochrane risk of bias tool [10]. The most helpful systematic reviews would also GRADE [11] the certainty of evidence made, and as such, provide the reader with an objective assessment of strength of recommendation that can be made based on the identified evidence, an approach adapted in this book for recommendations made by the authors (see section 1.7).

In examining a treatment in the field of infectious diseases, a few other caveats are in order. For many infections, there may be a very strong historic and biologic rationale to treat; in such cases, an RCT using placebo will be unethical. Furthermore, many infections may be too rare to study in RCTs, and some infected populations (such as injection drug users) may be difficult to enroll into treatment studies [12]. Observational methods, such as case-control or cohorts to examine therapies or durations associated with cure or relapse, may be the most appropriate methods in these circumstances. Second, while individual patient RCTs are held up as an ideal, it may be more sensible to study many infections through so-called "cluster randomization" in which the unit of randomization may be a hospital, school, neighborhood, or family. In particular, in large simple trials that involve a change in policies, for example, in infection prevention and control, this study design may be more appropriate than an individual-patient RCT because infections are transmissible between patients and there may be herd effects of prevention methods. Third, infectious diseases are more dynamic than other illnesses due to new emerging pathogens, and so we frequently encounter new illnesses with no direct body of evidence to guide management (e.g., Middle East respiratory syndrome coronavirus [MERS-CoV]). Furthermore, the effectiveness of antimicrobials is not static, but rather diminishes over time due to the development of antimicrobial resistance, and so the absolute risk reductions and numbers needed to treat in a trial may not be accurate in the future, which is in contrast to, for example, the effect of acetylsalicylic acid in the setting of stroke. Finally, decisions on prevention of infection during outbreaks by newly emerging pathogens must be made when little to nothing is known about this new urgent public health threat. As a consequence, the need for immediate implementation of prevention and treatment approaches often overrides the possibility of conducting studies in order to obtain high-level evidence.

1.6 Evidence-based Assessment of Prognosis

Many studies about risk factors and outcomes for infectious diseases are published, but the quality is variable. The best designs for assessing these are cohort studies in which a representative sample of patients is followed, either prior to developing the infection (to determine risk) or after being infected (to determine outcome). Patients should be assembled at a similar point in their illness ("inception cohort"), and follow-up should be sufficiently long and complete. Important potential confounding prognostic factors should be measured and adjusted for in the analysis. As with clinical trials, the outcome measures are a relative risk, absolute

risk, or hazard ratio associated with a particular infection or prognostic factor. For example, to assess the outcome of patients with MERS-CoV infection, we would optimally want an inception cohort of individuals with a laboratory confirmed diagnosis as early in the course of the disease as possible. These individuals would then be followed prospectively. In general, as diagnostic tests improve, our ability to detect early disease will improve.

A challenge unique to infectious diseases is that many infections are transmissible. Thus, a case of disease is, by definition, also a risk factor of disease for others, which complicates research in this field further.

1.7 Our Approach to Reflect the Level of Evidence in this Book

As outlined earlier, RCTs in infectious diseases research are still rare compared to other specialties such as cardiovascular and oncology. Optimally, we would conduct a systematic review for all prognostic factors of interest, diagnostic approaches as well as therapeutic interventions. By doing so, we would assess the risk of bias in included studies, and would be able to GRADE the certainty of evidence and strength of recommendation [11]. Obviously, such an approach would not be feasible; however, we aimed to consider systematic reviews and certainty of evidence assessments made in these reviews wherever possible, and—where no systematic review data was available—authors as content experts were asked to assess the level of evidence themselves based on their best knowledge of the evidence available. Finally, in order to reflect the level of evidence, we used specific wording to reflect the level of evidence of therapeutic or diagnostic recommendations made in this book.

If the evidence for a certain recommendation is backed up by several well-conducted RCTs, we are using statements such as "we recommend," "it is recommended," or "one should." If there is some evidence available, however, mostly observational studies or small RCTs with wide confidence intervals and/or at high risk of bias, we are making a weak suggestion using terms such as "we suggest," "one might," or "may be used." If the recommendation is based on expert opinion or guideline recommendations only, without a reasonable amount of supporting evidence, we are using terms such as "experts in the field suggest," "expert opinion is," or "some guidelines recommend." By using these terms, we are hoping to make it clearer how confident we are that a specific recommendation should be followed.

1.8 Other Major Changes in the Third Edition of this Book

In addition to consistent wording to reflect the level of evidence supporting our recommendations, the third edition has several new chapters to reflect what had been emerging in terms of important infectious diseases topics over the last few years. These new chapters discuss health-care associated pneumonia, *Clostridium difficile* infection, and antimicrobial stewardship. In order to fit these new chapters into the book, we needed to cut the other chapters significantly, which resulted in more concise and condensed text. The chapters on long-term care in special populations, diarrhea, and infections in thermally injured patients have been omitted from the current version.

Acknowledgements

We would like to acknowledge the two editors of the first and second edition, Mark Loeb and Marek Smieja, who were not involved in this third edition. Their contributions are still reflected in Chapter 1, where we left some of the previous content unchanged.

References

1 How to read clinical journals: I. Why to read them and how to start reading them critically. Can Med Assoc J. 1981;124(5):555–8.

2 Oxman AD, Sackett DL, Guyatt GH. Users' guides to the medical literature. I. How to get started. The Evidence-Based Medicine Working Group. JAMA. 1993;270(17):2093–5.

3 Sackett DL, Rosenberg WM, Gray JA, Haynes RB, Richardson WS. Evidence based medicine: what it is and what it isn't. BMJ. 1996;312(7023):71–2.

4 Dubos R. Pasteur and Modern Science. Washington: ASM Press; 1998.

5 Daniels M, Hill AB. Chemotherapy of pulmonary tuberculosis in young adults: an analysis of the combined results of three Medical Research Council trials. Br Med J. 1952;1(4769):1162–8.

6 Khan AR, Khan S, Zimmerman V, Baddour LM, Tleyjeh IM. Quality and strength of evidence of the Infectious Diseases Society of America clinical practice guidelines. Clin Infect Dis. 2010;51(10):1147–56.

7 Detsky AS, Abrams HB, Forbath N, Scott JG, Hilliard JR. Cardiac assessment for patients undergoing noncardiac surgery: A multifactorial clinical risk index. Arch Intern Med. 1986;146(11):2131–4.

8 de Gans J, van de Beek D. Dexamethasone in adults with bacterial meningitis. N Engl J Med. 2002;347(20):1549–56.

9 Devereaux PJ, Manns BJ, Ghali WA, Quan H, Lacchetti C, Montori VM, et al. Physician interpretations and textbook definitions of blinding terminology in randomized controlled trials. JAMA. 2001;285(15):2000–3.

10 Higgins JP, Altman DG, Gotzsche PC, Juni P, Moher D, Oxman AD, et al. The Cochrane Collaboration's tool for assessing risk of bias in randomised trials. BMJ. 2011;343:d5928.

11 Atkins D, Best D, Briss PA, Eccles M, Falck-Ytter Y, Flottorp S, et al. Grading quality of evidence and strength of recommendations. BMJ. 2004;328(7454): 1490.

12 Darenberg J, Ihendyane N, Sjolin J, Aufwerber E, Haidl S, Follin P, et al. Intravenous immunoglobulin G therapy in streptococcal toxic shock syndrome: a European randomized, double-blind, placebo-controlled trial. Clin Infect Dis. 2003;37(3):333–40.

Part 1

Specific Diseases

Chapter 2

Skin and Soft-tissue Infections
Douglas Austgarden and Guilio DiDiodato

2.1 Impetigo

Impetigo is a common skin infection distributed worldwide. *S. aureus* and β-hemolytic streptococci are invariably the pathogens [1]. Typically, streptococcal impetigo (non-bullous impetigo) starts as papules, turning to pustules that break down forming the characteristic "honey-colored" crust. Bullous impetigo is more commonly associated with staphylococci. In this form, vesicles first appear that evolve to larger bullae and eventually rupture leaving a shiny thin brown "varnish-like" crust. Usually the lesions are on exposed areas of the body, typically the face and extremities. Infection occurs most frequently in children of lower socioeconomic groups. Patients with impetigo rarely have systemic signs of infection. There is evidence from a systematic review and meta-analysis that treatment with topical antibiotics is more effective than placebo (odds ratio [OR] 2.69, 95% confidence interval [CI] 1.49–4.86) [2].

There is no significant difference between the effects of mupirocin and fusidic acid (OR 1.7, 95% CI 0.77–4.03), but topical mupirocin was superior to oral erythromycin (OR 1.22, 95% CI 1.05–2.97) [2]. It is recommended to treat with topical mupirocin or retapamulin twice daily for five days [3]. If there are signs of systemic toxicity, an outbreak involving several persons, or outbreaks of post-streptococcal glomerulonephritis, an oral antibiotic such as cloxacillin, a first-generation cephalosporin or a macrolide is recommended for seven days [3]. In a recent, outcome assessor-blinded, non-inferiority randomized controlled study comparing IM penicillin versus oral co-trimoxazole among children with non-bullous impetigo in a region with highly endemic impetigo, a three- or five-day course of co-trimoxazole was non-inferior to a single IM dose of benzathine benzylpenicillin (absolute difference 0.5%, 95% CI -6.2–7.3, with pre-specified non-inferiority margin 10%) [4]. *S aureus* was identified from 412 (81%) of 508 children, *S. pyogenes* from 455 (90%), and both from 377 (74%). MRSA was isolated in 19% of children. This may represent a novel approach in highly endemic regions.

In cases of a non-resolving impetigo, infection may be with community-acquired methicillin resistant *S. aureus* (MRSA) and doxycycline, clindamycin, or TMP/SMX should be considered [3].

2.2 Furuncles and Carbuncles

Furuncles, or "boils," are infections of hair follicles usually caused by *S. aureus*. Typically, lesions are painful, erythematous nodules with an overlying pustule. When several furuncles coalesce to form a larger abscess this is a carbuncle. Large furuncles and all carbuncles should be incised and drained [3]. Warm compresses may promote drainage. Antibiotics are rarely required unless there

Evidence-Based Infectious Diseases, Third Edition. Edited by Dominik Mertz, Fiona Smaill, and Nick Daneman.
© 2018 John Wiley & Sons Ltd. Published 2018 by John Wiley & Sons Ltd.

are systemic symptoms or an extensive cellulitis. If a patient has signs of systemic toxicity, you may consider Gram stain and culture of pus, and an oral antibiotic active against MRSA such as TMP/SMX or doxycycline is recommended [3]. If a patient has severe Systemic Inflammatory Response Syndrome (SIRS) or hypotension, parenteral antibiotics such as vancomycin, linezolid or daptomycin should be empirically initiated pending cultures [3].

Outbreaks can occur within families and individuals in close living quarters (e.g., in prisons). Sports teams, especially involving contact sports, can also experience outbreaks. Recurrent furunculosis seems to be associated with *S. aureus* nasal colonization [5]. Those most at risk for persistent colonization appear to express high avidity binding receptors for *S. aureus*, along with being at high risk of environmental exposure to *S. aureus* through poor living conditions due to poverty, homelessness, overcrowding, poor hygiene, hospitalization, residence in a long-term care facility, or incarceration.

Eradication with mupirocin (applied to the nares for five days each month), chlorhexidine washes, and frequent cleaning of personal items can be considered for recurrent infections [3].

2.3 Cellulitis and Erysipelas

Case Presentation 1

A healthy 45-year-old man hit his forearm while doing house renovations, causing a minor abrasion three days prior to his presentation. He noted minor swelling, pain, and erythema yesterday, but this morning there was much more pain. His right forearm was swollen and erythema covered most of the dorsal surface from wrist to elbow. He is afebrile, pulse rate of 78 per minute, and blood pressure of 134/75 mmHg. He has a small abrasion on his wrist with erythema extending to the elbow. The erythema is not raised, has indistinct borders, with no vesicles or bullae. The lesion is warm, tender to palpation, but there is no increase in pain on movement.

Cellulitis usually presents with pain, erythema with typically indistinct borders, and swelling. Fever and regional lymphadenitis are occasionally seen. Unfortunately, these signs and symptoms are not specific and many other processes can present with similar clinical findings, for example, superficial or deep vein thrombophlebitis, fasciitis, hematoma, dermatitis, and local reaction to a bite or sting.

Most commonly, *S. aureus* and *S. pyogenes* are the pathogens [6]. Less often and usually associated with underlying chronic disease, immunosuppression, or infection at a particular site (e.g., periorbital cellulitis with sinusitis), pathogens can include *Haemophilus influenzae, Pseudomonas aeruginosa*, other *Streptococcus* spp., Gram-negative bacilli, *Clostridium* spp., and other anaerobes. If there has been exposure to water, specific organisms should be considered. In salt water, *Vibrio vulnificus* can cause a cellulitis and a potentially life-threatening infection in patients with liver disease. In fresh water, *Aeromonas hydrophilia* is a possible pathogen.

Erysipelas is a distinctive form of cellulitis. The lesion is typically bright red, warm, painful (which differentiates it from more superficial infections) with a raised, clearly demarcated border (usually not seen in other forms of cellulitis). Facial erysipelas with the malar "butterfly" rash represents only 15–20% of cases and most infections involve the lower extremity [6]. Systemic symptoms, for example, fever, chills, sweats, and rigors, are common. Infants, young children, and older adults are most commonly affected. Erysipelas has a predisposition for areas of impaired lymphatic drainage, and in these patients, recurrent episodes can occur. Group A streptococcus (*S. pyogenes*) is primarily responsible for erysipelas, but groups B, C, and G as well as *S. aureus* have been described [7].

Surface cultures, aspiration, and blood cultures all have low diagnostic yield in identifying the infecting organism causing cellulitis. In the healthy patient without an unusual exposure, microbiologic testing is neither necessary nor cost-effective [3,8].

Laboratory investigations may be required in the management of patients with chronic diseases, such as diabetes, liver disease, or renal failure, where an infection may lead to acute deterioration of the underlying disease, influencing the choice and dose of antibiotics and the decision whether to admit to hospital. Plain radiographs to rule out a foreign body are sometimes needed. Often radiographs are obtained to screen for tissue air if necrotizing fasciitis is a concern, or for osteomyelitis in an infected diabetic foot ulcer.

In determining the choice of appropriate initial antibiotic coverage and route of administration, it is recommended to stratify cellulitis into purulent versus non-purulent, then further stratify into mild, moderate, or severe disease according to number of SIRS criteria present (temperature >38°C or <36°C, HR >90/min, RR >20/min, WBC count >12000 or <4000/mm^3) and presence of hypotension, immune compromise, or rapid progression [3,6].

In mild and localized cellulitis in the otherwise healthy, an oral agent covering *S. aureus* and *Streptococcus* spp. is sufficient, and there is no advantage to agents with broader spectrum antimicrobial activity [3]. A penicillinase-resistant penicillin, first- or second-generation cephalosporin, or clinda-mycin have appropriate activity, and there is no evidence from small heterogeneous studies demonstrating superiority of one agent over another [9]. A five-day course of treatment is suggested initially, but may be extended to 7–10 days if symptoms have not improved [3,6].

In patients with moderate or severe cellulitis, it is generally accepted that parenteral antibi-otics are required. Studies of moderate or severe cellulitis have included patients with cellulitis and one or more of the following: extensive area, ulceration, abscess, signs of SIRS, associated with surgical site, bite, for-eign body, trauma, intravenous drug injection site, diabetic foot or pressure ulcer, immuno-suppression (cancer and HIV), diabetes,

chronic corticosteroid use, or failure of pre-vious therapy.

Many antibiotic regimens evaluated in methodologically sound studies have dem-onstrated similar efficacy with inpatient populations and complicated skin infections, but there is no good evidence to support any one regimen over another [6]. Experts gener-ally agree β-lactam antibiotics are preferred over fluoroquinolones due to a more favora-ble side effect profile [3,10].

Many patients can be treated with paren-teral antibiotic therapy on an outpatient basis [3]. Prospective evaluations of outpa-tient antibiotic programs have shown that they are safe and effective, and a randomized controlled trial of intravenous antibiotics at home or in a hospital for treatment of celluli-tis demonstrated no difference in outcome between the two groups (mean difference in days to no advancement of cellulitis) [11]. Patient satisfaction was greater in patients treated at home. Intravenous ceftriaxone has been widely recommended for outpatient therapy owing to its once daily dosing, how-ever penicillin, cefazolin, and clindamycin are appropriate alternatives [3].

Case Presentation 1 (continued)

You decide this patient has cellulitis and unlikely has fasciitis. Since he is otherwise well with no history of unusual exposure, you feel no additional tests are required. Although you are concerned about the size and rapidity of spread, you are comfortable sending him home on IV ceftriaxone, and when you see him in follow-up two days later, he has responded well and you switch him to complete a course of oral cephalexin.

MRSA is an uncommon cause of cellulitis; however, MRSA should be considered for purulent infections in known high-risk popu-lations, such as athletes, children, men who have sex with men, prisoners, military recruits, residents of long-term care facilities, indi-viduals with previous MRSA exposure, and intravenous drug users. Oral clindamycin or combination of TMP/SMX or doxycycline with a β-lactam antibiotic is recommended for mild infection, and parenteral vancomycin, linezolid, or daptomycin may be considered if there are signs of systemic infection [3,6].

Recurrent cellulitis can occur typically in lower extremities of patients with obesity, chronic edema, venous insufficiency, eczema, or toe web abnormalities. Prophylactic penicillin or erythromycin can be considered for these patients [3,12,13].

2.4 Necrotizing Fasciitis

Case Presentation 2

A previously healthy carpenter presents to the Emergency Department with fever and a painful arm. Yesterday, he began to notice a sore right shoulder, was assessed in the Emergency Department later that evening, and diagnosed with a soft-tissue injury. Today, he has pain in his shoulder and upper arm as well as fever and lethargy. On examination, he is in moderate distress from the pain, his temperature is 38.9 °C, heart rate 122 per minute, and blood pressure of 90/60 mmHg. There is no obvious trauma or rash on his arm, but it is generally swollen and exquisitely tender to palpation and on movement of the shoulder or elbow. You begin to wonder if this man has a life-threatening infection.

Necrotizing fasciitis involves infection of the subcutaneous tissue with rapid spread and destruction of skin, subcutaneous fat, and fascia. Multiple names have been given to fasciitis depending on the causative agent, for example, gas gangrene with *Clostridium*, or location, such as Fournier's of the perineum. The mainstay of initial treatment, however, involves prompt recognition, resuscitation, surgical debridement, and broad spectrum antibiotics regardless of presumed bacteria or location.

The literature on necrotizing fasciitis is predominately empiric, based on retrospective reviews and small case series. Due to the relative rarity of cases and the complexity of the illness, randomized trials of management have been difficult to undertake. Recommendations are predominately expert consensus, based on common bacteriological etiologies.

Prospective surveillance of invasive group A streptococcus in the United States from 2005 to 2012 reported an incidence of 3.8 cases per 100,000 person-years and a death rate for necrotizing fasciitis of 29% [14]. Hypotension on presentation, age over 65, bacteremia, chronic illness, and multi-organ failure are associated with increased mortality [14,15].

Necrotizing fasciitis should be considered in any patient with "cellulitis" and SIRS or rapidly spreading infection. Toxic shock syndrome and multi-organ failure are present in 47% of patients with group A streptococcus necrotizing fasciitis [15]. Commonly, necrotizing fasciitis starts at a preexisting skin lesion, such as a surgical site, trauma, injection site of an intravenous drug user, chronic skin problems (e.g., pressure ulcer, diabetic foot, ischemic ulcer, or psoriasis), and in children varicella infection predisposes to necrotizing fasciitis [16]. A predisposing skin lesion was present in 74% of cases of group A streptococcus necrotizing fasciitis [15]. Any underlying medical condition, such as diabetes, alcohol abuse, immunosuppressive illness or treatment, cardiac disease, peripheral vascular disease, chronic lung disease, or chronic renal failure should increase the suspicion for necrotizing fasciitis [16].

The presentation of necrotizing fasciitis can vary from the appearances of a simple cellulitis or soft-tissue injury to the classic hemorrhagic bullae, presence of soft-tissue gas, septic shock, and multi-organ failure [17]. Most cases of necrotizing fasciitis initially present with a cellulitis, but progress over hours to days with spreading erythema and edema. A distinguishing clinical feature is the wooden-hard induration of the subcutaneous tissues. In cellulitis, the subcutaneous tissues are palpable and yielding; in fasciitis, the underlying tissues are firm, and the fascial planes and muscle groups cannot be discerned by palpation. Hemorrhagic bullae can form as a result of skin necrosis secondary to vessel thrombosis. Pain out of proportion to clinical findings is commonly reported as an important early sign. Anesthetic skin due to destruction of nerves can be a late sign. Soft-tissue gas is a classic finding especially with clostridial infection. Estimates of the frequency of these signs and symptoms are not available.

Necrotizing fasciitis can be caused by many organisms and usually is polymicrobial with a mixture of aerobic and anaerobic bacteria. One review showed that 85% of confirmed cases of necrotizing fasciitis were polymicrobial, while *S. aureus*, *S. pyogenes*, and *Clostridium* spp. were the most commonly isolated single pathogen [18]. Usual aerobic pathogens are *S. aureus*, *S. pyogenes*, and *E. coli*, while *Clostridium* spp., *Bacteroides fragilis*, and *Peptostreptococcus* spp. are predominate anaerobes.

The gold standard for diagnosis is surgical exploration to determine fascial involvement and to provide material for culture and microscopic examination [3,19]. Surgical exploration will also indicate the need for surgical debridement. Frozen section biopsy with urgent histopathologic analysis may be useful in diagnosis [17]. Fine-needle aspirate is positive for bacteria or pus 80% of the time. Soft-tissue gas observed clinically or with plain films is diagnostic, but not always present. Ultrasound, CT, and MRI have all been used to aid in the diagnosis of necrotizing fasciitis [20]. Imaging should not delay definitive surgical treatment in the unstable patient, but when available, CT or MRI might be used to assist in diagnosis and define the extent of infection. Laboratory investigations such as creatinine kinase, C-reactive protein, serum sodium, white blood cell count, serum calcium, creatinine, urea, and coagulation profiles have all been proposed to aid diagnosis, but in general, lack the specificity to reliably rule out necrotizing fasciitis [17].

Experts suggest in suspected cases a small exploratory incision be made to determine if there is fascial involvement.

Immediate resuscitation, including ventilatory and inotropic support, prompt surgical debridement or amputation, and broadspectrum parenteral antibiotics are the mainstay of management [3]. Owing to the diversity of potential pathogens and because the majority of cases of necrotizing fasciitis are associated with polymicrobial infection, the most commonly recommended initial antibiotic is vancomycin, linezolid, or daptomycin plus pipercillin-tazobactam or a carbapenem or ceftriaxone and metronidazole, or in truly severe penicillin allergic patients, a fluoroquinolone and metronidazole.

Once a pathogen(s) has been identified, antibiotics should be tailored to the pathogen(s). The addition of clindamycin to penicillin may improve outcomes in streptococcal infections, and for group A streptococcus necrotizing fasciitis, penicillin and clindamycin is recommended [3]. In penicillin-allergic patients, a second- or third-generation cephalosporin can usually be safely substituted for penicillin. If a patient has a true penicillin/cephalosporin allergy, then vancomycin, linezolid, or daptomycin may be alternatives.

For MSSA, cloxacillin or cefazolin are recommended options and clindamycin if penicillin allergic, with vancomycin, linezolid, or daptomycin for MRSA. Clindamycin and penicillin are recommended for *Clostridium* species; doxycycline plus ciprofloxacin or ceftriaxone for *Aeromonas hydrophilia* and doxycycline plus third generation cephalosporin, for *Vibrio vulnificus* [3].

Intravenous immunoglobulin (IVIG) has been proposed as a treatment for group A fasciitis associated with toxic shock syndrome by mitigating the super-antigen response to group A streptococcus exotoxins, but its benefit is unclear. In a large retrospective cohort study of 4,127 cases, there was no significant difference in mortality nor hospital stay with IVIG [21]. Experts currently do not recommend the use of IVIG pending further research [3]. IVIG use in other forms of necrotizing fasciitis has not been studied and its use is not recommended in these settings.

Hyperbaric oxygen therapy (HBO) has been used as an adjunct for necrotizing fasciitis, but there are have been no randomized trials [22]. There is very weak evidence from multiple small, retrospective studies in both clostridial and nonclostridial necrotizing fasciitis of benefit [23]. While HBO should not delay surgical debridement and unstable patients should not be transferred, this treatment might be considered in centers with expertise.

For a discussion of post-operative necrotizing fasciitis, see Chapter 19, Infections in General Surgery.

2.5   Diabetic Foot Infections

Case Presentation 3

A 63-year-old man with a long-standing history of type 2 diabetes, complicated by peripheral neuropathy, presents with a two-day history of increasing drainage from an ulcer on his right foot. Today, redness and swelling in his foot was noted. On examination, he is afebrile, with a normal heart rate and blood pressure. On his right foot, he has a 2-cm ulcer on the sole between the first and second metatarsal heads, with swelling and erythema to the mid-foot dorsally. His blood sugar is 18 mmol/liter and his WBC count is normal.

Due to the triad of vascular insufficiency, peripheral neuropathy, and impaired immune function, foot ulceration and infection are common among diabetic patients. Foot infections are among the most common cause for hospital admission in such patients. Osteomyelitis is present in an estimated 20% of complicated infections, and diabetic foot infection accounts for 50% of lower extremity amputations. Diabetic foot infections need a multidisciplinary team approach involving endocrinologist, podiatrist, wound care specialist, diabetic educators, plastic, orthopedic, and vascular surgeons, and infectious disease specialists for their care [24,25]. However while the treatment of many patients is not in line with current guidelines [26], the evidence on the performance of diagnostic tests and interventions is weak and further research is needed [27].

Usually, diabetic foot infections occur in a preexisting ulcer and prior trauma is common [28]. Peripheral neuropathy is the greatest risk factor for foot ulcers and infection, and patients often have no complaints of pain. Patients will usually have discharge from the ulcer, erythema, swelling, and unexplained hyperglycemia. If there is no draining ulcer but the foot is erythematous and swollen, a Charcot foot (diabetic neuroarthropathy) should be considered.

Diabetic foot infections should be classified using a valid classification system based on the extent of local infection (swelling or induration, erythema, warmth, pain, and discharge), involvement of deeper tissues and systemic inflammatory response [25]. Patients with limb-threatening infections, however, often have no fever, chills, or elevated white blood cell count [25].

Surface cultures from wounds are not recommended for identifying infection in chronic wounds. Curettage of the base following debridement or aspiration from non-necrotic tissue is recommended and may yield more dependable results to identify the infecting pathogen(s) [25]. In non-limb-threatening infection, *S. aureus* and group B streptococcus are considered the major pathogens. *Enterococcus* spp., Gram-negatives and anaerobes are often cultured, but it is unclear if they are colonizers or pathogens. In moderate to severe diabetic foot infections, Gram-negatives such as *E. coli*, *Proteus* spp., *P. aeruginosa*, *Serratia* spp., and *Enterobacter* spp., and anaerobes, such as *Bacteroides* and *Peptostreptococcus* spp., are often isolated and usually considered pathogenic.

For non-limb-threatening infections, initial antimicrobial therapy should be directed toward *S. aureus* and streptococci, and a first-generation cephalosporin, for example, cefazolin, is an appropriate choice [25]. For limb-threatening diabetic foot infections, broad-spectrum antibiotics are recommended [25] and many of the trials of complicated or moderate to severe cellulitis included diabetic foot infections. Randomized trials specifically performed on diabetic foot infections included use of ampicillin/sulbactam, imipenem/cilastin, cefoxitin, ceftizoxime, ofloxacin, moxifloxacin, and ertapenem. All the trials had similar results with clinical cure or improvement in the range of 80–90%. A systematic review concluded that the evidence was too weak to recommend any particular antimicrobial agent for foot ulcers in diabetes [29]. In certain circumstances, outpatient therapy would be appropriate depending on diabetic control, extent of infection, and availability of follow-up.

There are other interventions that can be considered in the management of diabetic foot infections. While there is no evidence to support one type of wound dressing over another, experts suggest the selection of wound dressing should be based on the characteristics of the wound: if dry, it should be hydrated; if draining, the exudate should be absorbed; if necrotic, it should be debrided [25]. Relieving pressure is an important part of wound care and "off-loading pressure" with either a removable device or rigid immobilization is suggested to improve wound healing.

Negative pressure wound therapy and hyperbaric oxygen may be considered as adjunctive therapies based on very low-level evidence. Urgent vascular bypass surgery can be an option if ischemia is a major contributor to a non-healing ulcer or infection.

For a further discussion on the management of complicated infections and osteomyelitis in diabetic patients, refer to Chapter 3, Bone and joint infections.

2.6 Animal Bites

Animal bites are very common, but the vast majority of people never seek medical attention. Dogs account for around 60% of all bites, with another 10–20% of bites from cats [30]. An estimated 10,000 hospitalizations and 20 deaths per year occur secondary to dog bites, most being in children [31,32]. Deaths are usually due to the attack itself and only rarely from secondary infectious complications. Most bites are from family pets and a minority from stray animals.

Patients with bites have a bimodal pattern of presentation. If children are bitten, if the injury is significant, or if there are concerns over the potential for infection, or for tetanus and rabies, medical attention is sought immediately. Later, patients will present with signs and symptoms of secondary infection. An estimated 3–18% of dog bites and 28–80% of cat bites become infected [33].

Important historical information to focus on include the past medical history of the patient, especially any history of immunosuppression or significant chronic disease, status of tetanus immunization, time of and circumstances surrounding the event (provoked or unprovoked), and details concerning the animal, for example health, ownership, and location. The wound should be assessed for site and potential for nerve, tendon, bone, or joint involvement, especially on the hands and feet. Any wound over a metacarpophalangeal joint should be considered a clench fist injury (punch injury). If the patient presents with established infection, systemic signs, site and extent of infection, lymphadenopathy, and possibility of tenosynovitis, osteomyelitis, and septic arthritis should be considered.

Copious irrigation, debridement of necrotic tissue, and removal of foreign bodies are essential in early management of bite wounds [3,30]. Puncture wounds should be irrigated with a needle or plastic tip catheter inserted into the wound. Infected wounds should be opened if previously sutured, eschar removed and abscesses drained, then irrigated copiously. Closure of bite wounds is controversial as there are no randomized studies of this intervention. Wounds less than 24 hours old, with no signs of infection, on the face, trunk, or proximal extremities can probably be closed safely. All wounds on hands or feet, should be left open, especially if caused by cat or human [3,32].

Pathogens responsible for 50 dog bites and 57 cat bites were evaluated [34]. There was a mean of five pathogens per wound with a range of 0–16. For dogs, the most common aerobic bacteria were *Pasteurella* spp. (50% of patients), especially *Pasteurella canis*, *Streptococcus* spp. (46%), *Staphylococcus* spp. (46%), *Neisseria* spp. (16%), and *Corynebacterium* spp. (12%), while the most frequent anaerobes were *Fusobacterium* spp. (32%), *Bacteroides* spp. (30%), *Porphyromonas* spp. (28%), and *Prevotella* spp. (28%). Cats had similar bacteria, with the exception that *Pasteurella* spp. grew in 75% of cases with *P. multocida* being the most frequent species.

For an infected animal bite, it is recommended to use oral amoxicillin-clavulanate or parenteral pipercillin-tazobactam if signs of systemic toxicity [3]. In penicillin allergic patients, a second or third generation cephalosporin (PO or IV) with anaerobic coverage using either metronidazole or clindamycin is recommended; other alternatives could include a carbapenem, moxifloxacin, or doxycycline [3]. There are no prospective trials nor comparative studies of different antibiotic regimens for treating infected animal bites.

In human bites, the usual organisms are *S. aureus*, *Streptococcus* spp., and anaerobes as well as an organism specific to the oral flora of humans, a fastidious Gram-negative rod, *Eikenella corrodens*. It has an unusual sensitivity profile in that it is sensitive to penicillin and β-lactam/β-lactamase inhibitors, but relatively resistant to cloxacillin, first-generation cephalosporins, erythromycin, and clindamycin [32]. A β lactam/β-lactamase inhibitor combination is the recommended initial choice with doxycycline or moxifloxacin in the penicillin allergic patient [3].

The majority of patients with infected bite wounds can be managed as outpatients with oral antibiotics. Alternatively, parenteral antibiotics could be initiated with stepdown to oral therapy when the infection is resolving.

Antibiotic prophylaxis of animal bites is controversial. A Cochrane Library systematic review showed a favorable odds ratio for prophylaxis of cat and human bites, but not dogs, and for prophylaxis in hand wounds, but not face/neck or trunk wounds [35]. Current expert opinion suggests a three- to five-day course of amoxicillin-clavulanate or moxifloxacin for penicillin allergic for prophylaxis in patients with immunosuppression, asplenic, advanced liver disease, pre-existing or resultant edema of affected area, and for moderate to severe injuries, especially to the hand, feet, and face or involving the joint capsule such as clenched fist injury [3].

Animal bites can potentially transmit rabies, and many patients will seek medical attention for fear of rabies infection. Local public health authorities can be a valuable resource in ascertaining the risk of rabies transmission in an individual case and the need for post-exposure prophylaxis.

References

1 Darmstadt GL, Lane AT. Impetigo: an overview. Pediatr Dermatol. 1994 Dec;11(4):293–303. PubMed PMID: 7899177.

2 Koning S, van der Sande R, Verhagen AP, van Suijlekom-Smit LW, Morris AD, Butler CC, et al. Interventions for impetigo. Cochrane Database Syst Rev. 2012 Jan 18;1:CD003261. PubMed PMID: 22258953.

3 Stevens DL, Bisno AL, Chambers HF, Dellinger EP, Goldstein EJ, Gorbach SL, et al. Practice guidelines for the diagnosis and management of skin and soft tissue infections: 2014 update by the infectious diseases society of America. Clin Infect Dis. 2014 Jul 15;59(2):147–59. PubMed PMID: 24947530.

4 Bowen AC, Tong SY, Andrews RM, O'Meara IM, McDonald MI, Chatfield MD, et al. Short-course oral co-trimoxazole versus intramuscular benzathine benzylpenicillin

for impetigo in a highly endemic region: an open-label, randomised, controlled, non-inferiority trial. Lancet. 2014 Dec 13;384(9960):2132–40. PubMed PMID: 25172376.

5   Hedstrom SA. Recurrent staphylococcal furunculosis. Bacteriological findings and epidemiology in 100 cases. Scand J of Infect Dis. 1981;13(2):115–9. PubMed PMID: 7313565.

6   Raff AB, Kroshinsky D. Cellulitis: a review. JAMA. 2016 Jul 19;316(3):325–37. PubMed PMID: 27434444.

7   Bisno AL, Stevens DL. Streptococcal infections of skin and soft tissues. N Engl J Med. 1996 Jan 25;334(4):240–5. PubMed PMID: 8532002.

8   Perl B, Gottehrer NP, Raveh D, Schlesinger Y, Rudensky B, Yinnon AM. Cost-effectiveness of blood cultures for adult patients with cellulitis. Clin Infect Dis. 1999 Dec;29(6):1483–8. PubMed PMID: 10585800.

9   Kilburn SA, Featherstone P, Higgins B, Brindle R. Interventions for cellulitis and erysipelas. Cochrane Database Syst Rev. 2010 Jun 16(6):CD004299. PubMed PMID: 20556757.

10 Falagas ME, Matthaiou DK, Vardakas KZ. Fluoroquinolones vs beta-lactams for empirical treatment of immunocompetent patients with skin and soft tissue infections: a meta-analysis of randomized controlled trials. Mayo Clinic Proc. 2006 Dec;81(12):1553–66. PubMed PMID: 17165634.

11 Corwin P, Toop L, McGeoch G, Than M, Wynn-Thomas S, Wells JE, et al. Randomised controlled trial of intravenous antibiotic treatment for cellulitis at home compared with hospital. BMJ. 2005 Jan 15;330(7483):129. PubMed PMID: 15604157. Pubmed Central PMCID: 544431.

12 Oh CC, Ko HC, Lee HY, Safdar N, Maki DG, Chlebicki MP. Antibiotic prophylaxis for preventing recurrent cellulitis: a systematic review and meta-analysis. J of Infect. 2014 Jul;69(1):26–34. PubMed PMID: 24576824.

13 Mason JM, Thomas KS, Crook AM, Foster KA, Chalmers JR, Nunn AJ, et al. Prophylactic antibiotics to prevent cellulitis of the leg: economic analysis of the PATCH I & II trials. PloS One. 2014;9(2):e82694. PubMed PMID: 24551029. Pubmed Central PMCID: 3925077.

14 Nelson GE, Pondo T, Toews KA, Farley MM, Lindegren ML, Lynfield R, et al. Epidemiology of Invasive Group A Streptococcal Infections in the United States, 2005-2012. Clin Infect Dis. 2016 Aug 15;63(4):478–86. PubMed PMID: 27105747.

15 Kaul R, McGeer A, Low DE, Green K, Schwartz B. Population-based surveillance for group A streptococcal necrotizing fasciitis: Clinical features, prognostic indicators, and microbiologic analysis of seventy-seven cases. Ontario Group A Streptococcal Study. Am J Med. 1997 Jul;103(1):18–24. PubMed PMID: 9236481.

16 Hunter J, Quarterman C, Waseem M, Wills A. Diagnosis and management of necrotizing fasciitis. Brit J Hosp Med. 2011 Jul;72(7):391–5. PubMed PMID: 21841612.

17 Morgan MS. Diagnosis and management of necrotising fasciitis: a multiparametric approach. J Hosp Infect. 2010 Aug;75(4):249–57. PubMed PMID: 20542593.

18 Elliott D, Kufera JA, Myers RA. The microbiology of necrotizing soft tissue infections. American J Surg. 2000 May;179(5):361–6. PubMed PMID: 10930480.

19 Hussein QA, Anaya DA. Necrotizing soft tissue infections. Crit Care Clinics. 2013 Oct;29(4):795–806. PubMed PMID: 24094377.

20 Malghem J, Lecouvet FE, Omoumi P, Maldague BE, Vande Berg BC. Necrotizing fasciitis: contribution and limitations of diagnostic imaging. Joint, Bone, Spine: Revue du Rhumatisme. 2013 Mar;80(2):146–54. PubMed PMID: 23043899.

21 Kadri SS, Swihart BJ, Bonne SL, Hohmann SF, Hennessy LV, Louras P, et al. Impact of intravenous immunoglobulin on survival in necrotizing fasciitis with vasopressor-

dependent shock: a propensity score-matched analysis from 130 US hospitals. Clin Infect Dis. 2017 Apr 01;64(7):877–85. PubMed PMID: 28034881.

22 Levett D, Bennett MH, Millar I. Adjunctive hyperbaric oxygen for necrotizing fasciitis. Cochrane Database Syst Rev. 2015 Jan 15;1:CD007937. PubMed PMID: 25879088.

23 Kaide CG, Khandelwal S. Hyperbaric oxygen: applications in infectious disease. Em Med Clinics of N Amer. 2008 May;26(2):571–95, xi. PubMed PMID: 18406988.

24 Gottrup F, Holstein P, Jorgensen B, Lohmann M, Karlsmar T. A new concept of a multidisciplinary wound healing center and a national expert function of wound healing. Arch of Surg. 2001 Jul;136(7): 765–72. PubMed PMID: 11448387.

25 Lipsky BA, Berendt AR, Cornia PB, Pile JC, Peters EJ, Armstrong DG, et al. 2012 Infectious Diseases Society of America clinical practice guideline for the diagnosis and treatment of diabetic foot infections. Clinical Infect Dis. 2012 Jun;54(12):e132–73. PubMed PMID: 22619242.

26 Prompers L, Huijberts M, Apelqvist J, Jude E, Piaggesi A, Bakker K, et al. Delivery of care to diabetic patients with foot ulcers in daily practice: results of the Eurodiale Study, a prospective cohort study. Diabetic Med. 2008 Jun;25(6):700–7. PubMed PMID: 18544108.

27 Nelson EA, O'Meara S, Craig D, Iglesias C, Golder S, Dalton J, et al. A series of systematic reviews to inform a decision analysis for sampling and treating infected diabetic foot ulcers. Health Tech Assess. 2006 Apr;10(12):iii–iv, ix–x, 1–221. PubMed PMID: 16595081.

28 Lavery LA, Armstrong DG, Wunderlich RP, Mohler MJ, Wendel CS, Lipsky BA. Risk factors for foot infections in individuals with diabetes. Diabetes Care. 2006 Jun;29(6):1288–93. PubMed PMID: 16732010.

29 Selva Olid A, Sola I, Barajas-Nava LA, Gianneo OD, Bonfill Cosp X, Lipsky BA. Systemic antibiotics for treating diabetic foot infections. Cochrane Database Syst Rev. 2015 Sep 04(9):CD009061. PubMed PMID: 26337865.

30 Oehler RL, Velez AP, Mizrachi M, Lamarche J, Gompf S. Bite-related and septic syndromes caused by cats and dogs. Lancet Infect Dis. 2009 Jul;9(7):439–47. PubMed PMID: 19555903.

31 Weiss HB, Friedman DI, Coben JH. Incidence of dog bite injuries treated in emergency departments. JAMA. 1998 Jan 07;279(1):51–3. PubMed PMID: 9424044.

32 Fleisher GR. The management of bite wounds. N Engl J Med. 1999 Jan 14;340(2):138–40. PubMed PMID: 9887167.

33 Goldstein EJ. Bite wounds and infection. Clin Infect Dis. 1992 Mar;14(3):633–8. PubMed PMID: 1562653.

34 Talan DA, Citron DM, Abrahamian FM, Moran GJ, Goldstein EJ. Bacteriologic analysis of infected dog and cat bites. Emergency Medicine Animal Bite Infection Study Group. N Engl J Med. 1999 Jan 14;340(2):85–92. PubMed PMID: 9887159.

35 Medeiros I, Saconato H. Antibiotic prophylaxis for mammalian bites. Cochrane Database Syst Rev. 2001 (2): CD001738. PubMed PMID: 11406003.

Chapter 3

Bone and Joint Infections

Nora Renz and Andrej Trampuz

3.1 Introduction

The evidence base for diagnosis and management of musculoskeletal infections has become stronger in the last years with publication of a substantial number of new articles. This chapter covers three of the most important entities of musculoskeletal infection: septic arthritis, prosthetic joint infection (PJI), and osteomyelitis.

3.2 Septic Arthritis

Case Presentation 1

A 76-year-old woman presents to her family practitioner with a 72-hour history of increasing pain in the left knee associated with fever and has been unable to walk for 12 hours prior to presentation. She has a five-year history of osteoarthritis progressively affecting both knees, for which she had taken non-steroidal anti-inflammatory agents. She has had no surgery to the knee. There is no history of gout, injury, or other recent illness. Physical examination reveals a temperature of 39 °C. The left knee is held in 30 degrees of flexion; any movement from that position is extremely uncomfortable. There is a tense and tender effusion in the knee, which is warm to the touch. She is admitted to hospital for investigation of acute arthritis of the left knee.

3.2.1 Background

Acute septic arthritis is a medical and surgical emergency because of the rapid destruction of the joint. A delay between symptom onset and initiation of adequate therapy is the major determinant of outcome. In native joints, septic arthritis is most commonly caused by hematogenous seeding of microorganisms from a distant infection focus [1,2]. Because the synovial membrane is highly vascularized and contains no limiting basement membrane, microorganisms can more easily pass from the blood into the joint space, resulting in an acute onset of purulent joint inflammation. Patients at highest risk for hematogenous seeding are intravenous drug users, patients with indwelling vascular catheters and devices, and patients with infective endocarditis. However, bacteremia may be only transient, and blood cultures are positive in only 50% of cases. Other mechanisms of septic arthritis are direct inoculation of microorganisms into the joint as a result of intraarticular injections, surgical interventions, open joint injury, or trauma [3].

Microorganisms in the joint space trigger an acute synovial inflammatory response. Within a few hours, activated inflammatory cells fill the closed synovial space. The inflammatory cells release enzymes and cytokines and the microorganisms produce in addition toxins that can kill eukaryotic cells. The consequences are chemical toxic damage to the cartilage and underlying subchondral bone,

Evidence-Based Infectious Diseases, Third Edition. Edited by Dominik Mertz, Fiona Smaill, and Nick Daneman.
© 2018 John Wiley & Sons Ltd. Published 2018 by John Wiley & Sons Ltd.

but also pressure damage due to the increased joint pressure secondary to the large accumulated inflammatory effusion [1,2].

Septic arthritis is diagnosed in 2–10 per 100,000 patients per year, and is considerably more common in patients suffering from rheumatoid arthritis (28–38 patients per 100,000 patients per year). The incidence is increasing because of the aging population and the increasing use of immunosuppressive treatments as well as of the growing numbers of joint interventions. The risk of post-interventional septic arthritis is one case per 22,000 interventions, and after arthroscopy, one case per 250–1,000 interventions [4]. Despite adequate therapy, 25–50% of patients with septic arthritis experience permanent joint damage with impaired joint function.

3.2.2 Diagnosis of Septic Arthritis

3.2.2.1 Clinical Signs
Most patients (80–85%) present with an acute onset of joint swelling and pain. The pain is present at rest, aggravated with weight bearing, and the joint motion is limited. Joint erythema and excess heat are present in most cases. Fever is present in about 50% of patients. In 90% of patients with septic arthritis, only one joint is involved, and 10% suffer from multiple joint involvement, mainly found in patients with underlying rheumatoid arthritis [5]. Predominantly weight-bearing joints are affected, such as knee joints in 45–55% and hip joints in 15–25%, followed by shoulder, wrist, ankle, and elbow joints (together in 5–10%) [6].

3.2.2.2 Laboratory Studies
Leukocyte count and serum C-reactive protein (CRP) concentration should be determined. The sensitivity of leukocyte count >10,000 cells/µL is 90% and for CRP >100 mg/l is 77%, but both parameters are nonspecific [7]. As the predominant route of infection is hematogenous seeding from a distant infectious focus, two to three pairs of blood cultures should be drawn.

The examination of the synovial fluid is the most important diagnostic tool in patients with suspected septic arthritis. Analysis of the synovial fluid should include differential leukocyte count (using an EDTA tube to avoid coagulation), microbiological culture, and the presence of crystals (using native tube). Immediate incubation of the aspirate in blood culture bottles appears to increase the culture sensitivity.

A synovial fluid leukocyte count of >20,000 cells/µL or granulocyte percentage >90% is highly suggestive for septic arthritis and should prompt immediate arthroscopic lavage. Typically, only crystal-induced arthritis may present with such high synovial fluid leukocyte counts mimicking septic arthritis [7].

3.2.2.3 Microbiology
Staphylococcus aureus is the predominant causative microorganism in 40–60% followed by streptococci in 20–30% of cases. Gram-negative bacilli are found in 4–20%, especially in intravenous drug users, immunocompromised hosts, elderly patients, or after trauma [1]. Other organisms may assume some importance in particular groups (e.g., tuberculous infection in immigrants from developing world and in people with HIV infection). Culture-negative septic arthritis cases are described in 10–20% as a consequence of antimicrobial pretreatment or fastidious to grow microorganisms. Polymicrobial infections are often associated with penetrating trauma.

The Gram stain has a sensitivity of only about 50%. The microbiological diagnostic yield can be increased if the synovial fluid is inoculated into blood culture bottles [8]. If culture results are negative because patients were pretreated with antimicrobials or because of fastidious to grow or atypical microorganisms, bacterial DNA can be identified by polymerase chain reaction [9]. Crystals can be detected by polarized light microscopy of the synovial fluid. The presence of crystals does not rule out septic arthritis as coexistence of crystals has been described.

3.2.2.4 Imaging
Conventional x-ray detects pre-existing joint diseases (i.e., osteoarthritis, rheumatoid

arthritis, osteomyelitis, or chondrocalcinosis). Ultrasound can be useful to guide joint aspiration. Bone scintigraphy is usually positive after 10 days, which is not specific but may be helpful in the diagnosis of sacroiliac joint infection. Computed tomography is sensitive for the detection of bone erosions, joint effusion, and soft tissue infections. Magnetic resonance imaging is even more sensitive; however, it is only required for the diagnosis of sternoclavicular or sacroiliac arthritis, symphysitis, or post-operative arthritis following cruciate ligament reconstruction.

Case Presentation 1 (continued)

Initial laboratory tests have shown a white cell count (WBC) in blood of 15,000/μL with 85% polymorph nuclear cells (PMN), and a CRP of 230 mg/l. Blood cultures were collected. Radiographic examination of the knee confirms the presence of osteoarthritis. Urinalysis is negative for sugar and protein. Synovial fluid analysis of the joint puncture indicates WBC of 65,000/μL, with 92% PMN. No organisms were identified on Gram stain.

3.2.3   Treatment and Outcomes

The natural history of an untreated case is destruction of the infected joint. Therefore, the main treatment goal is the restoration of a painless full joint function by the eradication of infection with antimicrobial agents and by joint decompression by removal of the effusion. The key to successful management is early recognition of the diagnosis, the rapid surgical intervention and initiation of appropriate antimicrobial therapy. The mortality rate ranges between 5–15%.

3.2.3.1   Surgical Treatment

For the mechanical and surgical treatment of septic arthritis, different strategies can be considered: repetitive needle aspirations, arthroscopy, or arthrotomy. The use of irrigation-suction drainage systems may increase the risk of secondary infections and is therefore not recommended. Joint irrigation with antiseptics is contraindicated because most antiseptics such as chlorhexidine or octenidine may lead to chondrolysis and destruction of the joint [10]. The administration of intra-articular antimicrobial treatment is also contraindicated because a chemical synovitis can be induced.

3.2.3.2   Antimicrobial Treatment

In patients with a high suspicion, empiric therapy should begin as soon as synovial fluid had been obtained, or once the results of synovial fluid microscopy are available and are supportive of the diagnosis. As empiric treatment, we recommend intravenous amoxicillin/clavulanic acid, piperacillin/tazobactam, cefazolin, or cefuroxime. For the latter two, gentamicin can be added if broader Gram-negative coverage is deemed necessary—depending on the local epidemiology. In a setting with high rates of methicillin-resistant *Staphylococcus aureus* (MRSA) or in patients with risk factors for MRSA infections, we suggest adding vancomycin for empiric treatment until MRSA can be ruled out. Definitive choice of antimicrobial agent is determined by the susceptibility of the etiologic microorganism. The administration of high-dose and bactericidal systemic antimicrobial therapy is mandatory. Systemic antimicrobial therapy achieves excellent drug levels in the infected joint as the inflamed synovia is well perfused. There are no randomized controlled studies evaluating the efficacy of different antimicrobial treatments.

We suggest a duration of antimicrobial therapy of four weeks [2,11]. Dependent on the causing microorganism, the initial two weeks of intravenous therapy can be switched to oral therapy for the remaining treatment course. An earlier switch to oral therapy is possible if the microorganisms are susceptible to bactericidal oral treatment regimens with good bioavailability such as rifampin-fluoroquinolone or rifampin-trimethoprim/sulfamethoxazole (cotrimoxazole) combination for staphylococci, and ciprofloxacin monotherapy for Enterobacteriaceae.

Case Presentation 1 (continued)

An arthroscopic lavage of the left knee with 14 liters of normal saline was performed on the day of admission. Empiric intraoperative therapy with cefuroxime and gentamicin was started. Blood cultures and synovial fluid cultures grew *Staphylococcus aureus*, susceptible to methicillin/oxacillin, clindamycin, trimethoprim/sulfamethoxazole (cotrimoxazole), ciprofloxacin, and rifampin. Transesophageal echocardiography showed no vegetations on the heart valves. The regimen was adjusted to intravenous flucloxacillin for two weeks followed by oral rifampin in combination with cotrimoxazole for another two weeks.

3.2.3.3 Implications for Practice

- A high index of suspicion for septic arthritis allows for a rapid initiation of therapy and better outcomes. Early signs of infection should prompt diagnostic workup that includes synovial fluid aspiration.
- The examination of the synovial fluid is the most important diagnostic tool in patients with suspected septic arthritis. A synovial leukocyte count >20,000 cells/µl or >90% granulocytes should prompt arthroscopic lavage.

3.3 Prosthetic Joint Infection (PJI)

Case Presentation 2

A 67-year-old woman with a 14-year history of rheumatoid arthritis received a primary right total hip replacement two years ago. Although she has been generally well with satisfactory control of her rheumatoid arthritis, she reported increasing pain in the right hip over the last 1.5 years, and radiographs show loosening of the implant. WBC and CRP were in normal range. No percutaneous sinus tract was present.

3.3.1 Background

Joint replacement surgery is the major procedure to alleviate pain and to improve mobility in patients with destructed joints. It is one of the most successful surgeries and less than 10% of recipients develop a complication during their lifetime [12]. PJI represents an important complication, associated with high morbidity, need for complex treatment and substantial healthcare costs. In addition to prolonged hospitalization, PJI can lead to unsatisfactory functional result or even permanent disability, including arthrodesis or leg amputation [13]. The incidence of infection after arthroplasty has decreased since the late 1960s, when infection rates were as high as 10%. The introduction of antimicrobial prophylaxis and better infection prevention measures in the operating room led to infection rates <2%.

Implant-associated infections are typically caused by microorganisms growing in structures known as biofilms, a highly hydrated extracellular matrix ("slime") attached to a surface. Depletion of metabolic substances or waste product accumulation in biofilms causes microbes to enter a slow- or non-growing (stationary) state. Therefore, biofilm microorganisms are up to 1,000 times more resistant to growth-dependent antimicrobial agents than their planktonic (free-living) counterparts.

3.3.2 Diagnosis of Prosthetic Joint Infection

3.3.2.1 Definition and Classification

Despite several criteria for diagnosing PJI were published [14,15], many authors rely on simple definitions [13] according to which infection is diagnosed when at least of one of the following criteria is present: (a) cutaneous sinus tract communicating with the prosthesis, (b) visible purulence around the prosthesis, (c) histopathological characteristics of inflammation, (d) increased WBC and differential in the synovial fluid, or (e) positive culture of the synovial fluid, periprosthetic tissue or sonication fluid.

PJI can be classified according to the route of infection (perioperative, hematogenous or contiguous) and the time from implantation to the onset of symptoms [13]. *Acute PJI* occurs either within one month after surgery or through hematogenous spread anytime thereafter, whereas *chronic PJI* is typically caused by low-virulent organisms introduced into the surgical site during surgery and typically present 3–36 months after surgery.

Leading clinical signs of early infections are systemic (fever) and local signs of inflammation (pain, erythema, edema, wound healing disturbance). Persisting or increasing joint pain and early loosening (within 2–3 years after implantation) are the hallmarks of a delayed infection, but clinical signs of infection may also completely lack. Low-grade infections are difficult to distinguish from aseptic failure, often presenting only with early loosening and persisting pain. Late hematogenous infections present either with a sudden onset of systemic symptoms or as subacute infection following unrecognized bacteremia. The most frequent primary foci causing hematogenous PJI are infections of the skin, respiratory, intestinal and urinary tract as well as dental and intravascular infections [16].

3.3.2.2 Preoperative Diagnostic Tests

No single routinely used clinical or laboratory test has been shown to achieve ideal accuracy for the diagnosis of PJI [17]. A combination of laboratory, histopathology, microbiology, and imaging studies is usually required. Ideally, the infection is diagnosed (or excluded) before surgery. Therefore, preoperative joint aspiration with determination of leukocyte count and culture of synovial fluid is the first step in differentiating a septic from an aseptic process. Routine blood tests include inflammatory markers such as white leukocyte count and CRP. None of these tests is sufficiently sensitive or specific to diagnose or exclude PJI with high accuracy [18]. Normal inflammatory markers do not exclude PJI, especially not low-grade infections. Importantly, inflammatory markers are increased in the first days after surgery in the absence of an infection, reflecting postinterventional, healing-associated aseptic inflammation. In the absence of an infection, inflammatory markers continuously decrease and typically normalize within one to two weeks post-surgery.

Synovial fluid leukocyte count and differential represents a simple, rapid, and accurate test for differentiating PJI from aseptic failure. In a prospective study of 133 patients with total knee arthroplasty revision, synovial fluid leukocyte count was investigated [19]. Patients with underlying inflammatory joint disease were excluded. Aseptic failure was diagnosed in 99 patients and PJI in 34 patients. A leukocyte count of >1700/μl had a sensitivity of 94% and a specificity of 88% for diagnosing PJI; a differential of >65% granulocytes had a sensitivity of 97% and a specificity of 98%. Subsequent studies used various other synovial fluid leukocyte cut-off values of 3,000 [20], 4,200 [21], 1,590 [22], and 1,100 [23].

Unfortunately, no uniform definition criteria and various diagnostic methods were used and there is currently no gold standard for diagnosing PJI based on leucocyte counts [13–15]. As an average of the synovial fluid leucocyte counts used in the studies above, we recommend to use a cut-off of >2000/μl or >70% granulocytes for diagnosing PJI given its good balance of sensitivity and specificity. Culture of synovial fluid detects the infecting microorganism in 45%–100% and may be further improved by inoculation into a pediatric blood culture bottle [24]. Therefore, we recommend to perform synovial fluid aspiration before revision surgery on any prosthetic joint, which should be sent for microbiology and determination of leukocyte count and differential. New biomarkers such as alpha-defensin in synovial fluid showed high specificity, but low sensitivity for diagnosing PJI. This test is therefore more suitable as confirmatory than screening tool [25].

3.3.2.3 Intraoperative Diagnostic Tests

Periprosthetic tissue cultures are standard specimens for detecting the infecting microorganism [24]. At least three tissue specimens should be obtained for culture. Swabs have a low sensitivity and should be avoided. It is important to discontinue any antimicrobial therapy at least two weeks prior tissue sampling for culture whenever possible [26]. Intraoperative samples should be cultured on agar plates and inoculated into enrichment broths and should be incubated for at least two weeks [27,28].

Sonication of removed prosthesis, followed by culture of the sonication fluid, significantly improved the diagnosis of PJI. The removed implant is transported to the microbiological laboratory in a sterile container. After addition of Ringer's solution or normal saline covering about 80% of the implant, the container is vortexed during 30 seconds and sonicated (40 kHz) during one minute before plating the sonication fluid. In a study with 331 patients with total knee or hip prostheses [26], 252 were reported aseptic failure and 79 had PJI. The sensitivities of periprosthetic tissue and sonication fluid cultures were 61% and 79% ($p < 0.001$) and the specificities were 99.2% and 98.8%, respectively. Fourteen cases of PJI were detected by sonication fluid culture but not by periprosthetic tissue culture. In patients receiving antimicrobial therapy within 14 days before surgery, the sensitivities of periprosthetic tissue and sonication fluid culture were 45% and 75% ($p < 0.001$), respectively. The sonication procedure was validated also for other implants, including spine hardware, intravascular devices, and breast implants [29–31].

A novel approach for the diagnosis of PJI is the combination of two complementary diagnostic methods, namely sonication of the removed implants and multiplex real time PCR of the resulting sonication fluid. Interestingly, this combined method can improve the diagnosis of PJI, particularly among patients who had previously received antibiotic therapy (sensitivity of 100% with multiplex PCR versus 42% for sonication fluid culture) [32].

Histopathological examination of periprosthetic tissue samples has a sensitivity of >80% and a specificity of >90%. Recently, histopathological criteria for a standardized evaluation of the periprosthetic membrane were defined [33]; wear particle induced type (type 1; detection of foreign body particles, macrophages, and multinucleated giant cells occupy at least 20% of the area); infectious type (type 2; granulation tissue with neutrophils, plasma cells and few, if any, wear particles); combined type (type 3; aspects of type 1 and type 2 occur simultaneously); and indeterminate type (type 4; neither criteria for type 1 nor type 2 are fulfilled).

3.3.2.4 Imaging

Plain radiographs after implantation are helpful to determine the implant position and evaluate the bone stock, but are neither sensitive nor specific to diagnose PJI [13]. A rapid development of a continuous radiolucent line of greater than 2 mm or severe focal osteolysis within the first one to two years is often associated with infection. Ultrasonography may detect fluid effusions around the prosthesis and can be used to guide joint aspiration and drainage procedures. It is especially helpful in prosthetic hip infection. Nuclear imaging techniques are sensitive, but their specificity in the evaluation of arthroplasty-associated infection is still controversial. Computed tomography (CT) is more sensitive than plain radiography in the imaging of the joint space. In addition, it may assist in guiding joint aspiration and selecting the surgical approach. Magnetic resonance imaging (MRI) displays greater resolution for soft tissue abnormalities than CT or radiography and greater anatomical detail than radionuclide scans. Positron emission tomography (PET) needs further evaluation for implant imaging.

Based on these data, we suggest to perform plain radiograph in all patients with suspected PJI before surgery (evaluation of possible periprosthetic fracture, loosening or migration of the implant, osteolysis) as well as after surgery to determine the implant position and generate a baseline image. We recommend additional imaging only in exceptional situations, for example, CT for search of sequestra, PET for search of bone metastasis.

Case Presentation 2 (continued)

The right prosthetic hip was preoperatively aspirated. The synovial fluid showed 3,500 leukocytes/μl with 76% granulocytes. Cultures of synovial fluid grew Cutibacterium (formerly *Propionibacterium*) *acnes* after 10 days of incubation in anaerobic conditions. The patient was scheduled for an exchange of all prosthetic components.

3.3.3 Treatment and Outcomes

During the last two decades, new management concepts have evolved based on in vitro experiments, animal models, and clinical experience. A concerted interdisciplinary cooperation among orthopedic surgeons, infectious diseases specialists, and microbiologists is essential to achieve an optimal treatment outcome of PJI.

3.3.3.1 Surgical Treatment

No data are available from randomized controlled studies. Antimicrobial recommendations are suggestions, which showed in several retrospective studies that the treatment outcome is improved when the algorithm originally published by Zimmerli et al. [13] is followed [34–38].

The discrimination between acute and chronic infection is crucial for the choice of the adequate treatment. In acute PJI, we recommend debridement, retention of fixed components, and exchange of only mobile parts as the least invasive option. For successful treatment with retention of the prosthesis, soft tissue and bone should be intact, isolated microorganisms should be susceptible to biofilm-active antimicrobials and the prosthesis should be fixed (without implant loosening). This approach was validated for orthopedic implant-related infections in a

prospective observational cohort study [34]. In this study, the primary outcome was treatment failure after a two-year follow-up. Causative pathogens were mainly *Staphylococcus aureus* (41.6%) and coagulase-negative staphylococci (33.9%). Among 233 patients with orthopedic implant-related infections related to prostheses, failure was documented in 10.8% (12 of 111) and when related to osteosyntheses, failure occurred in 9.8% (12 of 122) after two years of follow-up. In all, 90% of orthopedic implant-related infections were successfully cured with surgical debridement and implant-retention in addition to long-term antimicrobial therapy according to a predefined treatment algorithm: if patients fulfilled strict selection criteria, and there was susceptibility to rifampin for Gram-positive pathogens and ciprofloxacin for Gram-negative pathogens.

In other cases, we recommend exchange of the entire prosthesis, including the bone cement (if present). In patients with intact soft tissue, good bone stock, and in the absence of previous revision surgery, a one-stage (direct) exchange is suggested. Otherwise a two-stage exchange with a short (2–3 weeks) or long interval (6–8 weeks) is recommended [13]. During the prosthesis-free interval, we recommend the use of antibiotic-loaded spacers for dead space management, stability, some degree of mobility and local antibiotic treatment [39]. Longer intervals (>8 weeks) should be avoided especially if spacers are in situ, as the antibiotic concentration in the cement eventually falls below the minimal inhibitory concentration for most bacteria, allowing for persistence of biofilm bacteria on cement [40]. Difficult-to-treat infections caused by pathogens resistant to biofilm-active antimicrobials usually require a multi-stage-procedure. Adding an additional debridement and exchange of the spacer improves the surgical and local antibiotic treatment. For a small number of patients with PJI, restoration of joint function is not achievable, and permanent prosthesis removal without replacement or long-term suppressive antimicrobial therapy is the only rational choice.

3.3.3.2 Antimicrobial Treatment

To treat biofilm-associated bone infections, several factors should be considered when selecting antibiotics: good penetration into bone, bactericidal activity, and excellent biofilm-activity. For oral treatment, high oral bioavailability is also required.

The optimal antimicrobial therapy is best defined in staphylococcal foreign body-associated infections, and we suggest the routine use of rifampin for susceptible staphylococci. The clinical efficacy of a rifampin combination was evaluated in staphylococcal infections associated with stable orthopedic devices in a randomized, placebo-controlled, double-blind trial [41]. A total of 33 patients with staphylococcal infection associated with stable orthopedic implants and with <21 days duration of symptoms of infection were included. Initial debridement and two-week intravenous course of flucloxacillin or vancomycin with rifampin or placebo, followed by either ciprofloxacin-rifampin or ciprofloxacin-placebo long-term therapy. The cure rate was 12 (100%) of 12 in the ciprofloxacin-rifampin group compared to 7 (58%) of 12 in the ciprofloxacin-placebo group ($p = .02$). In conclusion, among patients with stable implants, short duration of infection, and initial debridement, patients able to tolerate long-term (3 months) therapy with rifampin-ciprofloxacin experienced cure of the infection without removal of the implant.

Fluoroquinolones are good combination drugs because of their good bioavailability [13]. Because of increasing resistance to fluoroquinolones, other antistaphylococcal drugs such as trimethoprim/sulfamethoxazole (cotrimoxazole), doxycycline, or fusidic acid have been combined with rifampin. Streptococcal PJI results in frequent relapses and often results from hematogenous spread from the mouth or from infective endocarditis [42,43]. In vitro data showed no effect of rifampin on adherent streptococci. For enterococci, in vitro and animal models showed biofilm-activity for fosfomycin, especially in combination with gentamicin, which needs to be proven in clinical trials. For susceptible Gram-negative organisms, ciprofloxacin as a monotherapy is sufficient.

Case Presentation 2 (continued)

Based on the treatment algorithm, a one-stage exchange of the right hip prosthesis was chosen. In 4 of 7 periprosthetic tissue samples and in the sonication fluid of the removed prosthesis *C. acnes* (>1,000 CFU/ml) has grown. Empiric therapy with cefuroxime was adjusted to intravenous penicillin G and oral rifampin for two weeks, followed by oral amoxicillin and rifampin for additional 10 weeks. At two-year-follow-up, the patient was pain-free, fully mobile, and with good function of the prosthesis.

3.3.3.3 Implications for Practice

- Although PJI is a rare event after arthroplasty, it represents an important complication, associated with high morbidity, need for complex treatment, and substantial healthcare costs.
- An accurate and rapid diagnosis of PJI is crucial for the treatment success. Although randomized-controlled trials are lacking in this field, existing data supports published management algorithms as outlined above that should be followed.

3.4 Osteomyelitis

Case Presentation 3

A 62-year-old man presents to his family practitioner with pain and redness in the absence of a skin lesion, at the plate osteosynthesis at the right tibia, which was implanted one year ago after a closed tibia fracture suffered from a traffic accident. Radiological examination showed a nonunion (pseudarthrosis) at the site of the previous fracture. Blood leukocyte count and CRP are normal.

3.4.1 Background

Osteomyelitis is an inflammatory condition of the bone caused by an infecting microorganism. Osteitis describes infection affecting only cortical bone; osteomyelitis implies that the cortex and medulla are involved. Normal healthy bone is quite resistant to infection; in experimental models, it is necessary to cause injury or bone death prior to inoculation with a large number of bacteria to induce osteomyelitis.

Osteomyelitis is classified by the route of infection. Hematogenous osteomyelitis is due to blood-borne spread of bacteria from a distant infectious focus such as soft tissue, respiratory tract, urogenital tract infection, infective endocarditis or other intravascular device-associated infections. Contiguous osteomyelitis is secondary to either (a) a contiguous focus of infection (after trauma or surgery), or (b) secondary to vascular insufficiency (in diabetic foot infections) [44]. The various types of osteomyelitis require differing antimicrobial and surgical strategies. We recommend using the classification for chronic osteomyelitis designed by Cierny and Mader, taking into account the anatomical spread and the general physiological status of the patient [45]. It emphasizes the importance of considering the whole patient not just the local disease.

3.4.2 Diagnosis of Osteomyelitis

3.4.2.1 Clinical Findings

Acute hematogenous osteomyelitis is usually seen in prepubertal children or the elderly. It has been postulated that minor bone injury may cause intramedullary hemorrhage, predisposing to the deposition of bacteria in hematogenous osteomyelitis. Hematogenous osteomyelitis has a rapid onset of symptoms, with localized pain, fever, and malaise. 30% of children have a history of recent minor injury to the site of infection. Signs of bacteremia (rigors, vomiting, and prostration) are present in half of the patients. The infection is most often in the metaphysis of a long bone (distal femur and proximal tibia are common), beginning in the medulla but spreading rapidly to involve the cortex with sinus formation, sub-periosteal abscess formation, and soft-tissue extension. In young children, the infection may spread to the adjacent joint and present as septic arthritis. Spread of the infection with periosteal stripping causes local ischemia and further microvascular thrombosis and tissue death.

Contiguous osteomyelitis occurs when a pathogen enters the bone from an adjacent infective source. This may follow an open fracture, surgery, a skin ulcer, or a pressure sore. It can occur in any bone and is more commonly seen in adults, particularly in those with concomitant diseases such as diabetes with foot ulcers, paraplegia with pressure sores, peripheral arterial or venous insufficiency with ulceration, or fracture with internal fixation. Contiguous osteomyelitis may present acutely, within days of an injury or surgery, or may have a more insidious onset producing extensive bone involvement over many weeks or months in a debilitated patient. Unlike hematogenous osteomyelitis, contiguous osteomyelitis always compromises the surrounding soft tissues and may cause cortical bone death prior to medullary infection.

3.4.2.2 Blood Investigations

The blood leukocyte count is not a reliable indicator and can be normal despite the presence of an infection [46]. The concentration of CRP appears more reliable and can be especially used for follow-up of the response to treatment [47]. Concentrations of calcium, phosphate, and alkaline phosphatase are normal in osteomyelitis, in contrast to metastatic or some metabolic bone diseases [48].

3.4.2.3 Microbiological Investigations

Intraoperative bone biopsies are the most representative microbiological samples and their importance cannot be overemphasized. Material taken from an open sinus tract or superficial wounds by swabbing may give misleading results because the isolates can include colonizing microorganisms at the wound site [24]. Bone biopsy samples should be processed for aerobic and anaerobic cultures. In case of presence of foreign material, the osteosynthetic material should be sent for sonication (see earlier section on PJI).

Tissue specimens obtained for histopathology either by biopsy or during surgery as frozen sections can be used as an additional diagnostic criterion, in particular in patients on antimicrobial treatment prior to obtaining the samples; more than five neutrophils per high-power field indicate an infection with high sensitivity and specificity [48].

3.4.2.4 Imaging

The diagnosis of skeletal infection entails a variety of imaging methods, but conventional radiography is necessary at both initial presentation and follow-up. Plain films show soft-tissue swelling, narrowing or widening of joint spaces, bone destruction, and periosteal reaction. Bone destruction, however, is not apparent on plain films until after 10–21 days of infection.

Both CT and MRI have excellent resolution power and can reveal the destruction of the medulla as well as periosteal reaction, cortical destruction, articular damage, and soft-tissue involvement, even when conventional radiographs are normal. In addition, CT provides excellent definition of cortical bone and a basic assessment of the surrounding soft tissues. It is especially useful in identification of sequestra. MRI, however, is more useful than CT for soft-tissue assessment. MRI also reveals early bony edema and is therefore most useful for early detection of infection.

Various radiopharmaceuticals are currently used for bone scintigraphy. Methylene diphosphonate binds to sites of increased bone metabolic activity and is highly sensitive in the early detection of acute osteomyelitis. Leucocyte scanning with radiolabeled blood cells (leukocytes or granulocytes labelled

with indium-111 or technetium-99m) or specific antibodies has been used for imaging of infection with reported high sensitivity, and especially specificity, but it is less commonly used [49].

Case Presentation 3 (continued)

The clinical findings are consistent with chronic osteomyelitis after fracture fixation. Removal of the plate was performed and the removed plate was sent for sonication. Sonication fluid culture and two of three peri-implant tissue samples grew *Staphylococcus epidermidis*, resistant to oxacillin/methicillin and fluoroquinolones, but susceptible to rifampin, doxycycline, and trimethoprim/sulfamethoxazole (cotrimoxazole). The histologic findings of bone samples showed inflammation consistent with chronic osteomyelitis.

3.4.3 Treatment and Outcomes

3.4.3.1 Surgical Treatment

In contrast to acute osteomyelitis, chronic osteomyelitis and osteosynthesis-associated infections are unlikely to be eradicated without surgical treatment. The goal of surgery is to achieve a viable vascularized environment and elimination of dead bone and fixation devices, which act as a nidus for the infection and biofilm development. Radical debridement down to living bone is required to achieve this aim in many cases. Inadequate debridement is one cause of high recurrence rates in chronic osteomyelitis [47]. Surgery for chronic osteomyelitis consists therefore of removal of sequestra and resection of scarred and infected bone and soft tissue [44]. Adequate debridement can leave a large dead space that must be managed to prevent recurrence and a significant bone loss that might result in bone instability. Appropriate reconstruction of both the bone and soft-tissue defects may be needed. If an implant is present, surgical procedures follow an algorithm similar to the one of prosthetic joint infections with retention of the hardware in acute and exchange of the implant in chronic infections.

3.4.3.2 Antimicrobial Treatment

A combined antimicrobial and surgical approach is recommended in chronic osteomyelitis, whereas for acute haematogenous osteomyelitis surgery is generally unnecessary and antimicrobial therapy alone is sufficient [48]. We suggest antimicrobial therapy of 6 weeks for osteomyelitis and 12 weeks in case of presence of osteosynthetic material [47].

In most cases, intravenous antibiotics can be switched to the oral route after two weeks of initial therapy. Several studies have shown that oral treatment with rifampin in combination with fluoroquinolone, trimethoprim/sulfamethoxazole (cotrimoxazole), doxycycline or fusidic acid is effective in staphylococcal bone infections [50]. The main advantage of oral antibiotic combinations is their excellent bioavailability, good intracellular penetration and activity against intracellular staphylococci. Fluoroquinolones inhibit fracture healing, but the clinical significance is negligible.

> **Clinical Presentation 3 (continued)**
>
> After removal of the plate, the affected bone and soft tissue were debrided. During the same surgery, an intramedullary nail was implanted. Intravenous vancomycin was initiated and oral rifampin was added after four days when the wound showed no drainage. After 2 weeks, intravenous treatment was switched to oral combination of rifampin and cotrimoxazol for 10 additional weeks. After surgery, the patient showed radiologically good bone formation with complete consolidation after six months.

3.4.3.3 Implications for Practice

- The key to successful management is early diagnosis, including bone sampling for microbiological and histopathological examination to allow for adequate diagnosis and targeted antimicrobial therapy.
- Chronic osteomyelitis is associated with avascular necrosis of bone and formation of sequestra (dead bone), and surgical debridement is necessary in addition to antibiotic therapy. By contrast, acute osteomyelitis can respond to antibiotics alone.
- Antimicrobial therapy for osteomyelitis should last 6 weeks, but 12 weeks are necessary in the presence of osteosynthetic material.

References

1 Goldenberg DL. Septic arthritis. Lancet. 1998;351(9097):197–202.
2 Mathews CJ, Weston VC, Jones A, Field M, Coakley G. Bacterial septic arthritis in adults. Lancet. 2010;375(9717):846–55.
3 Ross JJ. Septic Arthritis of Native Joints. Infect Dis Clinics N Am. 2017;31(2):203–18.
4 Geirsson AJ, Statkevicius S, Vikingsson A. Septic arthritis in Iceland 1990–2002: increasing incidence due to iatrogenic infections. Ann of the Rheumat Dis. 2008;67(5):638–43.
5 Dubost JJ, Fis I, Denis P, Lopitaux R, Soubrier M, Ristori JM, et al. Polyarticular septic arthritis. Med. 1993;72(5):296–310.
6 Gupta MN, Sturrock RD, Field M. A prospective 2-year study of 75 patients with adult-onset septic arthritis. Rheum. 2001;40(1):24–30.
7 Margaretten ME, Kohlwes J, Moore D, Bent S. Does this adult patient have septic arthritis? JAMA. 2007;297(13):1478–88.
8 Hughes JG, Vetter EA, Patel R, Schleck CD, Harmsen S, Turgeant LT, et al. Culture with BACTEC Peds Plus/F bottle compared with conventional methods for detection of

bacteria in synovial fluid. J Clin Microbiol. 2001;39(12):4468–71.

9 Bonilla H, Kepley R, Pawlak J, Belian B, Raynor A, Saravolatz LD. Rapid diagnosis of septic arthritis using 16S rDNA PCR: a comparison of 3 methods. Diagnost Microbiol Infect Dis. 2011;69(4):390–5.

10 van Huyssteen AL, Bracey DJ. Chlorhexidine and chondrolysis in the knee. J Bone Joint Surg Brit Vol. 1999;81(6):995–6.

11 Weston V, Coakley G. Guideline for the management of the hot swollen joint in adults with a particular focus on septic arthritis. J Antimicrob Chemother. 2006;58(3):492–3.

12 Kurtz S, Ong K, Lau E, Mowat F, Halpern M. Projections of primary and revision hip and knee arthroplasty in the United States from 2005 to 2030. J Bone Joint Surg Am Vol. 2007;89(4):780–5.

13 Zimmerli W, Trampuz A, Ochsner PE. Prosthetic-joint infections. N Engl J Med. 2004;351(16):1645–54.

14 Parvizi J, Gehrke T, International Consensus Group on Periprosthetic Joint I. Definition of periprosthetic joint infection. J Arthroplasty. 2014;29(7):1331.

15 Osmon DR, Berbari EF, Berendt AR, Lew D, Zimmerli W, Steckelberg JM, et al. Diagnosis and management of prosthetic joint infection: clinical practice guidelines by the Infectious Diseases Society of America. Clin Infect Dis. 2013;56(1):e1–e25.

16 Tande AJ, Palraj BR, Osmon DR, Berbari EF, Baddour LM, Lohse CM, et al. Clinical Presentation, Risk Factors, and Outcomes of Hematogenous Prosthetic Joint Infection in Patients with Staphylococcus aureus Bacteremia. Am J Med. 2016;129(2):221 e11–20.

17 Gomez-Urena EO, Tande AJ, Osmon DR, Berbari EF. Diagnosis of Prosthetic Joint Infection: Cultures, Biomarker and Criteria. Infect Dis Clinics Nh Am. 2017;31(2):219–35.

18 Moran E, Byren I, Atkins BL. The diagnosis and management of prosthetic joint infections. J Antimicrob Chemother. 2010;65 Suppl 3:iii45–54.

19 Trampuz A, Hanssen AD, Osmon DR, Mandrekar J, Steckelberg JM, Patel R. Synovial fluid leukocyte count and differential for the diagnosis of prosthetic knee infection. Am J Med. 2004;117(8):556–62.

20 Zmistowski B, Restrepo C, Huang R, Hozack WJ, Parvizi J. Periprosthetic joint infection diagnosis: a complete understanding of white blood cell count and differential. J Arthroplasty. 2012;27(9):1589–93.

21 Schinsky MF, Della Valle CJ, Sporer SM, Paprosky WG. Perioperative testing for joint infection in patients undergoing revision total hip arthroplasty. J Bone Joint Surg Am Vol. 2008;90(9): 1869–75.

22 Dinneen A, Guyot A, Clements J, Bradley N. Synovial fluid white cell and differential count in the diagnosis or exclusion of prosthetic joint infection. Bone Joint J. 2013;95-b(4):554–7.

23 Ghanem E, Parvizi J, Burnett RS, Sharkey PF, Keshavarzi N, Aggarwal A, et al. Cell count and differential of aspirated fluid in the diagnosis of infection at the site of total knee arthroplasty. J Bone Joint Surg Am Vol. 2008;90(8):1637–43.

24 Corvec S, Portillo ME, Pasticci BM, Borens O, Trampuz A. Epidemiology and new developments in the diagnosis of prosthetic joint infection. Int J Artif Organs. 2012;35(10):923–34.

25 Renz N, Yermak K, Perka C, Trampuz A. Alpha defensin lateral flow test for diagnosis of periprosthetic joint infections – not a screening but a confirmatory test. J Bone Joint Surg Am 2018 May 2;100(9):742–50.

26 Trampuz A, Piper KE, Jacobson MJ, Hanssen AD, Unni KK, Osmon DR, et al. Sonication of removed hip and knee prostheses for diagnosis of infection. N Engl J Med. 2007;357(7):654–63.

27 Portillo ME, Salvado M, Alier A, Martinez S, Sorli L, Horcajada JP, et al. Advantages of sonication fluid culture for the diagnosis of

prosthetic joint infection. J Infect. 2014;69(1):35–41.

28 Portillo ME, Salvado M, Trampuz A, Siverio A, Alier A, Sorli L, et al. Improved diagnosis of orthopedic implant-associated infection by inoculation of sonication fluid into blood culture bottles. J Clin Microbiol. 2015;53(5):1622–7.

29 Piper KE, Jacobson MJ, Cofield RH, Sperling JW, Sanchez-Sotelo J, Osmon DR, et al. Microbiologic diagnosis of prosthetic shoulder infection by use of implant sonication. J Clin Microbiol. 2009;47(6):1878–84.

30 Oliva A, Pavone P, D'Abramo A, Iannetta M, Mastroianni CM, Vullo V. Role of Sonication in the Microbiological Diagnosis of Implant-Associated Infections: Beyond the Orthopedic Prosthesis. Adv Exp Med Biol. 2016;897:85–102.

31 Janz V, Wassilew GI, Kribus M, Trampuz A, Perka C. Improved identification of polymicrobial infection in total knee arthroplasty through sonicate fluid cultures. Arch Orthop Trauma Surg. 2015;135(10):1453–7.

32 Achermann Y, Vogt M, Leunig M, Wust J, Trampuz A. Improved diagnosis of periprosthetic joint infection by multiplex PCR of sonication fluid from removed implants. J Clin Microbiol. 2010;48(4):1208–14.

33 Krenn V, Morawietz L, Perino G, Kienapfel H, Ascherl R, Hassenpflug GJ, et al. Revised histopathological consensus classification of joint implant related pathology. Pathol Res Pract. 2014;210(12): 779–86.

34 Tschudin-Sutter S, Frei R, Dangel M, Jakob M, Balmelli C, Schaefer DJ, et al. Validation of a treatment algorithm for orthopaedic implant-related infections with device-retention-results from a prospective observational cohort study. Clin Microbiol Infect. 2016;22(5):457 e1–9.

35 Achermann Y, Vogt M, Spormann C, Kolling C, Remschmidt C, Wust J, et al.

Characteristics and outcome of 27 elbow periprosthetic joint infections: results from a 14-year cohort study of 358 elbow prostheses. Clin Microbiol Infect. 2011;17(3):432–8.

36 Betsch BY, Eggli S, Siebenrock KA, Tauber MG, Muhlemann K. Treatment of joint prosthesis infection in accordance with current recommendations improves outcome. Clin Infect Dis. 2008;46(8):1221–6.

37 Giulieri SG, Graber P, Ochsner PE, Zimmerli W. Management of infection associated with total hip arthroplasty according to a treatment algorithm. Infect. 2004;32(4):222–8.

38 Ilchmann T, Zimmerli W, Ochsner PE, Kessler B, Zwicky L, Graber P, et al. One-stage revision of infected hip arthroplasty: outcome of 39 consecutive hips. Int Orthop. 2016;40(5):913–8.

39 Campoccia D, Montanaro L, Speziale P, Arciola CR. Antibiotic-loaded biomaterials and the risks for the spread of antibiotic resistance following their prophylactic and therapeutic clinical use. Biomaterials. 2010;31(25):6363–77.

40 Esteban J, Gadea I, Perez-Jorge C, Sandoval E, Garcia-Canete J, Fernandez-Roblas R, et al. Diagnosis of spacer-associated infection using quantitative cultures from sonicated antibiotics-loaded spacers: implications for the clinical outcome. Eur J Clin Microbiol Infect Dis. 2016;35(2):207–13.

41 Zimmerli W, Widmer AF, Blatter M, Frei R, Ochsner PE. Role of rifampin for treatment of orthopedic implant-related staphylococcal infections: a randomized controlled trial. Foreign-Body Infection (FBI) Study Group. JAMA. 1998;279(19):1537–41.

42 Akgun D, Trampuz A, Perka C, Renz N. High failure rates in treatment of streptococcal periprosthetic joint infection: results from a seven-year retrospective cohort study. Bone Joint J. 2017;99-b(5):653–9.

43 Lora-Tamayo J, Senneville E, Ribera A, Bernard L, Dupon M, Zeller V, et al. The not-so-good prognosis of streptococcal

periprosthetic joint infection managed by implant retention: the results of a large multicenter study. Clinical Infect Dis. 2017.

44 McNally M, Nagarajah K. (iv) Osteomyelitis. Orthopaed Trauma. 2010;24(6):416–29.

45 Cierny G, 3rd, Mader JT, Penninck JJ. A clinical staging system for adult osteomyelitis. Clin Orthopaed and Rel Research. 2003(414):7–24.

46 Hunziker S, Hugle T, Schuchardt K, Groeschl I, Schuetz P, Mueller B, et al. The value of serum procalcitonin level for differentiation of infectious from noninfectious causes of fever after orthopaedic surgery. J Bone Joint Surg Am Vol. 2010;92(1):138–48.

47 Metsemakers WJ, Kuehl R, Moriarty TF, Richards RG, Verhofstad MH, Borens O, et al. Infection after fracture fixation: current surgical and microbiological concepts. Injury. 2016.

48 Lew DP, Waldvogel FA. Osteomyelitis. Lancet. 2004;364(9431):369–79.

49 Jutte P, Lazzeri E, Sconfienza LM, Cassar-Pullicino V, Trampuz A, Petrosillo N, et al. Diagnostic flowcharts in osteomyelitis, spondylodiscitis and prosthetic joint infection. Quart J Nuclear Med Molecular Imaging. 2014;58(1):2–19.

50 Trampuz A, Widmer AF. Infections associated with orthopedic implants. Curr Opin Infect Dis. 2006;19(4):349–56.

Chapter 4

Infective Endocarditis

Bahareh Ghadaki and Deborah Yamamura

Case Presentation 1

A 29-year-old woman presents to the emergency room with a three-day history of fever, malaise, nausea, vomiting, myalgia, and headache. The patient is previously well except for a remote history of inguinal hernia repair. She denies any intravenous drug use and is a non-smoker and non-drinker. There is no significant family history. She had a pedicure one week before her symptoms and had noticed some bleeding at the time. She currently works as a registered practical nurse at a community hospital.

Physical examination reveals a temperature of 38.5 °C, pulse of 110 per minute, and blood pressure of 110/70 mmHg. Cardiac examination reveals a normal S1 and S2 without any audible murmur. Neurological examination is normal. Conjunctivae reveal small petechiae. Non-tender erythematous nodules are present on her hands. Initial laboratory results are significant for a hemoglobin of 127 x 10^9/L, platelets 92 x 10^9/L, white blood count 3.2 g/L with 1.6 x 10^9/L absolute neutrophils with toxic granulation. HIV 1/2 Ag/Ab Combo Screen is non-reactive.

The differential diagnosis includes native valve infective endocarditis. The patient is admitted and three sets of blood cultures are obtained 30 minutes apart. You determine the clinical likelihood that the patient has endocarditis and consider what investigations are required.

4.1 Clinical Diagnosis

The pre-test probability that the patient has endocarditis should consider the epidemiology of infective endocarditis (IE). Patient demographics, the clinical presentation, and presence of risk factors help inform the clinical diagnosis.

4.1.1 Epidemiology

The epidemiology of IE is best derived from population-based studies, which are less likely to be influenced by referral bias. A comprehensive systematic review identified 17 population-based studies from four major world regions. The crude annual incidence of IE was in the range of 1.5 to 11.6 cases per 100,000 people [1]. Much of the variation in incidence rates was attributable to differences in case definition, disease misclassification, and differences in populations at risk. Several studies have highlighted the changing epidemiology of IE, including higher rates seen in the aging population, male gender, those with underlying heart disease including prosthetic valves and intra-vascular devices, and multiple co-morbidities [2–4].

Evidence-Based Infectious Diseases, Third Edition. Edited by Dominik Mertz, Fiona Smaill, and Nick Daneman.

Furthermore, the proportion of healthcare associated (or nosocomial) IE has increased and now represents 7–33% of IE cases [2,3,5,6].

The five most common organisms causing IE are *S. aureus* (MRSA median percentage 28%), Viridans group streptococci (VGS), other Streptococcus species, coagulase negative staphylococci (CoNS), and *Enterococcus* species [7]. *S. aureus* remains the predominant pathogen causing native valve IE, while CoNS is associated more commonly with prosthetic valve IE [7]. Similar to the temporal changes in patient characteristics, important changes have also occurred in the pathogens associated with IE. A recent systematic review of both population and hospital-based studies demonstrated that the global proportion of cases attributed to *Staphylococcus aureus* has increased from 18.1% in the 1960s to 29.7% in the 2000s with current percentages in North America as high as 52% [4]. CoNS and *Enterococcus* species are now seen in up to 10% of cases, likely owing to increases in intra-vascular catheters and prosthetic valves. Conversely, the proportions of IE attributed to VGS and culture negative endocarditis have decreased from 27.4% to 17.6% and 23% to 14.2%, respectively [4].

4.1.2 Clinical Presentation and Risk Factors

Diagnosing IE involves both a clinical assessment of associated risk factors, and a physical examination focusing on the cardiac, immunological, and vascular manifestations of endocarditis (Table 4.2).

A large multi-national prospective observational study demonstrated common predisposing conditions for IE, including degenerative valvular heart disease, presence of prosthetic valves, chronic intravenous access, co-morbid conditions such as diabetes, hemodialysis dependency, and history of injection drug use (IDU) [5]. Geographic analyses demonstrate a significantly higher proportion of patients with co-morbidities, chronic intravenous access and IDU among IE patients in North America, and more con-

genital heart disease among patients in South America [5].

While the clinical manifestations of IE can be quite variable, the two most common features that have been identified are fever and a new murmur, which are present in 62–96% and 36–48% of patients respectively [3,5]. In addition, vascular embolism (17–58%), splenomegaly (11–15%), and signs of heart failure (44%) can support the diagnosis, while the classic "stigmata of endocarditis" such as Osler nodes, Janeway lesion, and Roth spots are rare (<5%) [3,5]. When clinical suspicion is high, a lack of physical findings does not rule out IE.

4.2 Laboratory Investigations

4.2.1 Blood Cultures

Blood cultures should be obtained prior to the initiation of empiric antimicrobial treatment. At least three blood culture sets should be obtained 30 minutes apart over a 24-hour period for optimal detection of bacteremia and candidemia. Increasing the number of blood culture sets from two to three reduces the false negative rates from 10–18% to 2–4% [8]. Blood culture volume is one of the most important pre-analytic factors that optimize detection of pathogens. For adults, 8–10 ml per bottle (16–20 ml per venipuncture) is generally recommended (depending on the manufacturer) and a weight-based algorithm to guide pediatric blood culture volumes is recommended [9]. With the improvement of continuous monitoring blood culture systems, 98–99% of organisms are detected using a 5–7 day incubation protocol compared to the traditional 21-day incubation protocol for suspected endocarditis [8]. The HACEK group of organisms (*Haemophilus, Aggregatibacter, Cardiobacterium, Eikenella,* and *Kingella*) are readily detected with the shortened protocol [10]. *Candida spp.* are detected within five to seven days by most continuous monitoring blood culture systems. Other fungal pathogens such as dimorphic fungi and molds other than

Fusarium spp. require a lysis-centrifugation blood culture system [11].

Organism specific protocols (serology, specialized media, or molecular methods) to detect difficult to culture (*Bartonella*, *Legionella*) or non-culturable (*Coxiella*, *Tropheryma*) pathogens is recommended [12,13]. *Coxiella* (Q-fever) serology is a major criterion in the Modified Duke Criteria and should be obtained if blood cultures are negative.

4.2.2 Molecular Advances in Microbiology

Early diagnosis of IE and rapid identification of the causative organism is paramount for guiding antimicrobial management. Unfortunately, culture negative endocarditis, while decreasing in incidence still remains common (3.8–14%) [4,6]. This proportion is influenced by administration of antibiotics prior to obtaining cultures in addition to presence of atypical or difficult to culture organisms. Culture-independent molecular techniques such as polymerase chain reaction (PCR) and DNA sequencing are therefore gaining increasing attention. Evidence supporting the use of these molecular diagnostic approaches shows that heart valve PCR improves microbiological diagnosis of IE in 20–30% of cases, with a sensitivity of 92% compared to 44% for culture for diagnosis of definite IE [14,15]. Its primary role at this time remains restricted to patients to patients with culture negative IE who have undergone valve surgery [16,17].

4.3 Echocardiography

In addition to microbiological diagnosis, echocardiography is essential for the confirmation of IE. Most studies that used pathologic specimens or long-term follow-up as the reference standard for diagnosis of IE are more than two decades old. These studies consistently established that transesophageal echocardiography (TEE) has better operating characteristics than transthoracic echocardiography (TTE). In these case series, the sensitivity and specificity of TTE/TEE for diagnosing IE was 44–63%/87–100%, and 91/98%/91–100%, respectively [18,19]. Although advances in echocardiographic technology have improved TTE, two recent large prospective studies have demonstrated that it still remains an insensitive test [20,21]. TEE remains superior (sensitivity 82–95%) for the detection of IE on prosthetic valves, and in the presence of specific complications such as perivalvular abscesses and periannular complications [22,23].

Despite the superiority of TEE, it should not be used first-line for every patient with suspected IE as a negative or normal TTE in patients without an underlying valvular abnormality and/or prosthetic material, has a high negative predictive value of 97% [20]. Although TEE improves the sensitivity of the Duke Criteria (discussed later) for diagnosing both culture-positive [24] and culture-negative [25] endocarditis compared to classifications based on TTE results, this improvement is largely confined to (a) patients with intermediate probabilities of IE on clinical grounds, and (b) patients with prosthetic valves [24,26].

AHA and European guidelines support initial echocardiography in all cases of suspected IE. When clinical suspicion remains low and a good quality TTE is negative, then other diagnoses should be considered. If TTE reveals vegetations and the likelihood of complications is low, then subsequent TEE is unlikely to add incremental value. On the other hand, if clinical suspicion remains high, especially in the setting of a prosthetic valve or high-risk features for complication (valvular dysfunction, suggestion of peri-valvular extension), TEE should be performed following TTE regardless of its result [16,17,27].

4.4 Diagnostic Criteria

Incorporating clinical, laboratory, and echocardiographic information, the Duke Criteria remain the final step in the diagnosis of endocarditis. The Duke Criteria were originally proposed in 1994 as a research tool in order to stratify patients suspected of IE into three categories: definite, possible and rejected [28]. Since their development, observational studies in 1,700 geographically and clinically diverse patients have demonstrated superior operating characteristics, with moderate sensitivity and high specificity, compared with the earlier Beth Israel criteria [29]. In 2000, several refinements were made to both the major and minor criteria resulting in the new Modified Duke Criteria (see Table 4.1) [30].

The new criteria incorporated four major changes including the redefinition of major criteria with the inclusion of all types of *S. aureus* bacteremia, including community and hospital acquired as well as the inclusion of *Coxiella* serologic diagnostic testing. In addition, echocardiographic findings not meeting major criteria were removed from

---

Table 4.1 The Modified Duke Criteria* for diagnosis of infective endocarditis.

Major criteria

I Positive blood culture for infective endocarditis

A Typical microorganism for IE from 2 separate blood cultures

    1 Viridans group streptococci, *Streptococcus bovis*, HACEK group, *Staphylococcus aureus*, or

    2 Community-acquired enterococci, in the absence of a primary focus, or

B Persistently positive blood cultures, defined as recovery of a microorganism consistent with IE from:

    1 At least 2 positive blood cultures drawn more than 12 hours apart, or

    2 All of 3 or a majority of 4 or more separate blood cultures, with first and last drawn at least 1 hour apart

C A Single positive blood culture for *Coxiella burnetii* or anti-phase 1 IgG antibody titer ≥1:800

II Evidence of endocardial involvement

A Positive echocardiogram for IE

    1 Oscillating intra-cardiac mass, on valve or supporting structures, or in the path of regurgitant jets, or on implanted material, in the absence of an alternative anatomic explanation, or

    2 Abscess, or

    3 New partial dehiscence of prosthetic valve, or

B New valvular regurgitation (increase or change in preexisting murmur not sufficient)

Minor criteria

  I Predisposition: predisposing heart condition or injection drug use

  II Fever: ≥38.0 °C (100.4 °F)

III Vascular phenomena: major arterial emboli, septic pulmonary infarcts, mycotic aneurysm, intracranial hemorrhage, conjunctival hemorrhages, Janeway lesions

IV Immunologic phenomena: glomerulonephritis, Osler nodes, Roth spots, rheumatoid factor

  V Microbiologic evidence: positive blood culture but not meeting major criterion as noted previously,[†] or serologic evidence of active infection with organism consistent with IE

---

*Adapted from reference [27]. The diagnosis of "definite endocarditis" is made on pathologic grounds when appropriate pathologic specimens from surgery or autopsy reveal positive histology and/or culture. The diagnosis of "definite endocarditis" is made on clinical grounds when two major criteria, one major and three minor criteria, or five minor criteria are met. The diagnosis of "possible endocarditis" is given when one major and one minor criteria, or three minor criteria are met. The diagnosis of endocarditis is "rejected" if there is a firm alternative diagnosis to explain the clinical manifestations, if there is resolution of the manifestations suggesting IE with ≤4 days of antibiotic therapy, or if no pathologic evidence of IE is found at surgery or autopsy, in patients who received ≤4 days of antibiotic therapy.

[†]Excluding single positive cultures for coagulase-negative staphyloccoci and organisms that do not cause IE.

the minor criteria and the possible category was further restricted as noted in Table 4.1 [27,30]. Since their publication, few studies have evaluated the modified criteria. The sensitivity of the "definite" classification is 63–83% using surgical or autopsy data as a gold standard [31,32]. As such, further validation studies are required to establish the clinical utility of the Modified Duke Criteria in the diagnosis of IE.

In addition, clinicians should note that the Duke Criteria are meant to be a guide for diagnosing IE and must not replace clinical judgment. This is especially true in settings where the sensitivity of the Duke Criteria is diminished such as culture negative endocarditis, prosthetic valves, or cardiac devices [32,33].

4.5 Future Diagnostic Modalities

Non-invasive imaging modalities have recently been explored to improve the diagnosis of IE especially in situations where TEE is shown to have decreased sensitivity. These include patients with prosthetic valves or with cardiac or extra-cardiac complications. In a recent systematic review, the diagnostic value of electrocardiogram (ECG)-gated multidetector CT angiography (MDCTA) and F-fluorodeoxyglucose (F-FDG) PET/CT was compared to that of traditional echocardiography [34]. Although the studies included in this review were graded as low quality, the diagnostic advantage of these tests was supported. MDCTA showed increased sensitivity for identifying both native and prosthetic valve IE (97% and 93%) and perivalvular extension, whereas F-FDG PET/CT had added value for detection and exclusion of extra-cardiac complications such as systemic embolism [34]. Further studies looking at the risk and benefits, and exact role of each modality are required however before they can be recommended for their routine use in the diagnosis of IE.

Case Presentation 1 (continued)

The patient is placed empirically on vancomycin and ceftriaxone. Two blood culture sets are positive after eight hours for Gram-positive cocci in clusters. Cloxacillin is added empirically. The next day, the blood culture isolate is identified as *Staphylococcus aureus*. Trans-esophageal echocardiography reveals a mobile mass on the mitral valve leaflet, and color Doppler study shows mitral regurgitation with no evidence of extension of the intracardiac lesion. Susceptibility testing confirms the isolate is susceptible to cloxacillin. Repeat blood cultures at 72 hours are persistently positive for *S. aureus*. The patient develops left leg weakness and visual field deficits. Fundoscopic examination reveals multiple micro-haemorrhages and Roth spots. While deciding on the most appropriate course of antibiotics, you wonder which cerebral imaging modality to order to assess for cerebrovascular complications.

4.6 Diagnostic Criteria

This patient meets two major criteria in the Duke classification—isolation of a typical organism for IE in two blood culture sets, and echocardiographic detection of an oscillating mass attached to a valvular leaflet. Accordingly, the patient is classified as having "definite endocarditis." Determination of the most appropriate antibiotic regimen requires consideration of the appropriate agent(s), their dose, and duration of treatment.

4.7 Antimicrobial Management

Successful management of IE hinges on microbial eradication and sterilization of heart valves with antimicrobial therapy. The nature of the vegetation environment (high bacterial load, biofilm formation, low metabolic activity) often poses challenges to effective therapy [27]. To overcome these inherent characteristics, general management principals can be applied to all patients. These include the use of bactericidal antibiotics, combination therapy for synergistic effect—especially in the treatment of enterococcal IE, and prolonged antibiotic therapy [27,35].

In all cases of suspected IE, empiric antibiotics should be initiated once blood cultures are drawn. Although there are no randomized controlled trials evaluating empiric therapy for infective endocarditis, the European Society of Cardiology (ECS) cites Level C evidence for empiric treatment of community acquired native valve IE with ampicillin plus cloxacillin with gentamicin [17]. Once blood culture results become available, antibiotics can be selected to target the specific organism.

The AHA has provided thorough treatment recommendations for IE caused by specific organisms (see Table 4.2) [27]. Few randomized trials of these regimens have been

Table 4.2 Selected native valve endocarditis treatment regimens.*

Organism	Regimen	Duration	Comments
Viridans group streptococci (VGS)/S. *gallolyticus* with penicillin (PCN) MIC ≤ 0.12 μg/mL	Penicillin G 12–18 million U IV per 24 h OR Ceftriaxone 2 g IV/IM q24h	4 weeks 4 weeks	For penicillin/ceftriaxone allergy, vancomycin 15 mg/kg IV q12h
VGS/S. *gallolyticus* with PCN MIC > 0.12 to ≤ 0.5 μg/mL	Penicillin G 24 million U IV per 24 h PLUS Gentamicin 3 mg/kg IV/IM q24h	4 weeks 2 weeks	Ceftriaxone may be a reasonable alternative treatment option for VGS isolates that are susceptible For penicillin/ceftriaxone allergy, vancomycin 15 mg/kg IV q12h is a reasonable option.
VGS/S. *gallolyticus* or Nutritionally variant Streptococci with PCN MIC > 0.5 μg/mL	See treatment regimen for penicillin/ ampicillin-resistant enterococcal endocarditis (see reference [27])		
Oxacillin-sensitive Staphylococci	Oxacillin/nafcillin 2 g IV q4h OR Cefazolin 2 g IV q8h (for non-anaphylactictoid penicillin allergy)	6 weeks	For anaphylactoid penicillin allergy, substitute vancomycin 15 mg/kg IV q12h
Oxacillin-resistant Staphylococci	Vancomycin 15 mg/kg IV q12h OR Daptomycin ≥8 mg/kg/dose	6 weeks 6 weeks	
Enterococcus spp. susceptible to penicillin, ampicillin, gentamicin, and vancomycin (regimens for both native and prosthetic valve)	Ampicillin 2 g IV 4 h PLUS Gentamicin 3 mg/kg (ideal body weight) IV/IM in 2–3 equally divided doses OR Ampicillin 2 g IV 4 h PLUS Ceftriaxone 2 g IV q12h	4–6 weeks 6 weeks	Native valve: 4-wk therapy recommended for patients with symptoms of illness <3 mo; 6-wk therapy recommended for native valve symptoms >3 mo and for patients with prosthetic valve or prosthetic material. Recommended for patients with creatinine clearance >50 mL/min. For penicillin/ampicillin allergy, Vancomycin 15 mg/kg IV q12h for 6 weeks PLUS gentamicin 1 mg/kg IV/IM q8h for 6 weeks

*Adapted from Baddour LM et al. [27].

conducted because the disease itself is rare, and specific etiologies are rarer still [36]. We limit our discussion to reviewing the best and most recent available evidence on regimens for treating native valve *S. aureus*.

For methicillin susceptible native valve *S. aureus* IE, updated guidelines have removed the recommendation to add gentamicin for both right and left sided disease [27]. There is moderate evidence from a small number of prospective comparator clinical trials that adjunctive aminoglycoside therapy has no added value in clinical success, or reduction of mortality or relapse compared to monotherapy with a B-lactam [37]. In addition aminoglycosides are associated with increased harm (nephrotoxicity) [37].

Another option in the management of *S. aureus* IE is the use of daptomycin [27,38]. In a randomized controlled trial, the efficacy and safety of daptomycin was compared with standard therapy for *S. aureus* bacteremia and endocarditis. Results demonstrated non-inferiority of daptomycin for right sided endocarditis (RR 0.89 95% CI 0.42–1.89) secondary to both methicillin susceptible (MSSA) and resistant *S. aureus* (MRSA) [38]. For left sided IE, weaker evidence exists for the use of daptomycin [39]. Current guidelines have therefore incorporated daptomycin as an alternative treatment for both MSSA and MRSA IE [16,17,27].

There are no evidence-based data regarding the appropriate duration of therapy for *S. aureus* native valve IE. Based on consensus, the AHA recommends six weeks for uncomplicated infections and consideration of at least six weeks in those with complications such as perivalvular abscess [27].

4.8 Embolic Events

Embolic events affect 28–38% of patients with IE [2,40–42]. The most common sites for embolization are the central nervous system, spleen, lungs, kidneys, peripheral arteries, retinal arteries, and coronary vessels [2,40,42]. Large multi-center observational

studies demonstrate that most patients have evidence of embolism before or at the time of diagnosis of IE, with a smaller percentage (7–8.5%) developing new embolism after the initiation of antibiotic therapy [2,41,42]. In this subset of patients the incidence of embolic events is highest during the first two weeks of antibiotic therapy and then decreases rapidly [41,42].

Prediction of individual patient risk for embolization has been evaluated in a number of observational studies. Results from three contemporary prospective studies looking at patients with a diagnosis of IE demonstrate that *S. aureus* bacteremia and vegetation size >/= 10 mm are independently associated with risk of embolism [40–42]. In addition, a simple bedside prediction system has been developed and validated, which can quantify the embolism risk at admission of patients with IE [41]. The use of this tool can further facilitate treatment decisions, such as performing early surgery for those with a high embolism risk.

4.9 Cerebrovascular Imaging

Cerebrovascular complications such as ischemic and hemorrhagic stroke are not only common, seen in 10–40% of patients with IE, but are some of the most serious complications with associated poor outcomes [43]. IE patients with neurological symptoms should undergo imaging, preferably with MRI, which has superior sensitivity compared to CT in both symptomatic and asymptomatic patients [44]. In one large prospective series, clinically silent cerebral lesions, including ischemic stroke and cerebral micro-bleeds, were detected in up to 72% of patients at the acute phase of IE with MRI or MRA [45]. Mycotic aneurysm occur in 5–9%, although this is likely an underestimate. CT or MR angiography detect mycotic aneurysms, but have a lower sensitivity than cerebral angiography [46]. CTA or MRA is recommended for symptomatic patients, and if negative, angiography should be considered [17,27].

Despite the frequency of cerebral events, few studies have analyzed the impact of cerebral MRI in the management of IE. Low-level evidence suggests that cerebral MRI/MRA has clinical value in the diagnostic classification and treatment of patients with IE, particularly the timing of surgery and monitoring [44,47]. Whether these changes have any impact on clinical outcomes remains unclear and therefore routine use of cerebral MRI for patients without neurologic symptoms or signs cannot be endorsed at this time [27,44].

Case Presentation 1 (continued)

You start the patient on cloxacillin 2 g IV q4hours. An MRI head is ordered and reveals a small ischemic stroke. The patient's neurological symptoms improve over the following 48 hours. Unfortunately, however, the blood cultures remain persistently positive after six days of targeted therapy. A repeat TTE reveals extension of the mobile mass on the mitral valve with a new papillomatous lesion. A paravalvular abscess cannot be ruled out. You place a consultation to cardiovascular surgery for consideration of valve replacement surgery.

4.10 Surgical Intervention

4.10.1 Indications and Timing of Surgical Intervention

The proportion of patients with IE undergoing valve surgery is increasing [48]. Traditional indications include: valve dysfunction leading to heart failure, presence of heart block, perivalvular abscesses, or penetrating lesions, patients with fungal infection or highly resistant organisms, persistent bacteremia despite theoretically adequate antibiotic treatment, and possibly, persistent emboli despite appropriate therapy, or with echocardiographic detection of large (>10 mm) mobile vegetation(s) on the mitral valve [27].

Through decades of clinical experience supporting adherence to these indications, there has been only one randomized trial examining the role of valve surgery in the management of IE [49]. In this trial, early surgery (within 48 h) was compared with conventional treatment (including surgery if required) in patients with native valve endocarditis with severe left sided valve dysfunction and vegetations >10mm. Patients were excluded if they had heart failure, embolic stroke, prosthetic valve, or abscess. A significant reduction in the composite primary outcome of in-hospital death or embolism occurred in the early surgery group (3% vs. 23%, hazard ratio 0.10, 95% CI 0.01–0.82) primarily driven by a reduction in the rate of embolism [49]. Although the exclusion criteria of this study limit its generalizability, it spurred a re-interest in early surgical intervention for patients at high risk.

A recent systematic review and meta-analysis sought to determine the benefits of early surgery from available evidence [50]. In this review, a significant reduction in all cause mortality was seen in the early surgical group combining $\leq$7 days and 8–20 days (OR 0.61, 95% CI 0.5–0.74) compared to conventional therapy, in both the unmatched and propensity-matched group. Recurrence of endocarditis at follow-up was more common with early surgery, but this was not statistically significant [50]. This study is limited as the majority of the included studies were observational studies that are prone to selection bias and survivor bias.

In real-world settings, however, applicability of these recommendations to all patients can be challenging. This was highlighted in the International Collaboration on Endocarditis prospective cohort study, which enrolled 1,269 patients from across 29 centers and 16 countries [51]. In this study, 24% (202/863) of patients with a surgical indication were not operated on for a variety of reasons, including poor prognosis, hemodynamic instability, death, and evidence of stroke [51].

Decisions on the indication and timing of surgical intervention must therefore be tailored to the individual patient and should be determined through collaborative management with a multispecialty team, including expertise in cardiology, imaging, cardiothoracic surgery, and infectious diseases [27,52]. Finally, the use of a risk stratification tool that provides prognostic information regarding operative and long-term mortality should be used in order to facilitate decision making and council patients regarding operative risk [53].

4.10.2 Valve Surgery in Patients with Prior Emboli/Hemorrhage/Stroke

Due to the lack of randomized trials, controversy exists around the optimal timing of valve surgery in patients with stroke. Concerns surrounding early surgical intervention include risk of hemorrhagic transformation with anticoagulation during cardiopulmonary bypass or progression of cerebral ischemia due to episodes of perioperative hypotension. Newer evidence reveals that neurological deterioration post-surgery is lower than previously assumed [54,55].

Based on available evidence the decision around surgical timing must take into consideration the type and severity of the cerebrovascular complication. In patients with transient ischemic strokes, or silent cerebral emboli, the risk of post-operative neurological deterioration is low and as such surgical intervention is recommended without delay [17,54,55]. Conversely, in cases with intra-cranial hemorrhage, the neurological prognosis is likely to be poor and surgery must be postponed for at least one month [17,27,56]. For patients who present with a non-severe embolic stroke without evidence of hemorrhage, international guidelines suggest that early surgery is not contraindicated and can be undertaken safely [17,27]. After publication of these guidelines a meta-analysis of 14

observational trials evaluating patients with IE complicated by an ischemic stroke was published which demonstrated that early surgery (regardless of timing, <7 or <14 days) was associated with a 1.7 fold greater risk of mortality, with no observed benefit in one-year mortality [43]. Following this, a retrospective cohort study of 568 patients demonstrated that early surgery (within 7 days) is safe in IE patients with cerebral infarction [56]. The general consensus approach is therefore to consider early surgery for IE patients with non-severe ischemic stroke who have clear indications for surgical intervention such as heart failure, uncontrolled infection, or abscess [17,27]. In all others, delayed surgical management should be considered.

Case Presentation 1 (continued)

The patient underwent surgery eight days after presentation. At the time of surgery, the mitral valve vegetation was 1.5 cm and a paravalulvar abscess extending into the wall of the ventricle was confirmed. Debridement of the abscess and a mitral valve replacement with a mechanical valve was performed. The patient was continued on cloxacillin 2 g IV q4 hours for eight weeks following surgery and the first negative blood culture.

4.11 Duration of Antibiotic Therapy after Surgery

The duration of antibiotic therapy for IE are outlined in multiple international guidelines [16,17,27]. Duration depends on both causative organism and presence of prosthetic valve. Expert opinion suggests that the counting of days for the duration of therapy should begin on the first day on which blood cultures are negative in cases in which blood cultures were initially positive [27]. In situations where the patient undergoes valve surgery, limited evidence exists to help guide duration of therapy. In a small retrospective study, relapse did not occur in patients with negative valve cultures treated for less than two weeks after surgery. No statistically significant difference in relapse occurred with positive or negative cultures or Gram stain [57]. Given the small, retrospective nature of the study and the high frequency of *Streptococcus* spp. as the causative organism, further evaluation is required. The general consensus remains that if the resected tissue is culture negative, the total duration of post-operative treatment should remain as per native valve IE minus the number of days of treatment administered prior to valve surgery. For those with positive operative cultures, the total post-operative duration resets from the day of surgery [27].

4.12 Prognosis

4.12.1 Relapse and Reinfection

Two main types of recurrent endocarditis exist: relapse and reinfection. The term *relapse* generally refers to a repeat episode of IE within six months caused by the same organism, while r*einfection* describes an infection after six months and/or caused by a different organism [17,58]. Aside from using this general definition, molecular typing can be employed to differentiate between the two diagnoses [58]. This is often important given the implications of relapsed infection with respect to management and prognosis [58].

The risk of recurrent infection among survivors of IE ranges between 2–6% [17,59]. In the International Collaboration on Endocarditis—Prospective Cohort Study, re-infection was more common than relapse (81% vs. 19%) [59]. IE relapse occurs with specific groups of patients: IDUs (OR 2.9), history of previous IE (OR 2.8), and hemodialysis dependency (OR 2.5) [59]. Relapse also confers a worse prognosis with higher one-year mortality rates compared to those with a single episode of IE [59].

Patient counseling around the risk of recurrence should occur at follow-up highlighting that any new signs or symptoms of systemic toxicity require immediate evaluation, including ≥3 sets of blood cultures [27].

4.12.2 Mortality

Survival rates after the completion of antibiotic treatment in patients with IE is estimated to be 80–90% at one year, 70–80% at two years, and 60–70% at five years [17]. Among all patients with IE, independent risk factors for six-month mortality include variables related to: host factors (older age, dialysis), IE characteristics (prosthetic or nosocomial IE, *S. aureus* infection, left-sided valve vegetation), and IE complications (severe heart failure, stroke, paravalvular complication, and persistent bacteremia) [60].

Case Presentation 1 (continued)

The patient was seen in follow-up after completion of her antibiotic therapy. She had a repeat echocardiogram at one and three months, and is scheduled to have an echocardiogram at six and 12 months. CBC and CRP have been normal. She has a medical alert bracelet. The patient inquires what she should do in the future to prevent recurrence.

4.12.3 Antibiotic Prophylaxis

In 2008, AHA published an updated guideline on prophylaxis in the setting of infective endocarditis [61]. The highlights from the guidelines are presented in Table 4.3. Written instructions should be provided to the patient that include indications for prophylaxis and a standing prescription. Patients should be encouraged to obtain a medical alert bracelet.

Table 4.3 Recommendations regarding prophylaxis for infective endocarditis.

Indications for Prophylaxis	Recommended Procedures	Antibiotic regimen*
1. Patients with a prosthetic heart valve or prosthetic material used for valve repair	Dental work: manipulation of either gingival tissue or the periapical region of teeth or perforation of oral mucosa	Oral: Amoxicillin 2 g IV: Ampicillin 2 g IV OR cefazolin or ceftriaxone 1 g IV/IM
2. Patients with previous infective endocarditis	Respiratory tract: Incision or biopsy of the respiratory tract mucosa	Allergy to penicillin: ORAL: Cephalexin[†] 2 g OR
3. Patients with congenital heart disease (unrepaired or repaired with residual defects or completely repaired during the first six months)	Genitourinary and gastrointestinal tract: Only in the setting of active infection	Clindamycin 600 mg OR Azithromycin 500 mg IV: Cefazolin or ceftriaxone 1 g IV/IM OR Clindamycin 600 mg IV
4. Cardiac transplant recipients with valve regurgitation due to a structurally abnormal valve	Skin or musculoskeletal tissue: Only in the setting of active infection.	

*Regimen: Single Dose 30 to 60 min before procedure. Doses listed are for adults. Please refer to reference [61] for pediatric doses.
[†]Cephalosporins should not be used in an individual with a history of anaphylaxis, angioedema, or urticaria with penicillin or ampicillin.

References

1 Bin Abdulhak AA, Baddour LM, Erwin PJ, et al. Global and regional burden of infective endocarditis, 1990–2010: A systematic review of the literature. Glob Heart. 2014;9:131–43. doi:10.1016/j.gheart.2014.01.002

2 Hill EE, Herijgers P, Claus P, et al. Infective endocarditis: changing epidemiology and predictors of 6-month mortality: a prospective cohort study. Eur Heart J. 2007;28:196–203. doi:10.1093/eurheartj/ehl427

3 Cecchi E, Chirillo F, Castiglione A, et al. Clinical epidemiology in Italian Registry of Infective Endocarditis (RIEI): Focus on age, intravascular devices and enterococci. Int J Cardiol. 2015;190:151–6. doi:10.1016/j.ijcard.2015.04.123

4 Slipczuk L, Codolosa JN, Davila CD, et al. Infective endocarditis epidemiology over five decades: a systematic review. PLoS One. 2013;8. doi:10.1371/journal.pone.0082665

5 Murdoch DR, Corey GR, Hoen B, et al. NIH Public Access. 2013;169:463–73. doi:10.1001/archinternmed.2008.603.Clinical

6 Hoen B. DX. Supplementary Appendix to Infective endocarditis. N Engl J Med. 2013;1206782. doi:10.1056/NEJMoa1206782

7 Vogkou CT, Vlachogiannis NI, Palaiodimos L, et al. The causative agents in infective endocarditis: a systematic review comprising 33,214 cases. Eur J Clin Microbiol Infect Dis. 2016;:1–19. doi:10.1007/s10096-016-2660-6

8 Weinstein MP, Doern G V. A critical appraisal of the role of the clinical microbiology laboratory in the diagnosis of bloodstream infections. J Clin Microbiol. 2011;49:1–5. doi:10.1128/JCM.00765-11

9 Snyder JW. Blood cultures: the importance of meeting pre-analytical requirements in reducing contamination, optimizing sensitivity of detection, and clinical Relevance. Clin Microbiol Newsl. 2015;37: 53–7. doi:10.1016/j.clinmicnews.2015.03.001

10 Petti CA, Bhally HS, Weinstein MP, et al. Utility of extended blood culture incubation for isolation of haemophilus, and kingella organisms: a retrospective multicenter evaluation utility of extended blood culture incubation for isolation of and kingella organisms: a retrospective multicenter. J Clin Microbiol. 2006;44:1–4. doi:10.1128/JCM.44.1.257

11 Clinical and Laboratory Standards Institute. Principles and Procedures for Detection of Fungi in Clinical Specimens-Direct examination and Culture; Approved Guideline (M54A). 2012.

12 Houpikian P, Raoult D. Blood Culture-negative endocarditis in a reference center. 2005;84:162–73. doi:10.1097/01.md.0000165658.82869.17

13 Baron EJ, Scott JD, Tompkins LS. Prolonged incubation and extensive subculturing do not increase recovery of clinically significant microorganisms from standard automated blood cultures. Clin Infect Dis. 2005;41:1677–80. doi:10.1086/497595

14 Miller RJH, Chow B, Pillai D, et al. Development and evaluation of a novel fast broad-range 16S ribosomal DNA PCR and sequencing assay for diagnosis of bacterial infective endocarditis: multi-year experience in a large Canadian healthcare zone and a literature review. BMC Infect Dis. 2016;16:146. doi:10.1186/s12879-016-1476-4

15 Maneg D, Sponsel J, Müller I, et al. Advantages and limitations of direct PCR amplification of bacterial 16S-rDNA from resected heart tissue or swabs followed by direct sequencing for diagnosing infective endocarditis: A retrospective analysis in the routine clinical setting. Biomed Res Int. 2016. doi:10.1155/2016/7923874

16 Gould FK, Denning DW, Elliott TSJ, et al. Guidelines for the diagnosis and antibiotic treatment of endocarditis in adults: A report of the working party of the british society for antimicrobial chemotherapy. J Antimicrob Chemother. 2012;67:269–89. doi:10.1093/jac/dkr450

17 Habib G, Lancellotti P, Antunes MJ, et al. 2015 ESC Guidelines for the management of infective endocarditis. 2015. doi:10.1093/eurheartj/ehv319

18 Evangelista A, Gonzalez-Alujas MT. Echocardiography in infective endocarditis. Heart. 2004;90:614–7. doi:10.1136/hrt.2003.029868

19 Pedersen WR, Walker M, Olson JD, et al. Value of transesophageal echocardiography as an adjunct to transthoracic echocardiography in evaluation of native and prosthetic valve endocarditis. Chest. 1991;100:351–6. doi:10.1378/chest.100.2.351

20 Barton TL, Mottram PM, Stuart RL, et al. Transthoracic echocardiography is still useful in the initial evaluation of patients with suspected infective endocarditis: Evaluation of a large cohort at a tertiary referral center. Mayo Clin Proc. 2014;89:799–805. doi:10.1016/j.mayocp.2014.02.013

21 Cecchi E, Chirillo F, Faggiano P, et al. The diagnostic utility of transthoracic echocardiography for the diagnosis of infective endocarditis in the real world of the Italian registry on infective endocarditis. Echocardiography. 2013;30:871–9. doi:10.1111/echo.12173

22 Hostetter MK, Iverson S, Thomas W, et al. The New England Journal of Medicine Downloaded from nejm.org on October 21, 2011. For personal use only. No other uses without permission. Copyright © 1991 Massachusetts Medical Society. All rights reserved. 1991.

23 Habets J, Tanis W, Reitsma JB, et al. Are novel non-invasive imaging techniques needed in patients with suspected prosthetic heart valve endocarditis? A systematic review and meta-analysis. Eur Radiol. 2015;25:2125–33. doi:10.1007/s00330-015-3605-7

24 Roe MT, Abramson MA, Li J, et al. Clinical information determines the impact of transesophageal echocardiography on the diagnosis of infective endocarditis by the Duke Criteria. Am Heart J. 2000;139:945–51. doi:10.1067/mhj.2000.104762

25 Kupferwasser LI, Darius H, Müller AM, et al. Diagnosis of culture-negative endocarditis: the role of the Duke Criteria and the impact of transesophageal echocardiography. Am Heart J. 2001;142:146–52. doi:10.1067/mhj.2001.115586

26 Lindner JR, Case RA, Dent JM, et al. Diagnostic value of echocardiography in suspected endocarditis. Circulation. 1996;93:730 LP–736. http://circ.ahajournals.org/content/93/4/730.abstract

27 Baddour LM, Wilson WR, Bayer AS, et al. Infective endocarditis in adults: diagnosis, antimicrobial therapy, and management of complications: a scientific statement for healthcare professionals from the American Heart Association. 2015. doi:10.1161/CIR.0000000000000296

28 Durack DT, Lukes AS, Bright DK. New criteria for diagnosis of infective endocarditis: utilization of specific echocardiographic findings. Duke Endocarditis Service. Am J Med. 1994;96:200–9.

29 Bayer AS, Bolger AF, Taubert KA, et al. Heart and its complications. Heart. 1994;2936–48. doi:10.1016/S0031-398X(05)70273-3

30 Li JS, Sexton DJ, Mick N, et al. Proposed modifications to the Duke Criteria for the diagnosis of infective endocarditis. Fowler V Jr., Ryan T, Bashore T, Corey GR. Oxford University Press Stable. URL: http://www.jstor.org/stable/4461118 of Infective En. 2016;30:633–8.

31 der Vaart TW, der Meer JTM. P35 Scant support for use of the Duke Criteria in management decisions about patients suspected of infective endocarditis: a literature review. Int J Antimicrob Agents. 2013;41:S17. doi:10.1016/S0924-8579(13)70059-1

32 Topan A, Carstina D, Slavcovici A, et al. Assesment of the Duke Criteria for the diagnosis of infective endocarditis after twenty-years. An analysis of 241 cases. Clujul Med. 2015;88:321. doi:10.15386/cjmed-469

33 Prendergast BD. Diagnostic criteria and problems in infective endocarditis. Heart. 2004;90:611–3. doi:10.1136/hrt.2003.029850

34 Gomes A, Glaudemans AWJM, Touw DJ, et al. Diagnostic value of imaging in infective endocarditis: a systematic review. Lancet Infect Dis. 2016;0:269–89. doi:10.1016/S1473-3099(16)30141-4

35 Cahill TJ, Prendergast BD. Infective endocarditis. Lancet. 2016;387:882–93. doi:10.1016/S0140-6736(15)00067-7

36 Díez-Villanueva P, Muñoz P, Marín M, et al. Infective endocarditis: Absence of microbiological diagnosis is an independent predictor of inhospital mortality. Int J Cardiol. 2016;220:162–5. doi:10.1016/j.ijcard.2016.06.129

37 Falagas ME, Matthaiou DK, Bliziotis IA. The role of aminoglycosides in combination with a beta-lactam for the treatment of bacterial endocarditis: A meta-analysis of comparative trials. J Antimicrob Chemother. 2006;57:639–47. doi:10.1093/jac/dkl044

38 Fowler VG, Boucher HW, Corey GR, et al. Daptomycin versus standard therapy for bacteremia and endocarditis caused by Staphylococcus aureus. N Engl J Med. 2006;355:653–65. doi:10.1056/NEJMoa1208410

39 Carugati M, Bayer AS, Miro JM, et al. High-dose daptomycin therapy for left-sided infective endocarditis: a prospective study from the international collaboration on endocarditis. Antimicrob Agents Chemother. 2013;57:6213–22. doi:10.1128/AAC.01563-13

40 Rizzi M, Ravasio V, Carobbio A, et al. Predicting the occurrence of embolic events: an analysis of 1456 episodes of infective endocarditis from the Italian Study on Endocarditis (SEI). BMC Infect Dis. 2014;230:1–10.

41 Hubert S, Thuny F, Resseguier N, et al. Prediction of symptomatic embolism in infective endocarditis: Construction and validation of a risk calculator in a multicenter cohort. J Am Coll Cardiol. 2013;62:1384–92. doi:10.1016/j.jacc.2013.07.029

42 Thuny F, Disalvo G, Belliard O, et al. Risk of embolism and death in infective endocarditis: Prognostic value of echocardiography—A prospective multicenter study. Circulation. 2005;112:69–75. doi:10.1161/CIRCULATIONAHA.104.493155

43 Mihos CG, Pineda AM, Santana O. Original article: A meta-analysis of early versus delayed surgery for valvular infective endocarditis complicated by embolic ischemic stroke. 2016;11:187–92.

44 Champey J, Pavese P, Bouvaist H, et al. Value of brain MRI in infective endocarditis: a narrative literature review. Eur J Clin Microbiol Infect Dis. 2016;35:159–68. doi:10.1007/s10096-015-2523-6

45 Hess A, Klein I, Iung B, et al. Brain MRI findings in neurologically asymptomatic patients with infective endocarditis. AJNR Am J Neuroradiol. 2013;34:1579–84. doi:10.3174/ajnr.A3582

46 Hui FK, Bain M, Obuchowski NA, et al. Mycotic aneurysm detection rates with cerebral angiography in patients with infective endocarditis. J Neurointerv Surg. 2015;7:449–52. doi:10.1136/neurintsurg-2014-011124

47 Duval X, Iung B, Klein I, et al. Effect of early cerebral magnetic resonance imaging on clinical decisions in infective endocarditis: a prospective study. Ann Intern Med 2010;152:497–504, W175. doi:10.7326/0003-4819-152-8-201004200-00006

48 Tleyjeh IM, Abdel-Latif A, Rahbi H, et al. A systematic review of population-based studies of infective endocarditis. Chest. 2007;132:1025–35. doi:10.1378/chest.06-2048

49 Kang D-H, Kim Y-J, Kim S-H, et al. Early Surgery versus Conventional Treatment for Infective Endocarditis. N Engl J Med. 2012;366:2466–73. doi:DOI: 10.1056/NEJMoa1112843

50 Anantha Narayanan M, Mahfood Haddad T, Kalil AC, et al. Early versus late surgical intervention or medical management for infective endocarditis: a systematic review and meta-analysis. Heart.

2016;heartjnl-2015-308589. doi:10.1136/heartjnl-2015-308589

51 Chu VH, Park LP, Athan E, et al. Association between surgical indications, operative risk, and clinical outcome in infective endocarditis a prospective study from the international collaboration on endocarditis. Circulation. 2014;131:131–40. doi:10.1161/CIRCULATIONAHA.114.012461

52 Chirillo F, Scotton P, Rocco F, et al. Impact of a multidisciplinary management strategy on the outcome of patients with native valve infective endocarditis. Am J Cardiol. 2013;112:1171–6. doi:10.1016/j.amjcard.2013.05.060

53 Wang TKM, Oh T, Voss J, et al. Comparison of contemporary risk scores for predicting outcomes after surgery for active infective endocarditis. Heart Vessels. 2015;30:227–34. doi:10.1007/s00380-014-0472-0

54 Thuny F, Avierinos JF, Tribouilloy C, et al. Impact of cerebrovascular complications on mortality and neurologic outcome during infective endocarditis: A prospective multicentre study. Eur Heart J. 2007;28:1155–61. doi:10.1093/eurheartj/ehm005

55 Ruttmann E, Willeit J, Ulmer H, et al. Neurological outcome of septic cardioembolic stroke after infective endocarditis. Stroke. 2006;37:2094–9. doi:10.1161/01.STR.0000229894.28591.3f

56 Okita Y, Minakata K, Yasuno S, et al. Optimal timing of surgery for active infective endocarditis with cerebral complications: a Japanese multicentre study. Eur J Cardio-Thoracic Surg. 2016;50:ezw035. doi:10.1093/ejcts/ezw035

57 Morris AJ, Drinković D, Pottumarthy S, et al. Bacteriological outcome after valve surgery for active infective endocarditis: implications for duration of treatment after surgery. Clin Infect Dis. 2005;41:187–94. doi:10.1086/430908

58 Chu VH, Sexton DJ, Cabell CH, et al. Repeat infective endocarditis: differentiating relapse from reinfection. Clin Infect Dis. 2005;41:406–9. doi:10.1086/431590

59 Alagna L, Park LP, Nicholson BP, et al. Repeat endocarditis: analysis of risk factors based on the International Collaboration on Endocarditis—Prospective Cohort Study. Clin Microbiol Infect. 2013;1–10. doi:10.1111/1469-0691.12395

60 Park LP, Chu VH, Peterson G, et al. Validated Risk Score for Predicting 6-Month Mortality in Infective. J Am Hear Assoc. 2016;1–14. doi:10.1161/JAHA.115.003016

61 Nishimura RA, Carabello BA, Faxon DP, et al. ACC/AHA 2008 guideline update on valvular heart disease: focused update on infective endocarditis: a report of the American College of Cardiology/American Heart Association Task Force on Practice Guidelines endorsed by the Society of Cardiovascular Anesth. J Am Coll Cardiol. 2008;52:676–85. doi:10.1016/j.jacc.2008.05.008

Chapter 5

Meningitis and Encephalitis
Christopher E. Kandel and Wayne L. Gold

5.1 Meningitis

Case Presentation 1

A 30-year-old man presents to the emergency department with a 24-hour history of fever and headache. The patient's symptoms began abruptly and have worsened steadily over the course of the day. His partner reports that in the last six hours he has become confused. He does not report photophobia or neck stiffness. He has no significant past medical or surgical history. He does not take medications and denies alcohol, tobacco, or drug use. His family history is likewise non-contributory. Physical examination reveals a temperature of 38.5 °C, a pulse of 110 beats per minute, and a blood pressure of 130/70 mmHg. He has no localizing neurological deficits, but he is orientated only to person. Initial laboratory evaluation reveals a white blood cell count of 21.4×10^9/L. You admit the patient with the presumptive diagnosis of meningitis, order two sets of blood cultures, and plan to perform a lumbar puncture (LP). You wonder whether to order a computed tomography (CT) scan prior to the LP to rule out an intracranial mass lesion as well as whether antibiotics should be withheld until after the CT and LP have been performed.

5.1.1 Epidemiology

Acute meningitis may be caused by a wide variety of infectious pathogens as well as by non-infectious diseases (Box 5.1). Given its frequency and clinical impact, this chapter focuses specifically on acute bacterial meningitis. The annual incidence of bacterial meningitis varies by geographic region. In Western Europe and the United States, the incidence is less than 2 per 100,000 and has declined over time [1–3]. In contrast, the incidence is much higher in Africa [4].

Evidence-Based Infectious Diseases, Third Edition. Edited by Dominik Mertz, Fiona Smaill, and Nick Daneman.
© 2018 John Wiley & Sons Ltd. Published 2018 by John Wiley & Sons Ltd.

Box 5.1 Differential diagnosis of acute meningitis.

Bacteria

- *Streptococcus pneumoniae*
- *Neisseria meningitidis*
- *Listeria monocytogenes*
- *Haemophilus influenzae*
- *Streptococcus agalactiae*
- *Escherichia coli*
- *Klebsiella pneumoniae*
- *Pseudomonas aeruginosa*
- *Salmonella* spp.
- *Streptococcus suis*
- *Mycobacterium tuberculosis*

Rickettsiae

- *Rickettsia rickettsii*
- *Rickettsia conorii*
- *Rickettsia prowazekii*
- *Rickettsiae typhi*
- *Ehrlichia* and *Anaplasma* spp.

Spirochetes

- *Treponema pallidum*
- *Borrelia burgdorferi*
- *Leptospira* spp.

Protozoa and helminths

- *Acanthamoeba spp*
- *Naegleria fowleri*
- *Angiostrongylus cantonensis*
- *Baylisascaris procyonis*
- *Strongyloides stercoralis*

Viruses

- Non-polio enteroviruses (Echoviruses, Coxsackieviruses)
- Mumps virus
- Arboviruses
- Herpesviruses
- Lymphocytic choriomeningitis virus
- Human immunodeficiency virus
- Adenovirus
- Parainfluenza virus type 3
- Influenza virus
- Measles virus

Fungi

- *Cryptococcus neoformans*
- *Coccidioides immitis*
- *Histoplasma capsulatum*
- *Blastomyces dermatitidis*
- *Paracoccidioides brasiliensis*
- *Candida* spp.
- *Aspergillus* spp.
- *Sporothrix schenckii*

Neoplasms

- Lymphomatous meningitis
- Carcinomatous meningitis

Intracranial tumors and cysts

- Craniopharyngioma
- Dermoid/epidermoid cyst
- Teratoma

Medications

- Antimicrobial agents*
- Non-steroidal anti-inflammatory agents
- OKT3
- Azathioprine
- Cytosine arabinoside
- Immune globulin
- Ranitidine

Systemic illnesses

- Systemic lupus erythematosus
- Vogt–Koyanagi–Harada syndrome
- Sarcoidosis
- Behçet disease
- Rheumatoid arthritis
- Polymyositis
- Granulomatous polyangiitis
- Familial Mediterranean fever
- Kawasaki syndrome

Miscellaneous

- Seizures
- Migraine
- Serum sickness
- Heavy metal poisoning

- Syndrome of transient headache and neurological deficits with cerebrospinal fluid lymphocytosis (HaNDL)

*Trimethoprim, sulfamethoxazole, ciprofloxacin, amoxicillin, penicillin, cephalosporins, metronidazole.

As the majority of causative organisms of acute bacterial meningitis colonize the nasopharynx, it is unsurprising that immunization programs for *Streptococcus pneumoniae*, *Haemophilus influenzae* and *Neisseria meningitidis* have lowered the incidence of invasive diseases such as meningitis. Rates of invasive pneumococcal disease have declined in all age groups after the implementation of vaccination programs, with a more pronounced effect in infants [5–7]. Similar reductions have been observed following the introduction of *Neisseria meningitidis* type C and *Haemophilus influenzae* type B immunizations [8–10]. The expanding serotype coverage of recently licensed vaccines is likely to further reduce the incidence of bacterial meningitis [11].

5.1.2 Etiology of Bacterial Meningitis

The pathogens responsible for acute bacterial meningitis in adults over a 10-year period in the United States includes *S. pneumoniae* (70%), *N. meningitidis* (12%), *Streptococcus agalactiae* (7%), *H. influenzae* (6%), and *Listeria monocytogenes* (4%) [12]. The causative pathogens vary according to patient characteristics such as age, immunocompromising conditions or medications, neurosurgical procedures, recent head trauma and location of infection acquisition (nosocomial vs. community) [13]. Nosocomial meningitis often follows neurosurgical procedures or head trauma and as a result common pathogens include aerobic Gram-negative bacilli and *Staphylococcal spp* [14,15].

5.1.3 Clinical Presentation

Rapid recognition of meningitis is critical to ensure timely receipt of empiric antimicrobial therapy. Unfortunately, individual symptoms of meningitis are not sufficiently sensitive or specific to rule in or rule out the diagnosis. Fever is the most commonly found sign and is observed in 70–95% [16]. The classic triad of fever, neck stiffness, and altered level of consciousness occurs in less than 50% of patients, but the absence of all three of these features has a very high negative predictive value [17]. Physical examination findings with high specificity include Kernig's and Brudzinski's signs, but these are operator dependent [16,18]. Jolt accentuation of headache has a sensitivity approaching 100% and its absence effectively excludes the diagnosis of acute bacterial meningitis [16]. A history of symptoms referable to ear, sinuses or respiratory system infections should be elicited, if possible, as these commonly precede bacterial meningitis [17]. Rash is classically associated with meningococcal meningitis, but is a late manifestation and can be seen with other bacterial pathogens such as pneumococci [19].

5.1.4 Diagnosis

5.1.4.1 Lumbar Puncture and Neuroimaging

Prompt performance of a lumbar puncture is imperative in suspected cases of acute bacterial meningitis. Consideration should always be given for neuroimaging to identify those patients in whom cerebrospinal fluid (CSF) sampling is contraindicated. The chief risk of lumbar puncture in the setting of possible meningitis is brain herniation resulting from the increased pressure gradient accompanying the removal of CSF [11]. Indications for neuroimaging prior to lumbar puncture include new onset seizures, a history of central nervous system lesion(s), presence of a immunocompromising condition or therapies, or physical examination findings of papilledema, focal neurological deficits, or speech deficits [20,21]. Previous guidelines have recommended neuroimaging in those with an altered level of consciousness. However, this recommendation has been revised following the observation that its removal from guidelines in Sweden was associated with a decline in the development of neurologic sequelae and mortality that was correlated with a reduction in the time from presentation until administration of empiric antimicrobial therapy [22]. All patients for whom neuroimaging is requested prior to lumbar puncture should receive prompt empiric antimicrobial therapy prior to imaging.

Neuroimaging with CT or magnetic resonance imaging (MRI) once the diagnosis of meningitis is established is required for evaluation of persistent neurologic deficits. Patients with recurrent bacterial meningitis also require neuroimaging to assess for predisposing structural abnormalities with particular attention to the integrity of the dura and sinuses [23].

5.1.4.2 Cerebrospinal Fluid Culture

The gold standard for diagnosis of meningitis is CSF analysis. Prompt collection of CSF should be undertaken and sent for cell count with differential, protein concentration, glucose concentration (along with concurrent serum glucose), Gram stain, and bacterial culture. Initial clues for a bacterial etiology of meningitis include elevated opening pressure above 400 mm of water and a turbid or cloudy appearance of the CSF [24]. Typical findings for bacterial meningitis include CSF pleocytosis, hypoglycorrhachia, and elevated protein [17,25]. More than 90% of cases of bacterial meningitis will have CSF pleocytosis greater than 100 cells per microliter, the majority of which are comprised of polymorphonuclear cells in the acute setting

[17]. One prediction model found that the presence of any one of: CSF glucose less than 1.9 mmol/L, CSF-blood glucose ratio less than 0.23, CSF protein greater than 2.2 g/L, more than 2,000 cells/microliter in the CSF, or more than 1,180 cells/microliter of CSF polymorphonuclear cells was very specific for the diagnosis of community acquired bacterial meningitis [26]. *Listeria monocytogenes* infections frequently exhibit a CSF profile with a lower proportion of CSF polymorphonuclear cells along with a higher CSF-serum glucose ratio [27,28]. This is in contrast to viral pathogens, which characteristically have high proportions of lymphocytes [29].

Gram stain and bacterial culture of the CSF permit detection of the causative organism. The yield of a Gram stain varies markedly depending on the causative agent and degree of CSF pleocytosis with a range from 30–90%. This is higher in the case of *S. pneumoniae* and lower in the case of *N. meningitidis* [25]. Bacterial culture is positive in 80–90% of cases if collected prior to the administration of antibiotics [25]. Administration of antibiotics prior to CSF sampling reduces the yield of Gram stain and bacterial culture [30,31]; however, the CSF pleocytosis typically is unchanged for at least 24 hours [32–34]. Molecular testing may permit pathogen identification in such cases [35].

5.1.4.3 Blood Cultures

Blood cultures should be obtained in all cases of suspected meningitis, especially if a lumbar puncture is delayed, as the recovery of organisms is 50–80% [25]. If possible, these should be collected prior to the receipt of antibiotics, which lowers the yield considerably [36,37].

5.1.4.4 Molecular Testing Methods

The challenge of identifying organisms has led to the development of molecular methods such as polymerase chain reaction (PCR) to improve pathogen detection. Broad-range panels allowing for simultaneous testing of multiple pathogens have replaced PCR detection for specific pathogens such as *Streptococcus pneumoniae* [38–41]. The attraction of PCR-based techniques is the high sensitivity (85–100%) and specificity (95–100%) and enhanced yield after antibiotics have been administered [35,36,42]. The speed and cost of PCR-based testing has and will likely continue to improve [11].

Multi-target PCR testing can also identify viral pathogens such as herpes simplex virus and enterovirus, which may produce substantial cost savings by earlier cessation of antibiotics and shorter hospital stays [43,44]. PCR-based testing for viruses is more sensitive than viral culture or antibody detection [44].

Given that 16s rRNA is ubiquitous among bacteria, its detection has become an attractive means of identifying bacteria, with a sensitivity and specificity that approaches 90% [45]. Matrix-assisted laser desorption/ionization time of flight mass spectrometry (MALDI-TOF) is becoming commonplace in microbiology laboratories for the rapid identification of microorganisms and has successfully been applied directly to CSF [46]. Whole genome sequencing is an emerging technique currently used in outbreak settings [47]. As the cost and the time required for whole genome sequencing declines, this may have a role in the future for enhanced pathogen detection. These techniques have replaced rapid bacterial antigen testing, which has low sensitivity [25,48–50].

5.1.5 Therapy

> **Case Presentation 1 (continued)**
>
> The patient undergoes LP without prior CT scanning, which reveals an opening pressure of 250 mmH$_2$O. The patient is started on vancomycin 30 mg/kg IV every 12 hours and ceftriaxone 2 g IV every 12 hours. Subsequently, the CSF demonstrates a leukocyte count of $2,400\times10^6$/L (2,400/mm^3) with 70% neutrophils, protein concentration of 0.32 g/L (320 mg/ dL), and a glucose concentration of 3.4 mmol/L (62 mg/dL) with a serum glucose concentration of 7.2 mmol/L (130 mg/dL). The Gram stain reveals Gram-positive cocci in pairs and chains.

5.1.5.1 Antimicrobials

Antibiotics should be administered expediently in all suspected cases of bacterial meningitis. The selection of antibiotics requires an assessment of patient characteristics including age, immunosuppression, recent trauma, prior neurosurgical interventions, and unique epidemiologic exposures as well as knowledge of local resistance patterns [13]. Typical empiric antibiotic regimens include vancomycin in combination with a third-generation cephalosporin to cover common pathogens along with ampicillin in those older than age 50 or with immunocompromising conditions associated with an elevated risk of *L. monocytogenes* infection (Table 5.1) [24]. The addition of vancomycin provides empiric coverage against *S. pneumoniae* that may be resistant to both penicillin and cephalosporins [51]. Nosocomial meningitis requires coverage of gram-negative bacilli including *Pseudomonas aeruginosa* and *Staphylococcal spp.*, usually with an antipseudomonal cephalosporin or carbapenem in addition to vancomycin [14]. When treating cases of meningitis following neurosurgery, attention should be paid to local pathogens and known resistance patterns. If an organism is recovered then therapy should be targeted to the specific pathogen (Table 5.1).

5.1.5.2 Corticosteroids

The exuberant inflammatory response that accompanies bacterial lysis in meningitis has spawned numerous studies addressing the utility of adjuvant anti-inflammatory therapy with corticosteroids. A seminal trial of 301 adults with bacterial meningitis (defined by turbid CSF, bacteria visualized on Gram stain or CSF pleocytosis greater than 1,000 cells per cubic millimeter) randomized patients to receive placebo or intravenous dexamethasone at a dose of 10 mg every six hours with the first dose administered prior to or concurrent with the first dose of antibiotics [52]. This led to a significant reduction in mortality (relative risk 0.48; 95% confidence interval, 0.24–0.96) that was largely restricted to the subgroup with pneumococcal meningitis [52].

Table 5.1 Empiric treatment of bacterial meningitis.

Patient population	Likely pathogens	Antimicrobial	Dosage and route	Duration
Immunocompetent (Age 18–50 years)	*S. pneumoniae*	Vancomycin[†]	30 mg/kg IV every 12 hours[¶], *plus*	10–14 days
	N. meningitidis	Cefotaxime	2 g IV every 4-6 hours, or	7 days
		Ceftriaxone	2 g IV every 12 hours	7 days
Immunocompetent (Age >50 years)	*S. pneumoniae*	Vancomycin[†]	30 mg/kg IV every 12 hours[¶], *plus*	10–14 days
	N. meningitidis	Cefotaxime	2 g IV every 6 hours, or	7 days
	Gram-negative bacilli	Ceftriaxone	2 g IV every 12 hours, *plus*	21 days
	L. monocytogenes	Ampicillin	2 g IV every 4 hours	21 days
Nosocomial meningitis, post-neurosurgery, head trauma	Gram-negative bacilli	Ceftazidime	50–100 mg/kg IV every 8 hours[‡] *plus*	21 days
	Staphylococci	Vancomycin	30 mg/kg IV every 12 hours[¶]	21 days

Modified from references McGill et al. [11].
[†]Vancomycin provides activity against S. *pneumoniae* resistant to penicillin and cephalosporins.
[¶]Up to a maximum of 4 grams per day.
[‡]Up to a total of 2 grams every 8 hours.

A randomized trial in Vietnam of 217 adults and adolescents showed a possible mortality benefit (relative risk 0.79; 95% confidence interval, 0.45–1.39) among those with confirmed or suspected bacterial meningitis [53]. In contrast, a randomized trial of 465 patients from Malawi, where the prevalence of human immunodeficiency virus (HIV) infection is high, did not observe a beneficial effect of steroids (adjusted odds ratio of mortality 1.13, 95% confidence interval, 0.73–1.76) [54]. To evaluate whether the differences among the numerous randomized trials was due to patient characteristics such as underlying HIV, a meta-analysis of individual patient data was performed and found that dexamethasone was not beneficial [55]. A larger meta-analysis of 25 studies showed that corticosteroids reduced neurological sequelae—especially hearing loss—and possibly reduced mortality among those with pneumococcal meningitis [56]. These benefits did not extend to patients in low-income countries [56].

The dose of dexamethasone for the management of suspected bacterial meningitis is 10 mg intravenously every six hours for four days.

5.1.6 Preventive Therapy

5.1.6.1 *Haemophilus Influenzae*
There has been a marked shift in the causes of bacterial meningitis, which has been attributed to the introduction of childhood immunization programs. This effect has been most pronounced for *H. influenzae*, which was the leading cause of bacterial meningitis in the United States prior to vaccine availability [57]. *H. influenzae* type B (Hib) conjugate vaccines are highly immunogenic and have led to a substantial decline in the incidence of Hib meningitis [12]. Current recommendations are for infants to receive a primary series of Hib immunizations beginning at two months of age [58].

5.1.6.2 *Streptococcus Pneumoniae*
There are both conjugate and polysaccharide vaccines available for immunization against *S. pneumoniae* that cover an increasing

number of serotypes. These vaccines are efficacious in reducing invasive pneumococcal disease [59–61]. Immunization of infants has produced benefits in reducing invasive pneumococcal disease in adults, including pneumococcal meningitis. Current recommendations are for infants to receive a primary series of protein conjugate vaccine beginning at two months of age [58]. In adults who are immunocompromised, protein conjugate pneumococcal vaccine should also be administered followed by the administration of polysaccharide vaccine at a minimum of two months later. For adults 65 years of age or older without immunocompromising conditions, polysaccharide vaccine should be administered. [62,63].

5.1.6.3 *Neisseria Meningiditis*
There are 12 serogroups, of which six (A, B, C, W135, X, and Y) cause the majority of disease. Sporadic outbreaks of meningococcus that are propagated in areas of high population density continue to occur, defining the populations that derive maximal benefit from vaccination.

Currently, a vaccination series with meningococcal (serotypes A, C, W, and Y) immunizations is recommended for children at age 11 or earlier if specific conditions exist, including asplenia (functional or anatomic), persistent complement deficiency (acquired or congenital), or exposure to a hyperendemic area (travel or residence). In adults, until age 55, in the setting of these high-risk conditions vaccination is likewise indicated. Additionally, vaccination is recommended for adults who are military recruits, microbiologists routinely exposed to *N. meningitidis*, or first-year undergraduate students under the age of 21 and who reside in a dormitory and are incompletely immunized [63,64]. Recently, approval was granted for vaccines targeting serotype B, which are licensed for those 10 years of age and older, and is recommended for those at a heightened risk of infection [58,65]. In Canada, the recommendations are similar except for routine immunization against serotype C for all infants [66].

Meningococcal vaccinations can be used for the control of meningococcal outbreaks. While sufficient experience exists to recommend vaccination in controlling outbreaks due to serogroup C meningococcal disease only, use of existing vaccines may be applicable to control outbreaks due to other vaccine preventable serogroups [63].

5.1.7 Prognosis

Case Presentation 1 (continued)

The patient's CSF culture subsequently demonstrates growth of *S. pneumoniae*, which is resistant to penicillin but susceptible to ceftriaxone. Vancomycin therapy is discontinued. The patient's fever, headache, and confusion resolve by day three of therapy, although the patient now complains of mild ataxia. He completes 14 days of therapy with ceftriaxone and 4 days of therapy with dexamethasone, and his ataxia has resolved by the time of hospital discharge.

Case fatality rates of bacterial meningitis range from 10–30% in developed countries and have declined over time [11,12,17,22]. This risk of mortality varies by organism, and most recently in the United States, was 17.5% for *S. pneumoniae*, 20.5% for *L. monocytogenes*, 20.8% for Group B Streptococcus, 10.4% for *N. meningitidis*, and 7.2% for *H. influenzae* [12]. Predictors of mortality include advanced age, reduced level of consciousness, seizures, hypotension, thrombocytopenia, and a CSF pleocytosis above 1,000 cells per milliter [17,67]. Delay in administration of antibiotics has been associated with an increase in adverse events.

There is substantial morbidity in survivors of acute bacterial meningitis, including residual neurologic sequelae such as cognitive disturbance, hearing loss, seizures, and hydrocephalus [17,68]. Subtle neuropsychiatric abnormalities can be detected years later, but have minimal impact on function and are less than previously observed [69,70].

5.2   Encephalitis

Case Presentation 2

A 64-year-old woman is brought to the emergency department in the spring after a new onset seizure. The patient had been well until 48 hours prior, when she experienced the abrupt onset of fever and headache. Over the subsequent two days, she developed confusion and exhibited uncharacteristic behavior. She has no significant past medical history, she is not taking any medications and does not use alcohol, tobacco, or illicit drugs. The patient is retired, spends most of her time indoors and has not traveled recently. Her daughter does not report exposure of the patient to animals. On physical examination, she has a temperature of 38.9 °C, a pulse of 100 beats per minute, and a blood pressure of 140/64 mmHg. She is minimally responsive, does not have nuchal rigidity or focal neurologic findings. Her Glasgow Coma Scale score is 8. A serum white blood cell count is normal, as is a CT scan of the head. Evaluation of CSF demonstrates a leukocyte count of 500×10^6/L (500 cells/mm3) with lymphocyte predominance, an elevated protein concentration of 0.98 g/L (980 mg/dL, normal range 150–450 mg/dl), and a normal glucose concentration. You admit the patient with a diagnosis of acute encephalitis and institute intravenous acyclovir for the possibility of herpes simplex virus encephalitis. You consider other diagnostic testing.

Encephalitis refers to inflammation of the brain, and is distinguished from meningitis by the presence of abnormal brain function, which may manifest as altered mental status, motor, sensory or speech deficits, movement disorders, or seizures.

5.2.1   Diagnosis

Encephalitis is a pathological diagnosis reflecting inflammation of the brain parenchyma due to direct infection, post-infectious inflammation, or non-infectious etiologies [71]. In the absence of pathologic confirmation, which is rarely obtained pre-mortem, a scoring system has been devised based on clinical, biochemical, and radiographic testing that permits an estimation of the likelihood of encephalitis as a cause of neurologic dysfunction. Major and minor criteria are defined (Box 5.2) [71]. These criteria not only assist with diagnosis, but also standardize definitions to allow creation of data registries and cohort comparisons.

5.2.2   Epidemiology

The incidence of encephalitis varies according to geographic location and is estimated to

---

Box 5.2 Diagnostic criteria for encephalitis.

Major	
(required)	Altered mental status for ≥24 hours
	No alternative etiology found
Minor	
(2 = possible,	Body temperature ≥38.0C
≥3 = probable)	(100.4 F) within 72 hours of symptom onset
	Generalized or partial seizures
	New focal neurological deficits
	CSF white blood cells ≥5/cubic mm
	Suggestive neuroimaging
	Suggestive electroencephalography

Adapted from Venkatesan A et al. [71].

---

be between 5 and 10 cases per 100,000 population with approximately 20,000 cases occurring annually in the United States [72–74]. There are a multitude of causes of encephalitis that vary widely by geography, season, age, and host susceptibility factors, necessitating a complete history of potential exposures and vaccination status. An infection causing neuro-invasion or a post-infectious inflammatory phenomenon is found in 30–50%.

Box 5.3 Mimics of viral encephalitis.

- Brain abscess or subdural empyema
- Bacteria, including *Listeria monocytogenes, Neisseria meningitidis, Mycoplasma pneumoniae*
- Fungi, including *Cryptococcus neoformans, Aspergillus species,* agents of mucormycosis
- *Treponema pallidum*
- *Mycobacterium tuberculosis*
- Rickettsii
- *Toxoplasma gondii*
- Amoebas
- Tumor
- Subdural hematoma
- Systemic lupus erythematosus
- Adrenal leukodystrophy
- Toxic encephalopathy (including medications and illicit substances)
- Reye syndrome
- Vascular disease

Adapted from Whitley [75].

Box 5.4 Causative agents for acute viral encephalitis in the United States.

Arboviruses

- Eastern equine encephalitis virus
- Jamestown Canyon virus
- La Crosse virus
- Powassan virus
- Snowshoe Hare virus
- St. Louis encephalitis virus
- Venezuelan equine encephalitis virus
- Western equine encephalitis virus
- West Nile virus

Enteroviruses

- Coxsackievirus A and B
- Echoviruses
- Parechovirus
- Poliovirus

Herpesviruses

- Herpes simplex virus type 1
- Herpes simplex virus type 2
- Varicella zoster virus
- Epstein–Barr virus
- Cytomegalovirus
- Human herpes virus 6
- Simian herpes B virus

Other viruses

- Adenovirus
- Human immunodeficiency virus
- Influenza
- JC virus
- Lymphocytic choriomeningitis virus
- Measles virus
- Mumps virus
- Rabies virus

Adapted from Venkatesan et al. [71].

Improvements in diagnostic testing have allowed for diagnosis of previously uncharacterized cases. While viruses comprise the majority of the infectious etiologies, it is important to rule out potentially treatable mimickers of infectious or post-infectious encephalitis (Box 5.3) [75]. This chapter focuses primarily on viral encephalitis in adults in the United States.

5.2.3 Etiology of Viral Encephalitis

There are a multitude of viral causes of encephalitis (Box 5.4). Viruses may cause direct neuro-invasion and post-infectious autoimmune phenomenon, including anti-NMDA receptor antibody encephalitis [76]. The latter entity may be seen following herpes simplex encephalitis.

The most common cause of acute encephalitis in the United States is herpes simplex virus followed by enteroviruses, although there is likely an under-diagnosis of arboviral infections. Less common viral pathogens include other herpes group viruses, adenoviruses, measles, mumps, and HIV [77]. Other pathogens that require a high index of suspicion based on epidemiological risk include rabies virus, *Baylisascaris procyonis,* and *Balamuthia mandrillaris* [77]. Some pathogens demonstrate seasonal variation with the peak incidence of enteroviruses (including coxsackieviruses, echoviruses, parechoviruses,

---

Box 5.5 Seasonal preferences of selected viruses causing encephalitis.

Time of year	Virus
Summer/fall	Enteroviruses
	Eastern equine encephalitis virus
	La Crosse virus
	St Louis encephalitis
	Western equine encephalitis virus
	West Nile virus
Winter/spring	Influenza virus
	Measles virus
	Mumps virus
Any season	Herpes simplex virus type 1
	Human immunodeficiency virus
	Rabies virus
	Varicella zoster virus

Adapted from reference [76,79,84].

---

and polioviruses) occurring in the summer and fall (Box 5.5). Children and young adults are most commonly affected by these agents.

Arthropod-borne viruses (arboviruses) are a heterogeneous group of viruses transmitted by mosquitoes and ticks [78]. Encephalitis caused by these agents may be sporadic or epidemic, and peak in the late summer and early fall when the population of arthropod vectors is greatest [72]. As these viruses have restricted geographic distributions, a careful history to elucidate an epidemiologic exposure is crucial to target investigations [79]. The most common arbovirus is West Nile virus, which has expanded in number and geographic distribution in the United States since it was first discovered in New York City in 1999 [80]. Other arboviruses causing encephalitis include the California encephalitis (CE) serogroup (La Crosse, Jamestown Canyon, Snowshoe Hare, Tahyna), the togaviruses (Western equine encephalitis [WEE], Eastern equine encephalitis [EEE], Venezuelan equine encephalitis [VEE], and the flaviviruses [St. Louis encephalitis (SLE)]) [78]. Sporadic reports of deer tick encephalitis due to Powassan virus have been reported in the northeastern United States [81,82]. It is important to remain vigilant for the discovery of new viruses, including the Bourbon virus that caused a fatal illness in a man from Kentucky [83].

Imported viruses are an increasing cause of encephalitis and should be considered based on travel history with attention to locations visited and incubation periods from last possible exposure. The most common flavivirus causing encephalitis is the Japanese encephalitis virus. This entity should be considered among unvaccinated travelers to Southeast Asia who reside in a rural area for at least a month [84]. Zika virus has emerged as an important cause of encephalitis worldwide [85].

Two paramyxoviruses, measles and mumps, are rare causes of encephalitis because of effective childhood vaccination programs [76]. There continues to be multistate outbreaks of measles and mumps that are largely restricted to those who remain unvaccinated and should be considered in susceptible travelers to areas where herd immunity is sufficiently low to allow for virus circulation [86,87]. Subacute sclerosing panencephalitis (SSPE) is a rare progressive degenerative disease due to chronic measles infection of the central nervous system [88].

HIV, though commonly responsible for transient neurologic symptoms during acute infection, can rarely cause encephalitis and encephalopathy [89,90]. In those with HIV, consideration should be given to opportunistic infections including toxoplasmic encephalitis, cryptococcosis, tuberculosis, varicella zoster virus infection, cytomegalovirus infection, and JC polyoma virus causing progressive multifocal leukoencephalopathy [91].

Post-infectious disseminated encephalomyelitis is an acute inflammatory demyelinating disease that follows an infection or vaccination [92]. Many infectious agents and vaccines have been implicated as triggers, with molecular mimicry postulated to be the pathogenesis [92].

Rabies is transmitted by the bite of an infected animal and is a rare cause of encephalitis in the United States. Most human disease in the United States is due to bat transmission, although a history of bat bite is uncommon. Other animals that are most often infected include foxes, skunks, and raccoons [93].

5.2.4 Clinical Presentation

The sine qua non of encephalitis is altered level of consciousness [94]. This may be accompanied by fever, focal neurological deficits, or seizures [71]. Rarely, a rash may be present, which can be a clue to a viral etiology.

5.2.4.1 Herpes Simplex Type 1

Encephalitis due to herpes simplex is commonly due to HSV-1, which presents acutely in the majority of patients, but may also present with a subacute prodrome of fever, headache, and malaise. Fever is the most commonly observed sign, documented in over 90% of cases [95,96]. As the disease progresses, symptoms attributable to temporal lobe dysfunction, including altered level of consciousness, seizures, personality change, and focal neurological deficits are seen [95]. A vesicular eruption is uncommonly observed and its absence does not exclude the diagnosis [96,97]. Mortality approaches 10–20% at six months. Morbidity and mortality are increased with delays in initiation of antiviral therapy and disease severity at presentation [98].

5.2.4.2 Arboviruses

Encephalitis is an uncommon manifestation of arbovirus infection and typically occurs following a febrile prodrome [84]. The clinical spectrum of encephalitis ranges from mild neurological dysfunction to coma and may be abrupt or subacute in presentation [84,99]. CNS manifestations typically occur two to three days following the onset of fever and resolve over one to three weeks [84,99]. EEE is the most virulent of the arboviral encephalitides and produces symptomatic disease with a high frequency in all age groups with a mortality of approximately 30% [100,101].

West Nile Virus infection leads to an abrupt onset of fever, headache, and other non-specific symptoms that can progress to severe neurologic disease, which is estimated to occur in 1 in 150 of those infected. A morbilliform rash typically accompanies defervescence. Neurologic involvement may include parkinsonism, myoclonus, or cerebellar ataxia [80,99]. Case fatality rates are estimated to be 10% of those with neuroinvasive disease with advanced age being the strongest risk factor for death [80].

5.2.4.3 Enteroviruses

Most cases of enteroviral encephalitis are mild, with the majority of disease occurring in children. Patients with agammaglobulinemia may develop a chronic, lethal form of enteroviral encephalitis [102].

5.2.4.4 Other Herpes Viruses

Cytomegalovirus and Epstein-Barr virus rarely cause acute encephalitis, which most often occurs in the setting of profound immunosuppression [79]. Varicella zoster virus encephalitis, either secondary to primary infection or reactivation, may be complicated by encephalitis, typically occurring one to two weeks following the viral exanthem [103,104]. The absence of skin lesions does not reliably rule out infection. VZV infections can cause a small or large vessel vasculitis, in immunocompromised and immunocompetent patients, respectively, weeks to months after reactivation [103].

5.2.4.5 Rabies

Rabies encephalitis follows a prodrome of neuropathic pain occurring at the site of inoculation with progression to involve the central nervous system over the ensuing days [93]. The common form—furious rabies—manifests with fluctuating level of consciousness, hyperexcitability, aerophobia, hydrophobia, autonomic dysfunction, and stridor in the neurologic phase before progressing to coma [93].

5.2.4.6 Measles and Mumps

Acute encephalitis due to measles is most commonly a result of a post-infectious encephalomyelitis, which presents abruptly with fever, seizures, and altered level of consciousness [105]. This manifestation of measles occurs 3 to 10 days after the onset of the rash in 10 per 1,000 cases, and differs from SSPE that presents years after infection with the insidious development of behavior change. Manifestations also include myclonic seizures and death [105,106]. In immunocompromised patients, measles can cause encephalitis weeks to months after infection and manifests similarly to post-infectious encephalomyelitis aside from the absence of fever [105]. CNS manifestations in those infected with mumps usually occur in unvaccinated young adults irrespective of the presence of parotitis [107].

5.2.5 Laboratory Findings

In suspected cases of encephalitis, CSF should be sampled for glucose and protein concentrations, cell count and differential, Gram stain and bacterial culture, PCR for HSV 1/2 and VZV and enteroviruses, cryptococcal antigen, and syphilis in the appropriate clinical settings (Table 5.2) [71,79].

Demonstration of CSF pleocytosis, greater than 5 cells and less than 1,000 cells per cubic millimeter, with a lymphocyte predominance, satisfies a minor criteria for the diagnosis of encephalitis. This finding is not essential as encephalitis can be present in the absence of CSF pleocytosis, particularly in immunocompromised patients and early in the course of the disease [71]. Furthermore, early in the disease process, CSF may demonstrate a neutrophil predominance in up to 30–40% of cases.

Table 5.2 Recommended laboratory tests in the diagnosis of viral encephalitis.

Etiology	Diagnostic Tests
Herpes simplex virus type 1	PCR of CSF, viral culture of brain tissue
West Nile virus	PCR of CSF, IgM antibody of serum and CSF
Other arboviruses[†]	IgM and IgG antibody of serum and CSF
Enteroviruses	PCR of CSF
Varicella zoster virus	PCR of CSF, viral culture of brain tissue
Influenza	Nasopharyngeal swab
Cytomegalovirus	PCR of CSF
Epstein–Barr virus	PCR of CSF
Rabies virus	PCR of CSF, saliva or tissue, antigen testing of skin biopsy, brain tissue, serum and CSF serology
JC polyoma virus	PCR of CSF
Human immunodeficiency virus	PCR of CSF, plasma viral load, serology
Lymphocytic choriomeningitis virus	IgM and IgG antibody of serum and CSF
Herpes B virus	PCR of CSF
Post-infectious encephalitis[‡]	Document recent infection at primary site outside the CSF

Adapted from [79,109].

PCR, polymerase chain reaction; CSF, cerebrospinal fluid; IgM, immunoglobulin M; IgG, immunoglobulin G.

[†]Includes common arboviruses in North America, including St. Louis encephalitis, La Crosse encephalitis, Eastern equine encephalitis, and Western equine encephalitis.

[‡]Post-infectious encephalitis is usually caused by measles virus, varicella zoster virus, influenza virus, and vaccinia (pox) virus.

In HSV encephalitis, the median CSF WBC count is 50 cells per cubic millimeter, CSF RBC count is 48 cells per cubic millimeter, and median CSF protein is 75 mg per deciliter; however, in up to 5%, these tests are normal [97]. PCR testing for HSV is highly sensitive (above 95%) and specific (approaching 100%) [108,109]. Molecular-based testing has replaced viral culture, which is insensitive for HSV detection, and has reduced the need for brain biopsy in the diagnosis of HSV encephalitis [109]. Antecedent treatment with acyclovir only has minimal impact on the yield from molecular-based testing within the first week [110].

Additional testing for specific entities should be guided by the season, patient risk factors such as immunosuppression, travel and exposures, and neuroimaging findings [71]. West Nile serology in blood and CSF should be sent in summer and fall based on geographic prevalence. PCR of CSF for West Nile virus is often negative due to rapid viral clearance [71]. A nasopharyngeal swab for viral PCR testing should be requested during influenza season [71]. In most cases, serum and CSF samples should be collected and stored for future testing if needed [71].

Available laboratory tests for the causes of encephalitis are listed in Table 5.2 [71,109].

5.2.6 Other Diagnostic Modalities

5.2.6.1 Magnetic Resonance Imaging (MRI)

Neuroimaging in the form of MRI has become invaluable in helping to elucidate causes of encephalitis. Some pathogens have a predilection for specific regions of the brain. Early presentations of HSV encephalitis predominantly affect the temporal lobe unilaterally, as compared to other causes of temporal lobe encephalitis, with progression to bilateral involvement late in disease, while arboviruses tend to affect the basal ganglia and thalamus [97,111]. Respiratory viruses also tend to involve the basal ganglia and thalamus, and cause diffuse cerebral edema [71,111].

5.2.6.2 Electroencephalogram (EEG)

EEG abnormalities are often non-specific and can be seen with a multitude of causes. Specific findings of sharp wave discharges or lateralizing epileptiform discharges emanating from the temporal lobe are suggestive of HSV encephalitis [71]. Generalized stereotyped high-voltage periodic complexes can be observed in the setting of SSPE [112]. Generalized slowing in the anterior portion of the brain is suggestive of West Nile virus infection in the correct clinical context [99].

Case Presentation 2 (continued)

An MRI of the brain reveals unilateral temporal lobe enhancement. CSF was positive for HSV 1 by PCR.

5.2.7 Therapy

The mainstay of therapy for the majority of causes of encephalitis is supportive management. The exception is for HSV encephalitis and encephalitis due to other herpes group viruses, for which acyclovir at a dose 10 mg/kg intravenously every 8 hours for 14–21 days is efficacious [79]. Delayed therapy results in increased morbidity and mortality. A recent randomized controlled trial found no benefit with the addition of three months of oral valacyclovir following an initial course of acyclovir [113]. It is controversial as to whether a repeat lumbar puncture is indicated as PCR for HSV may remain positive in the CSF despite treatment [114].

Treatment of arboviral encephalitis remains supportive. Case series and animal studies have shown success with immune globulin, interferon, ribavirin, steroids, and antisense oligomers, but no controlled human studies have been conducted [80,99]. Attention to preventing the sequelae of prolonged hospitalization, such as venous thromboembolism and pressure ulceration, is important.

Enteroviral encephalitis in the setting of X-linked agammaglobulinemia has been treated with intra-ventricular gamma-globulin administration [79]. Pleconaril has been used successfully in clinical trials for enteroviral meningitis, but its efficacy in the setting of encephalitis remains unproven [115]. Intravenous immunoglobulin, ribavirin, and a number of investigational drugs remain under investigation [115].

Treatment of post-infectious encephalomyelitis frequently involves the administration of immunomodulatory medications such as corticosteroids, intravenous immunoglobulin, and plasma exchange, with the evidence limited to case series [79,116]. Anti-epileptic therapy is indicated for the control of seizures [116].

5.2.8 Preventive Therapy

With the absence of proven therapies for the majority of causes of encephalitis, the focus remains on prevention. Vaccinations are available for rabies and Japanese encephalitis and are indicated in specific populations. In the case of rabies, passive and active immunization can be used to abort infection following exposure [84,93]. The live, attenuated measles and mumps vaccines are extremely effective in preventing infection. Otherwise, prevention rests on the avoidance of vector exposure through population and person-level control measures [99]. Ongoing surveillance is important to catalog disease activity and identify new agents of encephalitis.

5.2.9 Prognosis

The causative organism strongly influences the outcome of encephalitis. Rabies and SSPE are almost uniformly fatal while arboviral infections are fatal in up to 20% of cases [93,99,105]. In the absence of therapy, mortality for HSV-1 exceeds 70% and even with treatment, residual neurocognitive disability is observed in 50% at one year [98,117]. Worse clinical outcomes with herpes simplex virus encephalitis are associated with more severe illness on presentation and delayed administration of acyclovir [98].

Case Presentation 2 (continued)

The patient received a 21-day course of intravenous acyclovir. She has a slow recovery over several weeks and is transferred to an acquired brain injury rehabilitation facility. Six months following presentation, she is living independently with a lower level of function than baseline and with mild short-term memory impairment and anosmia.

References

1 Okike IO, Ribeiro S, Ramsay ME, Heath PT, Sharland M, Ladhani SN. Trends in bacterial, mycobacterial, and fungal meningitis in England and Wales 2004-11: an observational study. Lancet Infect Dis. 2014;14(4):301–7.

2 Bijlsma MW, Brouwer MC, Kasanmoentalib ES, Kloek AT, Lucas MJ, Tanck MW, et al. Community-acquired bacterial meningitis in adults in the Netherlands, 2006-14: a prospective cohort study. Lancet Infect Dis. 2016;16(3):339–47.

3 Castelblanco RL, Lee M, Hasbun R. Epidemiology of bacterial meningitis in the USA from 1997 to 2010: a population-based observational study. Lancet Infect Dis. 2014;14(9):813–9.

4 Jafri RZ, Ali A, Messonnier NE, Tevi-Benissan C, Durrheim D, Eskola J, et al. Global epidemiology of invasive meningococcal disease. Popul Health Metr. 2013;11(1):17.

5 Harboe ZB, Dalby T, Weinberger DM, Benfield T, Mølbak K, Slotved HC, et al. Impact of 13-valent pneumococcal conjugate vaccination in invasive pneumococcal disease incidence and mortality. Clin Infect Dis. 2014;59(8):1066–73.

6   Feikin DR, Kagucia EW, Loo JD, Link-Gelles R, Puhan MA, Cherian T, et al. Serotype-specific changes in invasive pneumococcal disease after pneumococcal conjugate vaccine introduction: a pooled analysis of multiple surveillance sites. PLoS Med. 2013;10(9):e1001517.

7   Shigayeva A, Rudnick W, Green K, Chen DK, Demczuk W, Gold WL, et al. Invasive pneumococcal disease among immunocompromised persons: implications for vaccination programs. Clin Infect Dis. 2016;62(2):139–47.

8   Sadarangani M, Scheifele DW, Halperin SA, Vaudry W, Le Saux N, Tsang R, et al. The impact of the meningococcal serogroup C conjugate vaccine in Canada between 2002 and 2012. Clin Infect Dis. 2014;59(9):1208–15.

9   Bijlsma MW, Brouwer MC, Spanjaard L, van de Beek D, van der Ende A. A decade of herd protection after introduction of meningococcal serogroup C conjugate vaccination. Clin Infect Dis. 2014;59(9): 1216–21.

10 Adam HJ, Richardson SE, Jamieson FB, Rawte P, Low DE, Fisman DN. Changing epidemiology of invasive Haemophilus influenzae in Ontario, Canada: evidence for herd effects and strain replacement due to Hib vaccination. Vaccine. 2010;28(24): 4073–8.

11 McGill F, Heyderman RS, Panagiotou S, Tunkel AR, Solomon T. Acute bacterial meningitis in adults. Lancet. 2016;388(10063):3036–47.

12 Thigpen MC, Whitney CG, Messonnier NE, Zell ER, Lynfield R, Hadler JL, et al. Bacterial meningitis in the United States, 1998–2007. N Engl J Med. 2011;364(21): 2016–25.

13 Tunkel AR, Hartman BJ, Kaplan SL, Kaufman BA, Roos KL, Scheld WM, et al. Practice guidelines for the management of bacterial meningitis. Clin Infect Dis. 2004;39(9):1267–84.

14 van de Beek D, Drake JM, Tunkel AR. Nosocomial bacterial meningitis. N Engl J Med. 2010;362(2):146–54.

15 Conen A, Walti LN, Merlo A, Fluckiger U, Battegay M, Trampuz A. Characteristics and treatment outcome of cerebrospinal fluid shunt-associated infections in adults: a retrospective analysis over an 11-year period. Clin Infect Dis. 2008;47(1):73–82.

16 Attia J, Hatala R, Cook DJ, Wong JG. The rational clinical examination. Does this adult patient have acute meningitis? JAMA. 1999;282(2):175–81.

17 van de Beek D, de Gans J, Spanjaard L, Weisfelt M, Reitsma JB, Vermeulen M. Clinical features and prognostic factors in adults with bacterial meningitis. N Engl J Med. 2004;351(18):1849–59.

18 Thomas KE, Hasbun R, Jekel J, Quagliarello VJ. The diagnostic accuracy of Kernig's sign, Brudzinski's sign, and nuchal rigidity in adults with suspected meningitis. Clin Infect Dis. 2002;35(1):46–52.

19 Brouwer MC, Thwaites GE, Tunkel AR, van de Beek D. Dilemmas in the diagnosis of acute community-acquired bacterial meningitis. Lancet. 2012;380(9854):1684–92.

20 Hasbun R, Abrahams J, Jekel J, Quagliarello VJ. Computed tomography of the head before lumbar puncture in adults with suspected meningitis. N Engl J Med. 2001;345(24):1727–33.

21 Joffe AR. Lumbar puncture and brain herniation in acute bacterial meningitis: a review. J Intensive Care Med. 2007;22(4):194–207.

22 Glimåker M, Johansson B, Grindborg Ö, Bottai M, Lindquist L, Sjölin J. Adult bacterial meningitis: earlier treatment and improved outcome following guideline revision promoting prompt lumbar puncture. Clin Infect Dis. 2015;60(8):1162–9.

23 Bennett JE. Chronic Meningitis. In: Mandell, Douglas, and Bennett's Principles and Practice of Infectious Diseases, Updated ed, Eighth ed. Saunders; p. 1138–43.

24 van de Beek D, de Gans J, Tunkel AR, Wijdicks EFM. Community-acquired bacterial meningitis in adults. N Engl J Med. 2006;354(1):44–53.

25 Brouwer MC, Tunkel AR, van de Beek D. Epidemiology, diagnosis, and antimicrobial treatment of acute bacterial meningitis. Clin Microbiol Rev. 2010;23(3):467–92.

26 Spanos A, Harrell FE, Durack DT. Differential diagnosis of acute meningitis. An analysis of the predictive value of initial observations. JAMA. 1989;262(19):2700–7.

27 Brouwer MC, van de Beek D, Heckenberg SGB, Spanjaard L, de Gans J. Community-acquired Listeria monocytogenes meningitis in adults. Clin Infect Dis. 2006;43(10):1233–8.

28 Amaya-Villar R, García-Cabrera E, Sulleiro-Igual E, Fernández-Viladrich P, Fontanals-Aymerich D, Catalán-Alonso P, et al. Three-year multicenter surveillance of community-acquired Listeria monocytogenes meningitis in adults. BMC Infect Dis. 2010;10:324.

29 Ihekwaba UK, Kudesia G, McKendrick MW. Clinical features of viral meningitis in adults: significant differences in cerebrospinal fluid findings among herpes simplex virus, varicella zoster virus, and enterovirus infections. Clin Infect Dis. 2008;47(6):783–9.

30 Michael B, Menezes BF, Cunniffe J, Miller A, Kneen R, Francis G, et al. Effect of delayed lumbar punctures on the diagnosis of acute bacterial meningitis in adults. Emerg Med J. 2010;27(6):433–8.

31 Bohr V, Rasmussen N, Hansen B, Kjersem H, Jessen O, Johnsen N, et al. 875 cases of bacterial meningitis: diagnostic procedures and the impact of preadmission antibiotic therapy. Part III of a three-part series. J Infect. 1983;7(3):193–202.

32 Conly JM, Ronald AR. Cerebrospinal fluid as a diagnostic body fluid. Am J Med. 1983;75(1B):102–8.

33 Blazer S, Berant M, Alon U. Bacterial meningitis. Effect of antibiotic treatment on cerebrospinal fluid. Am J Clin Pathol. 1983;80(3):386–7.

34 Talan DA, Hoffman JR, Yoshikawa TT, Overturf GD. Role of empiric parenteral antibiotics prior to lumbar puncture in suspected bacterial meningitis: state of the art. Rev Infect Dis. 1988;10(2):365–76.

35 Kennedy WA, Chang S-J, Purdy K, Le T, Kilgore PE, Kim JS, et al. Incidence of bacterial meningitis in Asia using enhanced CSF testing: polymerase chain reaction, latex agglutination and culture. Epidemiol Infect. 2007;135(7):1217–26.

36 Bronska E, Kalmusova J, Dzupova O, Maresova V, Kriz P, Benes J. Dynamics of PCR-based diagnosis in patients with invasive meningococcal disease. Clin Microbiol Infect. 2006;12(2):137–41.

37 Nigrovic LE, Malley R, Macias CG, Kanegaye JT, Moro-Sutherland DM, Schremmer RD, et al. Effect of antibiotic pretreatment on cerebrospinal fluid profiles of children with bacterial meningitis. Pediatr. 2008;122(4):726–30.

38 Parent du Châtelet I, Traore Y, Gessner BD, Antignac A, Naccro B, Njanpop-Lafourcade B-M, et al. Bacterial meningitis in Burkina Faso: surveillance using field-based polymerase chain reaction testing. Clin Infect Dis. 2005;40(1):17–25.

39 Corless CE, Guiver M, Borrow R, Edwards-Jones V, Fox AJ, Kaczmarski EB. Simultaneous detection of Neisseria meningitidis, Haemophilus influenzae, and Streptococcus pneumoniae in suspected cases of meningitis and septicemia using real-time PCR. J Clin Microbiol. 2001;39(4):1553–8.

40 Tzanakaki G, Tsopanomichalou M, Kesanopoulos K, Matzourani R, Sioumala M, Tabaki A, et al. Simultaneous single-tube PCR assay for the detection of Neisseria meningitidis, Haemophilus influenzae type B and Streptococcus pneumoniae. Clin Microbiol Infect. 2005;11(5):386–90.

41 Bøving MK, Pedersen LN, Møller JK. Eight-plex PCR and liquid-array detection of bacterial and viral pathogens in cerebrospinal fluid from patients with suspected meningitis. J Clin Microbiol. 2009;47(4):908–13.

42 Richardson DC, Louie L, Louie M, Simor AE. Evaluation of a rapid PCR assay for

diagnosis of meningococcal meningitis. J Clin Microbiol. 2003;41(8):3851–3.

43 Tang YW, Hibbs JR, Tau KR, Qian Q, Skarhus HA, Smith TF, et al. Effective use of polymerase chain reaction for diagnosis of central nervous system infections. Clin Infect Dis. 1999;29(4):803–6.

44 Hukkanen V, Vuorinen T. Herpesviruses and enteroviruses in infections of the central nervous system: a study using time-resolved fluorometry PCR. J Clin Virol. 2002;25 Suppl 1:S87–94.

45 Srinivasan L, Pisapia JM, Shah SS, Halpern CH, Harris MC. Can broad-range 16S ribosomal ribonucleic acid gene polymerase chain reactions improve the diagnosis of bacterial meningitis? A systematic review and meta-analysis. Ann Emerg Med. 2012;60(5):609–20.e2.

46 Segawa S, Sawai S, Murata S, Nishimura M, Beppu M, Sogawa K, et al. Direct application of MALDI-TOF mass spectrometry to cerebrospinal fluid for rapid pathogen identification in a patient with bacterial meningitis. Clin Chim Acta Int J Clin Chem. 2014;435:59–61.

47 Litvintseva AP, Hurst S, Gade L, Frace MA, Hilsabeck R, Schupp JM, et al. Whole-genome analysis of Exserohilum rostratum from an outbreak of fungal meningitis and other infections. J Clin Microbiol. 2014;52(9):3216–22.

48 Finlay FO, Witherow H, Rudd PT. Latex agglutination testing in bacterial meningitis. Arch Dis Child. 1995;73(2):160–1.

49 Maxson S, Lewno MJ, Schutze GE. Clinical usefulness of cerebrospinal fluid bacterial antigen studies. J Pediatr. 1994;125(2):235–8.

50 Perkins MD, Mirrett S, Reller LB. Rapid bacterial antigen detection is not clinically useful. J Clin Microbiol. 1995;33(6):1486–91.

51 Auburtin M, Wolff M, Charpentier J, Varon E, Le Tulzo Y, Girault C, et al. Detrimental role of delayed antibiotic administration and penicillin-nonsusceptible strains in adult intensive care unit patients with

pneumococcal meningitis: the PNEUMOREA prospective multicenter study. Crit Care Med. 2006;34(11):2758–65.

52 de Gans J, van de Beek D. European Dexamethasone in Adulthood Bacterial Meningitis Study Investigators. Dexamethasone in adults with bacterial meningitis. N Engl J Med. 2002;347(20):1549–56.

53 Nguyen THM, Tran THC, Thwaites G, Ly VC, Dinh XS, Ho Dang TN, et al. Dexamethasone in Vietnamese adolescents and adults with bacterial meningitis. N Engl J Med. 2007;357(24):2431–40.

54 Scarborough M, Gordon SB, Whitty CJM, French N, Njalale Y, Chitani A, et al. Corticosteroids for bacterial meningitis in adults in sub-Saharan Africa. N Engl J Med. 2007;357(24):2441–50.

55 van de Beek D, Farrar JJ, de Gans J, Mai NTH, Molyneux EM, Peltola H, et al. Adjunctive dexamethasone in bacterial meningitis: a meta-analysis of individual patient data. Lancet Neurol. 2010;9(3):254–63.

56 Brouwer MC, McIntyre P, Prasad K, van de Beek D. Corticosteroids for acute bacterial meningitis. Cochrane Database Syst Rev. 2015;(9):CD004405.

57 Wenger JD, Hightower AW, Facklam RR, Gaventa S, Broome CV. Bacterial meningitis in the United States, 1986: report of a multistate surveillance study. The Bacterial Meningitis Study Group. J Infect Dis. 1990;162(6):1316–23.

58 Committee on Infectious Diseases, American Academy of Pediatrics. Recommended Childhood and Adolescent Immunization Schedule—United States, 2016. Pediatr. 2016;137(3):e20154531.

59 Black S, Shinefield H, Fireman B, Lewis E, Ray P, Hansen JR, et al. Efficacy, safety and immunogenicity of heptavalent pneumococcal conjugate vaccine in children. Northern California Kaiser Permanente Vaccine Study Center Group. Pediatr Infect Dis J. 2000;19(3):187–95.

60 Klugman KP, Madhi SA, Huebner RE, Kohberger R, Mbelle N, Pierce N, et al. A trial of a 9-valent pneumococcal conjugate vaccine in children with and those without HIV infection. N Engl J Med. 2003;349(14):1341–8.

61 O'Brien KL, Moulton LH, Reid R, Weatherholtz R, Oski J, Brown L, et al. Efficacy and safety of seven-valent conjugate pneumococcal vaccine in American Indian children: group randomised trial. Lancet. 2003;362(9381):355–61.

62 Moberley S, Holden J, Tatham DP, Andrews RM. Vaccines for preventing pneumococcal infection in adults. Cochrane Database Syst Rev. 2013;(1):CD000422.

63 Kim DK, Bridges CB, Harriman KH, Centers for Disease Control and Prevention (CDC), Advisory Committee on Immunization Practices (ACIP), ACIP Adult Immunization Work Group. Advisory committee on immunization practices recommended immunization schedule for adults aged 19 years or older--United States, 2015. MMWR Morb Mortal Wkly Rep. 2015;64(4):91–2.

64 Cohn AC, MacNeil JR, Clark TA, Ortega-Sanchez IR, Briere EZ, Meissner HC, et al. Prevention and control of meningococcal disease: recommendations of the Advisory Committee on Immunization Practices (ACIP). MMWR Recomm Rep. 2013;62(RR-2):1–28.

65 Folaranmi T, Rubin L, Martin SW, Patel M, MacNeil JR, Centers for Disease Control (CDC). Use of Serogroup B Meningococcal Vaccines in Persons Aged ≥10 Years at Increased Risk for Serogroup B Meningococcal Disease: Recommendations of the Advisory Committee on Immunization Practices, 2015. MMWR Morb Mortal Wkly Rep. 2015;64(22):608–12.

66 Canada PHA of, Canada PHA of. Page 13: Canadian Immunization Guide: Part 4 - Active Vaccines [Internet]. aem. 2007 [cited 2017 Sep 3]. Available from: https://www. canada.ca/en/public-health/services/ publications/healthy-living/canadian-immunization-guide-part-4-active-vaccines/ page-13-meningococcal-vaccine.html

67 Weisfelt M, van de Beek D, Spanjaard L, Reitsma JB, de Gans J. Attenuated cerebrospinal fluid leukocyte count and sepsis in adults with pneumococcal meningitis: a prospective cohort study. BMC Infect Dis. 2006;6:149.

68 Pfister HW, Feiden W, Einhäupl KM. Spectrum of complications during bacterial meningitis in adults. Results of a prospective clinical study. Arch Neurol. 1993;50(6):575–81.

69 Schmidt H, Heimann B, Djukic M, Mazurek C, Fels C, Wallesch C-W, et al. Neuropsychological sequelae of bacterial and viral meningitis. Brain J Neurol. 2006;129(Pt 2):333–45.

70 Weisfelt M, van de Beek D, Hoogman M, Hardeman C, de Gans J, Schmand B. Cognitive outcome in adults with moderate disability after pneumococcal meningitis. J Infect. 2006;52(6):433–9.

71 Venkatesan A, Tunkel AR, Bloch KC, Lauring AS, Sejvar J, Bitnun A, et al. Case definitions, diagnostic algorithms, and priorities in encephalitis: consensus statement of the international encephalitis consortium. Clin Infect Dis. 2013;57(8):1114–28.

72 Trevejo RT. Acute encephalitis hospitalizations, California, 1990-1999: unrecognized arboviral encephalitis? Emerg Infect Dis. 2004;10(8):1442–9.

73 Kulkarni MA, Lecocq AC, Artsob H, Drebot MA, Ogden NH. Epidemiology and aetiology of encephalitis in Canada, 1994-2008: a case for undiagnosed arboviral agents? Epidemiol Infect. 2013;141(11):2243–55.

74 Granerod J, Cousens S, Davies NWS, Crowcroft NS, Thomas SL. New estimates of incidence of encephalitis in England. Emerg Infect Dis. 2013;19(9).

75 Whitley RJ, Gnann JW. Viral encephalitis: familiar infections and emerging pathogens. Lancet. 2002;359(9305):507–13.

76 Whitley RJ. Viral encephalitis. N Engl J Med. 1990;323(4):242–50.

77 Glaser CA, Honarmand S, Anderson LJ, Schnurr DP, Forghani B, Cossen CK, et al. Beyond viruses: clinical profiles and etiologies associated with encephalitis. Clin Infect Dis. 2006;43(12):1565–77.

78 Calisher CH. Medically important arboviruses of the United States and Canada. Clin Microbiol Rev. 1994;7(1):89–116.

79 Tunkel AR, Glaser CA, Bloch KC, Sejvar JJ, Marra CM, Roos KL, et al. The management of encephalitis: clinical practice guidelines by the Infectious Diseases Society of America. Clin Infect Dis. 2008;47(3):303–27.

80 Petersen LR, Brault AC, Nasci RS. West Nile virus: review of the literature. JAMA. 2013;310(3):308–15.

81 El Khoury MY, Hull RC, Bryant PW, Escuyer KL, St George K, Wong SJ, et al. Diagnosis of acute deer tick virus encephalitis. Clin Infect Dis. 2013;56(4):e40–7.

82 Tavakoli NP, Wang H, Dupuis M, Hull R, Ebel GD, Gilmore EJ, et al. Fatal case of deer tick virus encephalitis. N Engl J Med. 2009;360(20):2099–107.

83 Kosoy OI, Lambert AJ, Hawkinson DJ, Pastula DM, Goldsmith CS, Hunt DC, et al. Novel thogotovirus associated with febrile illness and death, United States, 2014. Emerg Infect Dis. 2015;21(5):760–4.

84 Solomon T. Flavivirus encephalitis. N Engl J Med. 2004;351(4):370–8.

85 Petersen LR, Jamieson DJ, Powers AM, Honein MA. Zika Virus. N Engl J Med. 2016;374(16):1552–63.

86 Parker AA, Staggs W, Dayan GH, Ortega-Sánchez IR, Rota PA, Lowe L, et al. Implications of a 2005 Measles Outbreak in Indiana for Sustained Elimination of Measles in the United States. N Engl J Med. 2006;355(5):447–55.

87 Phadke VK, Bednarczyk RA, Salmon DA, Omer SB. Association between vaccine refusal and vaccine-preventable diseases in the united states: A review of measles and pertussis. JAMA. 2016;315(11):1149–58.

88 Bellini WJ, Rota JS, Lowe LE, Katz RS, Dyken PR, Zaki SR, et al. Subacute Sclerosing Panencephalitis: More Cases of This Fatal Disease Are Prevented by Measles Immunization than Was Previously Recognized. J Infect Dis. 2005;192(10):1686–93.

89 Hellmuth J, Fletcher JLK, Valcour V, Kroon E, Ananworanich J, Intasan J, et al. Neurologic signs and symptoms frequently manifest in acute HIV infection. Neurol. 2016;87(2):148–54.

90 Nzwalo H, Añón RP, Àguas MJ. Acute encephalitis as initial presentation of primary HIV infection. BMJ Case Rep. 2012;2012.

91 Tan IL, Smith BR, von Geldern G, Mateen FJ, McArthur JC. HIV-associated opportunistic infections of the CNS. Lancet Neurol. 2012;11(7):605–17.

92 Menge T, Hemmer B, Nessler S, Wiendl H, Neuhaus O, Hartung H-P, et al. Acute disseminated encephalomyelitis: an update. Arch Neurol. 2005;62(11):1673–80.

93 Hemachudha T, Ugolini G, Wacharapluesadee S, Sungkarat W, Shuangshoti S, Laothamatas J. Human rabies: neuropathogenesis, diagnosis, and management. Lancet Neurol. 2013;12(5):498–513.

94 Solomon T, Hart IJ, Beeching NJ. Viral encephalitis: a clinician's guide. Pract Neurol. 2007;7(5):288–305.

95 Sabah M, Mulcahy J, Zeman A. Herpes simplex encephalitis. BMJ. 2012;344:e3166.

96 Whitley RJ. Herpes simplex encephalitis: Adolescents and adults. Antiviral Res. 2006;71(2–3):141–8.

97 Chow FC, Glaser CA, Sheriff H, Xia D, Messenger S, Whitley R, et al. Use of Clinical and Neuroimaging Characteristics to Distinguish Temporal Lobe Herpes Simplex Encephalitis From Its Mimics. Clin Infect Dis. 2015;60(9):1377–83.

98 Raschilas F, Wolff M, Delatour F, Chaffaut C, De Broucker T, Chevret S, et al. Outcome of and prognostic factors for herpes simplex encephalitis in adult

patients: results of a multicenter study. Clin Infect Dis. 2002;35(3):254–60.

99 Davis LE, Beckham JD, Tyler KL. North American encephalitic arboviruses. Neurol Clin. 2008;26(3):727–ix.

100 Deresiewicz RL, Thaler SJ, Hsu L, Zamani AA. Clinical and neuroradiographic manifestations of eastern equine encephalitis. N Engl J Med. 1997;336(26):1867–74.

101 Przelomski MM, O'Rourke E, Grady GF, Berardi VP, Markley HG. Eastern equine encephalitis in Massachusetts: a report of 16 cases, 1970-1984. Neurol. 1988;38(5):736–9.

102 Webster AD, Rotbart HA, Warner T, Rudge P, Hyman N. Diagnosis of enterovirus brain disease in hypogammaglobulinemic patients by polymerase chain reaction. Clin Infect Dis. 1993;17(4):657–61.

103 Gilden DH, Kleinschmidt-DeMasters BK, LaGuardia JJ, Mahalingam R, Cohrs RJ. Neurologic Complications of the Reactivation of Varicella–Zoster Virus. N Engl J Med. 2000;342(9):635–45.

104 Peterslund NA. Herpes zoster associated encephalitis: clinical findings and acyclovir treatment. Scand J Infect Dis. 1988;20(6):583–92.

105 Orenstein WA, Perry RT, Halsey NA. The Clinical Significance of Measles: A Review. J Infect Dis. 2004;189 Suppl 1 S4–16.

106 Moss WJ. Measles. Lancet. 2017; epub ahead of print.

107 Bárcena-Panero A, de Ory F, Castellanos A, Echevarría JE. Mumps-associated meningitis and encephalitis in patients with no suspected mumps infection. Diagn Microbiol Infect Dis. 2014;79(2):171–3.

108 Leveque N, Van Haecke A, Renois F, Boutolleau D, Talmud D, Andreoletti L. Rapid virological diagnosis of central nervous system infections by use of a multiplex reverse transcription-PCR DNA microarray. J Clin Microbiol. 2011;49(11):3874–9.

109 Baron EJ, Miller JM, Weinstein MP, Richter SS, Gilligan PH, Thomson RB, et al. A Guide to Utilization of the Microbiology Laboratory for Diagnosis of Infectious Diseases: 2013 Recommendations by the Infectious Diseases Society of America (IDSA) and the American Society for Microbiology. Clin Infect Dis. 2013;57(4):e22–121.

110 Tang Y-W, Mitchell PS, Espy MJ, Smith TF, Persing DH. Molecular Diagnosis of Herpes Simplex Virus Infections in the Central Nervous System. J Clin Microbiol. 1999;37(7):2127–36.

111 Beattie GC, Glaser CA, Sheriff H, Messenger S, Preas CP, Shahkarami M, et al. Encephalitis With Thalamic and Basal Ganglia Abnormalities: Etiologies, Neuroimaging, and Potential Role of Respiratory Viruses. Clin Infect Dis. 2013;56(6):825–32.

112 Smith SJM. EEG in neurological conditions other than epilepsy: when does it help, what does it add? J Neurol Neurosurg Psychiatry. 2005;76 Suppl 2 ii8–12.

113 Gnann JW, Sköldenberg B, Hart J, Aurelius E, Schliamser S, Studahl M, et al. Herpes Simplex Encephalitis: Lack of Clinical Benefit of Long-term Valacyclovir Therapy. Clin Infect Dis. 2015;61(5):683–91.

114 DeBiasi RL, Tyler KL. Molecular Methods for Diagnosis of Viral Encephalitis. Clin Microbiol Rev. 2004;17(4):903–25.

115 Jain S, Patel B, Bhatt GC. Enteroviral encephalitis in children: clinical features, pathophysiology, and treatment advances. Pathog Glob Health. 2014;108(5):216–22.

116 Sonneville R, Klein I, de Broucker T, Wolff M. Post-infectious encephalitis in adults: diagnosis and management. J Infect. 2009;58(5):321–8.

117 Jouan Y, Grammatico-Guillon L, Espitalier F, Cazals X, François P, Guillon A. Long-term outcome of severe herpes simplex encephalitis: a population-based observational study. Crit Care. 2015;19:345.

Chapter 6

Community-acquired Pneumonia

Mark Downing and Jennie Johnstone

Case Presentation 1

A 63-year-old man presents to your office with fever and a productive cough. His symptoms began three days ago. He has a history of peptic ulcer disease and is on a proton pump inhibitor. Upon physical examination, the patient has a temperature of 38 °C (100.4 °F), respiratory rate of 32 breaths per minute, pulse of 100 beats per minute, and systolic blood pressure of 145 mmHg and diastolic pressure of 90 mmHg. The examination of the chest is normal. Based on the history, you suspect pneumonia. Are the history, physical examination, and any additional testing useful in determining if this patient has pneumonia?

6.1 Burden of Illness/Relevance to Clinical Practice

Community acquired pneumonia (CAP) is a common infection associated with significant morbidity and mortality, with an annual incidence of 25 cases per 10,000 adults and represents the eighth most common cause of death in the United States [1]. The objective of this chapter is to review the clinical evidence for the management of patients with CAP. The most important questions to answer are: What components of the history, physical exam, and additional testing are useful in determining whether this patient has pneumonia? If this patient has pneumonia, can he be treated as an outpatient or does he need admission to a hospital ward or the intensive care unit (ICU)? What empiric coverage should this patient receive? Does he need coverage for atypical pathogens? Is there a role for any adjunctive therapies? When can he be transitioned to oral antibiotics and how long should his duration of therapy be? Do vaccines prevent pneumonia?

6.2 History, Physical Examination, and Investigations

No individual element of the history or physical examination possesses a likelihood ratio high or low enough to rule CAP in or out. This conclusion was also supported by a 2003 systematic review of testing strategies for CAP [2]. Chest radiograph (CXR) is considered the gold standard for making a diagnosis of pneumonia. A prospective randomized study of patients with acute cough (lasting less than 1 month) found that physicians may miss pneumonia based on clinical findings alone and that the increased use of CXR may result in more frequent appropriate treatment [3]. One observational study of patients with suspected pneumonia showed that CXR findings influence medical management in 69% of cases [4]. Therefore,

Evidence-Based Infectious Diseases, Third Edition. Edited by Dominik Mertz, Fiona Smaill, and Nick Daneman.
© 2018 John Wiley & Sons Ltd. Published 2018 by John Wiley & Sons Ltd.

we recommend a CXR in the work-up of a patients with suspected pneumonia.

Chest computed topography (CT) has been suggested as a more sensitive test than CXR for the diagnosis of pneumonia. A recent prospective trial evaluated the utility of CT in guiding care for patients suspected of having pneumonia. CT was able to show an infiltrate in 33% of patients who did not have evidence of pneumonia on CXR as well excluding CAP in 30% of patients with an infiltrate on CXR. While CT may significantly impact treatment decisions, it is unclear whether its utility outweighs the risk of harm associated with radiation and whether the strategy is cost effective, and as such can not currently be recommended for routine use [5].

Case Presentation 1 (continued)

You decide to order a CXR, and the CXR demonstrates the presence of a left lower lung infiltrate without pleural effusion. Should you admit the patient to the hospital? Do you need to order any other tests to help you make this decision?

6.3 Admission Decision

Management stratification for CAP is largely based on treatment setting: the outpatient, inpatient, and intensive care populations

reflect different disease severities and prognoses. A number of prediction rules have been derived in an attempt to establish the patient's predicted morbidity and mortality, and therefore, where they should be most appropriately treated. The two most common scores are the CURB-65 and the PSI. Comparisons of their predicted mortality rates are listed in Table 6.1 [6, 7]. It should be noted that there are no randomized controlled trials that directly demonstrate the benefit of these prediction rules. While the PSI has been more extensively validated, the simple scoring system used in CURB-65 makes it much more practical at the bedside. We therefore suggest CURB-65 as an aid in guiding admission decisions, with the caveat that it should not overrule clinical judgement.

Case Presentation 1 (continued)

The complete blood count and serum chemistries are all within normal limits. You calculate that the patient has a CURB-65 score of 2 and consider admitting him to the hospital. If you admit the patient, what diagnostic tests should you order? What is the value of ordering a sputum stain and culture? What about blood cultures? Should you order tests to detect the presence of "atypical" pathogens (*Mycoplasma, Chlamydia, Legionella*)?

Table 6.1 Comparison of CURB-65 and PSI prediction scores.

CURB-65 Score		PSI Score	
One point each for: (a) **c**onfusion (b) **u**rea >7 mmol/L (c) **r**espiratory rate ≥30/min (d) **b**lood pressure; low systolic (<90 mmHg) or low diastolic (≤60 mmHg) (e) age ≥**65** years.		Age is often the most important risk factor, with one point given for each year of age (with 10 points subtracted for women). Other risk factors receive individual scores that range from 10 to 30 points. These include patient demographics, comorbid conditions, physical examination findings, and laboratory results.	
Score	*30-day mortality and management recommendation*	*Score*	*30-day mortality and management recommendation*
0–1	1.5% (outpatient)	<70	<1% (outpatient)
2	9.2% (inpatient or outpatient)	71–90	2.8% (inpatient or outpatient
3–5	22% (inpatient)	>91	8–27% (inpatient)

6.4   Additional Diagnostic Tests

Studies have generally shown that the yield of sputum Gram stain and culture in CAP is low. One prospective study of 74 inpatients with CAP failed to identify the pathogen in a single patient with ram stain alone, and only one patient (5%) had a pathogen identified by culture [8]. Another retrospective study [9] examined patients who did not respond to empiric therapy and found no difference in mortality in those who had regimens changed based on microbiologic studies and those who had antibiotics changed empirically (67% vs. 64%, respectively; p value not reported). The authors concluded that initial sputum cultures were not warranted except in high-risk patients who were more likely to harbor resistant organisms.

The incidence of positive blood cultures in adult patients hospitalized with CAP ranges from 5–27%, with higher yields in the critically ill population [10]. A large retrospective study ($n = 14,069$) found a non-significant association between drawing blood cultures prior to antibiotics and lower 30-day mortality rate (adjusted OR 0.92, 95% CI 0.82–1.02; $p = 0.10$) [11]. Another large retrospective analysis of a database ($n = 10,275$) [12] found that positive blood cultures for penicillin-susceptible *S. pneumoniae* in hospitalized patients did not have an impact on fluoroquinolone use. Blood cultures may change management, but there is minimal evidence to suggest they improve patient outcomes.

Since the yield from traditional microbiology culture techniques is low, molecular testing has provided additional diagnostic value in CAP. A recent prospective study of 2,488 patients in the United States incorporated multiplex PCR testing on sputum, urine antigen testing, and acute and convalescent serologies to identify a pathogen in cases of CAP [1]. Viral pathogens were detected in 27% of patients, highlighting the potential utility of molecular detection in guiding care and antimicrobial stewardship. Pneumococcal urine antigen was found to be much more sensitive than traditional culture techniques, identifying two thirds of cases of pneumococcal pneumonia in the study. However, a pathogen was detected in only 38% of all patients. Atypical organisms (*L. pneumophila*, *M. pneumonia*, and *C. pneumonia*) were uncommon in this study at 4%. However, urine legionella antigen testing is common practice in certain areas of the world where the prevalence is higher, and testing characteristics include a sensitivity of 70% and specificity of 100% for serogroup 1 [13].

Case Presentation 1 (continued)

What empiric antibiotics should you order if you decide to treat your patient in the ambulatory setting? What about the inpatient setting? For how long should a patient be treated?

6.5   Antibiotic Treatment

Since a pathogen is not identified in the vast majority of patients with CAP, the empiric choice of antibiotics is paramount. All empiric antibiotic regimens should target *S. pneumoniae* as this is the most common pathogen associated with the most morbidity and mortality. More debate surrounds the need to cover *H. influenzae* and the atypical pathogens. Higher rates of *S. pneumoniae* resistance to macrolides and doxycycline have made these options less appropriate as monotherapy, especially for inpatients. Guidelines from the Infectious Diseases Society of America (IDSA), British Thoracic Society (BTS), and Europe generally recommend either a betalactam alone or in combination with a macrolide or a fluoroquinolone as first line therapy [14–16].

6.6   Ambulatory Treatment

A 2014 Cochrane review of 11 RCTs showed no difference in terms of efficacy for outpatient antibiotic regimens; however, pooling of data was limited because most studies did not compare the same antibiotics. A 2005 meta-analysis [17] showed that there was no difference in treatment failure between patients with non-severe CAP who received a betalactam antibiotic alone versus those who received a regimen that included an antibiotic with activity against "atypical" pathogens. Furthermore, one prospective observational study [18] ($n = 864$) showed that ambulatory CAP patients who received antibiotics in accordance with 1993 ATS guidelines experienced no difference in outcomes (mortality, subsequent hospitalization, medical complications, symptom resolution, return to work and usual activities, health-related quality of life, and antimicrobial costs) as compared to those who received other antibiotics. The evidence indicates that ambulatory patients with CAP may be successfully treated with either a betalactam antibiotic or an antibiotic with activity against "atypical" pathogens.

6.7 Inpatient Treatment

The main question around inpatient coverage again concerns whether or not atypical coverage is needed. A 2012 Cochrane review looked at 28 trials involving 5,939 patients comparing regimens with atypical coverage to those without [19]. The authors found no difference in terms of efficacy (mortality and clinical improvement) or adverse events. They pointed out that only a single study looked at the addition of a second agent for atypical coverage. Furthermore, the majority of studies were open-label and funded by pharmaceutical companies.

Two recent studies have sought to answer the question of whether atypical coverage is needed for non-ICU inpatients with CAP. The first was a cluster randomized crossover trial where strategies were rotated at institutions every four months; betalactam monotherapy was compared to either combination therapy with a betalactam and a macrolide or monotherapy with a fluoroquinolone [20]. A total of 1,737 patients were enrolled. Non-inferiority was achieved for betalactam

monotherapy versus the other two treatment strategies in terms of 90-day mortality. In another open-label RCT, betalactam monotherapy was compared to combination therapy with a betalactam plus a macrolide [21]. The primary outcome was time to clinical stability as measured by vital signs. Non-inferiority was not achieved in this study as patients took longer to reach clinical stability and there were more 30-day readmissions in the single treatment group; however, there was no difference in mortality, ICU admission, or length of stay.

A systematic review incorporated these two studies with conflicting results into the previous data from eight observational studies, and determined that there was not enough evidence to change practice based on the 2007 IDSA guidelines [22], where atypical coverage is recommended for patients. The authors pointed out that 39% of patients in the betalactam monotherapy arm of the crossover study did still receive an antibiotic with atypical coverage at some point during their hospitalization, which may partly explain their results. However, some have argued that the study reflects the "real world," where many clinicians will use atypical coverage even if it is not in their algorithm. The study authors also pointed out that there was a very low rate of atypical infections (2%), which may not make this study applicable to other geographic regions.

In terms of severe CAP requiring ICU admission, there are no large RCTs. Retrospective studies have shown that there is reduced mortality associated with betalactam and macrolide combination therapy [23, 24]. Rates of atypical pathogens were low in these studies, so it is postulated that macrolides may be playing a different role, such as an anti-inflammatory or antitoxin effect.

There is still much debate over the choice of antibiotics in CAP, and given that there is no clear winner in terms of efficacy, it is reasonable to look at adverse events. The FDA has recently updated their warning for fluoroquinolone use, pointing to severe reactions such as tendonitis, tendon rupture, worsening of myasthenia gravis, central nervous system effects, and potentially irreversible neuropathy [25]. While CAP is not specifically addressed in the update, alternative agents are recommended whenever possible for acute bacterial sinusitis, acute bacterial exacerbation of COPD, and uncomplicated urinary tract infection. Azithromycin has been associated with a small but significant increase in cardiovascular mortality, although this has not been shown in other large cohort studies [26]. Antimicrobial stewardship programs will also take into account the ecological impact of antibiotic choices for CAP. Fluoroquinolone restriction has been a successful intervention to reduce *Clostridium difficile* rates [27]. Combination therapy with a betalactam and a macrolide may have more of an impact on antimicrobial resistance than a betalactam alone. Of note, doxycycline has been associated with a decreased risk of *C. difficile* infection compared to other antibiotics used for CAP in a retrospective cohort study, and has been suggested as an alternative agent to fluoroquinolones or macrolides if atypical coverage is needed [28].

In summary, betalactams and fluoroquinolones are the most reliable antipneumococcal agents and should be first-line therapy for CAP. Fluoroquinolones have several concerns with regards to adverse events and ecological impact that may make betalactam therapy more favorable. Both guidelines and evidence are conflicting on whether atypical coverage is needed for inpatients. Therefore, we recommend a betalactam as first-line therapy for CAP, with the addition of a macrolide in ICU patients and other select inpatients who are at high risk for an atypical infection.

6.8 Duration of Treatment

A recent multi-center RCT compared five days of antibiotics (if criteria for clinical stability were met as outlined in the IDSA guidelines) to a duration left to the physician's discretion after a minimum of five days of therapy, with the median duration in this group being 10 days [29]. A total of 312 inpatients were randomized. Clinical success rates and symptom scores were no different between the two groups in either the intention to treat or per protocol analyses. Based on the evidence, we recommend a treatment duration of five days if the patient has achieved clinical stability. Procalcitonin may help to determine duration of therapy in pneumonia. A prospective observational study of 1,759 patients in the United States demonstrated that those who followed a procalcitonin-based protocol required less antibiotics (5.9 vs. 7.4 days, p <0.001) with no difference in adverse outcomes [30]. A Cochrane review in 2012 assessed 14 trials that looked at procalcitonin-guided antimicrobial therapy, and found no difference in adverse outcomes with a significant reduction in antibiotic usage [31]. At this point, we cannot make a strong recommendation about procalcitonin testing.

6.9 Corticosteroids

A number of meta-analyses examined the data surrounding corticosteroid use in CAP [32–34]. A Cochrane review in 2011 identified six RCTs, and found that steroids may accelerate resolution of symptoms. However, only two of the studies were high quality [34], and evidence was not strong enough from the studies to make any specific recommendations.

6.10 Vaccines

A Cochrane review in 2013 evaluated the efficacy of the pneumococcal polysaccharide vaccine (PPV) in adults from 18 RCTs and 7 non-RCT studies [35]. The PPV was highly effective at preventing invasive pneumococcal disease with an odds ratio of 0.26 (0.14–0.45). There was efficacy at preventing all-cause pneumonia in low-income countries, but not high-income countries, and efficacy was reduced in patients with chronic illnesses. There was no improvement in mortality.

The efficacy of a conjugated pneumococcal vaccine was assessed in the CAPITA trial, published in 2015 [36]. This randomized, double-blind trial compared the efficacy of the 13-valent polysaccharide conjugate vaccine (PCV) to placebo in 84,496 patients over the age of 65. The vaccine was found to have significant efficacy at 45.6% for vaccine-type CAP and 75% for invasive pneumococcal disease. Hence, the Advisory Committee on Immunization Practices (ACIP) now recommends that adults aged greater than 65 receive a dose of PCV13 followed by PPV more than one year after [46].

Acknowledgements

We would like to acknowledge David C. Rhew for his contribution to the first edition version of this chapter.

References

1 Jain S, Self WH, Wunderink RG, et al. Community-acquired pneumonia requiring hospitalization among U.S. adults. N Engl J Med. 2015 Jul 30;373(5):415–27.

2 Metlay JP, Fine MJ. Testing strategies in the initial management of patients with community-acquired pneumonia. [Review] Ann of Intern Med. 2003;138:109–18.

3 Bushyhead JB, Wood RW, Tompkins RK, et al. The effect of chest radiographs on the management and clinical course of patients with acute cough. Medical Care. 1983;21: 661–73.

4 Speets AM, Hoes AW, van der Graaf Y, et al. Chest radiography and pneumonia in primary care: diagnostic yield and consequences for patient management. Eur Respir J. 2006;28:933–8.

5 Claessens YE, Debray MP, Tubach F, Brun AL, Rammaert B, Hausfater P, Naccache JM, Ray P, Choquet C, Carette MF, Mayaud C, Leport C, Duval X. Early chest computed tomography scan to assist diagnosis and guide treatment decision for suspected community-acquired pneumonia. Am J Respir Crit Care Med. 2015 Oct 15; 192(8):974–82.

6 Lim WS, van der Eerden MM, Laing R, et al. Defining community-acquired pneumonia severity on presentation to hospital: an international derivation and validation study. Thorax. 2003;58:377–82.

7 Metlay JP, Stafford RS, Singer DE. National trends in the management of acute cough by primary care physicians. J Gen Intern Med. 1997;12 Suppl 77.

8 Theerthakarai R, El Halees W, Ismail M, et al. Nonvalue of the initial microbiological studies in the management of nonsevere community-acquired pneumonia. Chest. 2001;119:181–4.

9 Sanyal S, Smith PR, Saha AC, et al. Initial microbiologic studies did not affect outcome in adults hospitalized with community-acquired pneumonia. Am J Respir Crit Care Med. 1999;160:346–8.

10 Waterer GW, Wunderink RG. The influence of the severity of community-acquired pneumonia on the usefulness of blood cultures. Respir Med. 2001;95:78–82.

11 Meehan TP, Fine MJ, Krumholz HM, et al. Quality of care, process, and outcomes in elderly patients with pneumonia. JAMA. 1997;278:2080–4.

12 Chang NN, Murray CK, Houck PM, et al. Blood culture and susceptibility results and allergy history do not influence fluoroquinolone use in the treatment of community-acquired pneumonia. Pharmacotherapy. 2005;25:59–66.

13 Formica N, Yates M, Beers M, et al. The impact of diagnosis by legionella antigen test on the epidemiology and outcomes of

Legionnaires' disease. Epidemiol Infect. 2001;127:275–80.

14 Mandell LA, Wunderink RG, Anzueto A, et al. Infectious Diseases Society of America/American Thoracic Society consensus guidelines on the management of community-acquired pneumonia in adults. Clin Infect Dis. 2007 Mar 1;44 Suppl 2:S27–72.

15 Lim WS, Baudouin SV, George RC, Lim WS, Baudouin SV, George RC, Hill AT, Jamieson C, Le Jeune I, Macfarlane JT, Read RC, Roberts HJ, Levy ML, Wani M, Woodhead MA; Pneumonia Guidelines Committee of the BTS Standards of Care Committee. Thorax. 2009 Oct;64 Suppl 3:iii1–55.

16 Woodhead M, Blasi F, Ewig S, et al. Guidelines for the management of adult lower respiratory tract infections—full version. Clin Microbiol Infect. 2011 Nov;17 Suppl 6:E1–59.

17 Mills GD, Oehley MR, Arrol B. Effectiveness of beta lactam antibiotics compared with antibiotics active against atypical pathogens in non-severe community acquired pneumonia: meta-analysis. BMJ. 2005;330:456.

18 Gleason PP, Kapoor WN, Stone RA, et al. Medical outcomes and antimicrobial costs with the use of the American Thoracic Society guidelines for outpatients with community-acquired pneumonia. JAMA. 1997;278:32–9.

19 Eliakim-Raz N, Robenshtok E, Shefet D, et al. Empiric antibiotic coverage of atypical pathogens for community-acquired pneumonia in hospitalized adults. Cochrane Database Syst Rev. 2012 Sep 12;(9):CD004418. doi: 10.1002/14651858. CD004418.pub4. Review.

20 Postma DF, van Werkhoven CH, van Elden LJ, et al. Antibiotic treatment strategies for community-acquired pneumonia in adults. N Engl J Med. 2015 Apr 2;372(14):1312–23.

21 Garin N, Genné D, Carballo S, et al. β-Lactam monotherapy vs β-lactam-macrolide combination treatment in

moderately severe community-acquired pneumonia: a randomized noninferiority trial. JAMA Intern Med. 2014 Dec;174(12):1894–901.

22 Lee JS, Giesler DL, Gellad WF, Fine MJ. Antibiotic therapy for adults hospitalized with community-acquired pneumonia: a systematic review. JAMA. 2016 Feb 9; 315(6):593–602.

23 Rodríguez A, Mendia A, Sirvent JM, et al. Combination antibiotic therapy improves survival in patients with community-acquired pneumonia and shock. Crit Care Med. 2007 Jun;35(6):1493–8.

24 Martin-Loeches I, Lisboa T, Rodriguez A, et al. Combination antibiotic therapy with macrolides improves survival in intubated patients with community-acquired pneumonia. Intensive Care Med. 2010 Apr;36(4):612–20.

25 US Food and Drug Administration. FDA Drug Safety Communication: FDA updates warnings for oral and injectable fluoroquinolone antibiotics due to disabling side effects. July 26, 2016.

26 Ray W, Murray K, Hall K, et al. Azithromycin and the risk of cardiovascular death. N Engl J Med. 2012; 366:1881–1890.

27 Dingle KE, Didelot X, Quan TP, et al. Effects of control interventions on Clostridium difficile infection in England: an observational study. Lancet Infect Dis. 2017 Apr;17(4):411–421.

28 Doernberg SB, Winston LG, Deck DH, Chambers HF. Does doxycycline protect against development of Clostridium difficile infection? Clin Infect Dis. 2012 Sep;55(5):615–20.

29 Uranga A, España PP, Bilbao A, et al. Duration of antibiotic treatment in community-acquired pneumonia: a multicenter randomized clinical trial. JAMA Intern Med. 2016 Sep 1;176(9):1257–65.

30 Albrich WC, Dusemund F, Bucher B, et al. Effectiveness and safety of procalcitonin-guided antibiotic therapy in lower respiratory tract infections in "real life": an

international, multicenter poststudy survey (ProREAL). Arch Intern Med. 2012 May 14;172(9):715–22.

31 Schuetz P, Müller B, Christ-Crain M, et al. Procalcitonin to initiate or discontinue antibiotics in acute respiratory tract infections. Cochrane Database Syst Rev. 2012 Sep 12;(9):CD007498.

32 Wan YD, Sun TW, Liu ZQ, et al. Efficacy and Safety of corticosteroids for community-acquired pneumonia: a systematic review and meta-analysis. Chest. 2016 Jan;149(1):209–19. doi: 10.1378/chest.15-1733. Epub 2016 Jan 6.

33 Siemieniuk RA, Meade MO, Alonso-Coello P, et al. Corticosteroid therapy for patients hospitalized with community-acquired pneumonia: a systematic review and meta-analysis. Ann Intern Med. 2015 Oct 6; 163(7):519–28.

34 Chen Y, Li K, Pu H, Wu T. Corticosteroids for pneumonia. Cochrane Database Syst Rev. 2011 Mar 16;(3):CD007720.

35 Moberley S, Holden J, Tatham DP, Andrews RM. Vaccines for preventing pneumococcal infection in adults. Cochrane Database Syst Rev. 2013 Jan 31;(1):CD000422.

36 Bonten MJ, Huijts SM, Bolkenbaas M, et al. Polysaccharide conjugate vaccine against pneumococcal pneumonia in adults. N Engl J Med. 2015 Mar 19;372(12):1114–25.

Chapter 7

Healthcare-associated Pneumonia

Jennie Johnstone and Mark Downing

Case Presentation 1

A 70-year-old woman presents to the emergency room with new onset fever, productive cough, and dyspnea. Her past medical history is significant for type 2 diabetes, end stage renal disease, and a myocardial infarction four years prior. She receives hemodialysis three times per week, but has not required admission to hospital since her myocardial infarction. On physical exam, the patient is febrile (38 °C [100.4 °F]), her respiratory rate is 32 breaths per minute, her pulse is 100 beats per minute, and her blood pressure is 145/90 mmHg. Respiratory exam reveals reduced air entry on the left side and associated crackles. A chest x-ray reveals a patchy infiltrate in the left lower lobe. You diagnose her with pneumonia. Although she is living in the community, she has extensive healthcare exposure related to her hemodialysis. Does her healthcare exposure influence the management of her pneumonia?

7.1 Introduction

Historically, community-dwelling patients who developed pneumonia were categorized as having community-acquired pneumonia (CAP). However, in 2005, the American Thoracic Society (ATS)/Infectious Disease Society of America (IDSA) guidelines introduced the concept of healthcare-associated

pneumonia (HCAP) as a way to identify patients with pneumonia from the community who may be at risk for infection with antimicrobial resistant pathogens [1]. The new classification system defined *HCAP* as patients with pneumonia ≤48 hours of hospital admission with ≥1 of the following risk factors for multidrug-resistant bacteria as a cause of infection: (a) hospitalization for ≥2 days in an acute-care facility within the preceding 90 days; (b) residence in a nursing home or long-term care facility; (c) antibiotic therapy, chemotherapy, or wound care within 30 days of current infection; (d) hemodialysis within 30 days; (e) home infusion therapy or home wound care; (f) a family member with infection due to multidrug-resistant bacteria [1].

The rationale for distinguishing HCAP from CAP was related to the fact that it was hypothesized that the pathogens associated with HCAP more closely resemble those seen with hospital-acquired pneumonia (HAP) and ventilator-associated pneumonia (VAP) rather than CAP [1]. Accordingly, the 2005 guidelines recommended that empiric therapy for patients with HCAP should more closely resemble HAP and VAP therapy rather than CAP therapy [1].

In the 2016 ATS/IDSA guidelines, HCAP was not included; the guidelines only focused on HAP and VAP. The authors reasoned that there were few data supporting the risk of multidrug-resistant pathogens in HCAP, and argued HCAP was more comparable to CAP

Evidence-Based Infectious Diseases, Third Edition. Edited by Dominik Mertz, Fiona Smaill, and Nick Daneman.
© 2018 John Wiley & Sons Ltd. Published 2018 by John Wiley & Sons Ltd.

than HAP and VAP [2]. The 2016 ATS/IDSA HAP/VAP guidelines suggested that HCAP may align better with CAP guidelines [2].

In this chapter, we review the epidemiology, microbiology, treatment, and outcomes for HCAP, and summarize how HCAP compares to CAP.

7.2 Epidemiology of Healthcare-associated Pneumonia

Studies have shown that HCAP consistently comprises approximately one-fifth of all pneumonia admitted to hospital, ranging from 17%–22% of included studies from the United States, Spain, Italy, and the United Kingdom [3–6]. In most observational studies, patients with HCAP are older than patients with CAP [3,4,7,8] and have more comorbidities [4]. Residence in a nursing home or long-term care facility is common, ranging from 25%–50% [3,4]. In general, the severity of pneumonia is higher in patients presenting with HCAP than CAP [5,8].

Case Presentation 1 (continued)

The patient is admitted to hospital, and you request a sputum culture and blood culture as part of the admission orders. Two days later, the sputum results are growing methicillin susceptible *Staphylococcus aureus*. What are the common pathogens associated with HCAP?

7.3 Microbiology of Healthcare-associated Pneumonia

The few studies that explored the microbiology of HCAP have had conflicting results [3,4,7,8]. In a large retrospective United States cohort study of HCAP, Kollef et al. found *S. aureus* to be the dominant pathogen,

accounting for almost half (47%) of all cases; *Pseudomonas* sp. was the second most common organism found (25%) [3]. A single-center retrospective United States cohort study comparing patients with HCAP to CAP found that patients with HCAP were significantly more likely to have methicillin resistant *S. aureus* (MRSA) (31% vs. 12% for CAP, $p < 0.001$) and *Pseudomonas aeruginosa* (26% vs. 5% for CAP, $p < 0.001$) and less likely to have *S. pneumoniae* (10% vs. 41% for CAP, $p < 0.001$) [7]. However, these results differed from European studies. In a Spanish prospective cohort study, *S. pneumoniae* was still the most common etiological agent in HCAP (28%), and the proportion was similar to CAP (34%) with no statistical difference between the two groups ($p = 0.18$). *S. aureus* and *Pseudomonas* sp. were not commonly identified, yet the differences between HCAP and CAP were statistically significant for both *S. aureus* (2% vs. 0%, respectively, $p = 0.005$) and *P. aeruginosa* (2% vs. <1%, respectively, $p = 0.03$) [4]. Similarly, a prospective cohort study of patients hospitalized with pneumonia in the United Kingdom found *S. pneumoniae* to be the most frequent pathogen in HCAP and CAP (49% vs. 60%, $p = 0.10$); MRSA and *P. aeruginosa* were infrequently identified in both HCAP and CAP (MRSA 2% vs. 0.6%, $p = 0.40$, *P. aeruginosa* 2% vs. 0.3%, $p = 0.2$) [8].

Given the conflicting results, a systematic review and meta-analysis was performed to summarize the comparison of microbiology in HCAP versus CAP. Twenty-four studies comprising n = 22,456 patients were included [9]; there were significant differences in the frequency of pathogens isolated in the HCAP group compared with the CAP group [9]. *S. pneumoniae* and atypical pathogens were less frequent in HCAP when compared to CAP ($p < 0.05$) and *S. aureus*, MRSA, *Enterobacericeae*, and *P. aeruginosa* were more frequent in the HCAP group compared with the CAP group ($p < 0.0001$). Specifically, HCAP was associated with an increased risk of MRSA (odds ratio [OR] 4.72, 95% confidence interval [CI] 3.69–6.04), and *P. aeruginosa* (OR 2.75, 95% CI 2.04–3.72) and a lower risk of *S. pneumoniae* (OR 0.61, 95% CI 0.49–0.75), *Legionella pneumophila* (OR 0.43, 95% CI 0.25–0.73), *Mycoplasma pneumoniae* (OR 0.26, 95% CI 0.26–0.55), and *Chlamydia pneumoniae* (OR 0.40, 95% CI 0.19–0.81) when compared to CAP [9]. A subgroup analysis comparing the risk of multidrug-resistant pathogens from Europe, North America, and Asia was performed; there was no significant difference between the risk based on geography (interaction $p > 0.05$). The authors note that, overall, the study quality was poor [9].

In the same systematic review and meta-analysis, the authors looked at the discriminatory ability of HCAP to predict resistant pathogens when compared to CAP and found it to be low; the sensitivity was 54% (95% CI 52%–55%), specificity was 71% (95% CI 71%–72%), and the area under the curve (AUC) was 0.70 (95% CI 0.69–0.71), thus raising questions about the ability of HCAP to identify patients with resistant pathogens [9].

In summary, although expert opinion suggests that the microbiology of HCAP is different than CAP [1] and may be more consistent with VAP/HAP, low-quality evidence suggests that although HCAP may be different than CAP [9], the ability for HCAP to predict the presence of multidrug-resistant pathogens is low [9].

Case presentation 1 (continued)

When writing admission orders, you are unsure whether to order antibiotics consistent with CAP guidelines or HAP/VAP guidelines. Ultimately, you decide to order renally adjusted intravenous piperacillin-tazobactam. What is the evidence supporting broad spectrum antibiotic use for HCAP?

7.4   Therapy of HCAP

The 2005 ATS/IDSA HCAP/HAP/VAP guidelines recommend that patients with HCAP should receive broad spectrum antimicrobial therapy, directed against antibiotic resistant pathogens [1], similar to the antibiotic choices for HAP. Recent HAP guidelines recommend that empiric HAP therapy should include coverage for methicillin susceptible *S. aureus*, *P. aeruginosa*, and other Gram-negative bacilli (e.g., piperacillin-tazobactam, cefepime, levofloxacin, meropenem), based on the local microbiology of HAP [2]; additional antibiotic coverage for MRSA should be considered when treating patients with risk factors for MRSA or for patients hospitalized on a unit where >20% of *S. aureus* isolates are MRSA, or those at high risk for mortality [2]. Additional antibiotic coverage for MRSA can include either vancomycin or linezolid based on data from two systematic reviews and meta-analyses showing similar efficacy when treating HAP and similar safety profiles [10,11]. In the first systematic review, eight randomized controlled trials (RCTs) were included and showed similar relative risk (RR) for clinical success between linezolid when compared to glycopeptides (including vancomycin) (RR 1.04, 95% CI 0.97–1.11, $p = 0.28$) and no difference in risk of adverse effects (RR 0.96, 95% CI 0.86–1.07, $p = 0.48$) [11]. The second systematic review included nine RCTs and the adjusted absolute clinical response difference was 0.9% (95% CI 1.2%–3.1%, $p = 0.41$); gastrointestinal side effects were more frequent with linezolid (risk difference 0.8%, 95% CI 0%–1.5%, $p = 0.05$), but there were no differences found for other adverse effects, including renal failure, thrombocytopenia, and drug discontinuation ($p > 0.5$ for all) [10]. Based on expert opinion and limited data, a second antipseudomonal agent from a separate class than the initial empiric antipseudomonal agent is recommended in this guideline to be added in patients with increased risk of Gram-negative infections (e.g., Gram-stain from a respiratory specimen with Gram-negative bacilli predominant or having structural lung disease associated with *Pseudomonas* infection) or increased risk of mortality [2]. The recommendations highlight the need for local antibiogram resistance data, as empiric treatment regimens will be informed by these data [2]. Empiric antibiotic for HAP does not include coverage for atypical bacteria (e.g., *L. pneumophila, M. pneumoniae, C. pneumoniae*) as they are seldom the cause of HAP [2]. Treatment duration for HAP is seven days based on indirect data from studies of VAP [2]; a systematic review and meta-analysis included four RCTs and there was no difference in mortality between short course (7–8 days) and long course (10–15 days) antibiotics (OR 1.20, 95% CI 0.84–1.72, $p = 0.32$), or between relapses, although there was a trend toward fewer relapses in the long-course arm (OR 1.67, 95% CI 0.99–2.83, $p = 0.06$) [12].

Whether HCAP should be treated the same as HAP is unclear. A United States study of patients with HCAP admitted to 150 ICUs within the Veterans Health Administration system found that patients receiving HCAP therapy concordant with the ATS/IDSA 2005 HCAP/HAP/VAP guidelines [1] had a *higher* 30-day patient mortality than patients with HCAP that received guideline concordant CAP therapy [13]. The authors speculate that the worse outcomes may have been related to fewer oral step-down options, and thus, longer length of stay. Alternatively, they suggest that the lack of atypical pathogen coverage within recommended HCAP therapeutic regimens could have had a role in the poorer outcomes [13]. Similar findings were identified in a cohort of 85,000 patients from 346 hospitals in the United States diagnosed with HCAP [14]. Therapy for HCAP based on ATS/IDSA HCAP/HAP/VAP 2005 guideline was associated with *increased* risk of death, even after adjustment for demographics, comorbidities, propensity score for treatment with guideline-based therapy, and initial pneumonia severity (OR 1.39, 95% CI 1.32–1.47) when compared to those receiving non-guideline based therapy [14]. Thus, there remains uncertainty as to the ideal way to treat HCAP.

Furthermore, the introduction of HCAP as a concept has been associated with an increase in broad spectrum antibiotic use. In a United States study in 128 Department of Veterans Affairs medical centers over five years, the antimicrobial use for over 95,000 patients admitted to hospital with pneumonia was examined [15]. Overall, during the study period, there was significant shift in the antimicrobial use; there was an increase in MRSA therapy ($p < 0.001$) and antipseudomonal therapy ($p < 0.001$), and a significant decrease in initial therapy with standard and atypical coverage ($p < 0.001$). Although there was a significant shift toward broad spectrum antibiotics, there was no increase in nosocomial pathogens [15].

HCAP was not included in the recent updated HAP/VAP ATS/IDSA guidelines [2]. Whether HCAP will be included in the revised CAP ATS/IDSA guidelines is unknown. In summary, although current expert opinion recommends broad spectrum antibiotics when treating HCAP, there is a paucity of data supporting this recommendation and is an important area of future research.

Case Presentation 1 (continued)

The clinical course is unremarkable, and after a week, the patient is well enough to be discharged home. Are clinical outcomes related to HCAP different than in patients with CAP?

7.5 Outcomes

A systematic review and meta-analysis summarized mortality associated with HCAP versus CAP [9]. Mortality from HCAP was higher than mortality from CAP in all 23 studies reviewed (OR 2.52, 95% CI 2.15–2.95) in unadjusted analyses [9]. However, patients with HCAP are generally older with more comorbidities than patients with CAP; an adjusted analysis using the four studies that included age and comorbid illness information, there was no significant increase in mortality associated with HCAP when compared to CAP (OR 1.20, 95% CI 0.85–1.70, $p = 0.30$). This suggests the associated higher mortality seen with HCAP when compared to CAP is related to fundamental differences between types of patients with HCAP and CAP, not because of differences in pathogenicity of bacteria or inadequate treatment regimens.

Two studies compared length of stay between patients with HCAP and CAP [3,4]. The United States study by Kollef et al. found patients with HCAP had a mean length of stay of 8.8 days versus 7.5 days for CAP ($p < 0.001$) [3]. In the Spanish study by Carratala et al., the median length of stay for HCAP was 9 days versus 8 days for CAP ($p = 0.003$) [4].

7.6 Summary

HCAP is a common cause of pneumonia in patients admitted to hospital, and generally affects older more comorbid patients than CAP. However, whether there are important microbiological differences between HCAP and CAP is controversial, particularly outside of the United States. Furthermore, the ideal therapy for HCAP is uncertain as guideline concordant HCAP therapy is not associated with improved outcomes. The concept of HCAP continues to develop, as was summarized in a HCAP Summit [16]. Future research is needed to better delineate patients with HCAP at highest risk of pneumonia due to antibiotic resistant pathogens [16,17]. Until more is known about the optimal management of HCAP, we suggest that physicians evaluate the risk of infection by atypical pathogens and/or resistant pathogens in each individual patient, when making treatment decisions. Some patients may benefit from antibiotic regimens consistent with CAP guidelines, whereas in other cases, antibiotics consistent with HAP guidelines may be more appropriate.

References

1 American Thoracic Society and Infectious Diseases Society of America. Guidelines for the management of adults with hospital acquired, ventilator-associated and healthcare associated pneumonia. Am J Respir Crit Care Med. 2005;171:388–416.

2 Infectious Diseases Society of America and the American Thoracic Society. Management of adults with hospital-acquired and ventilator-associated pneumonia: 2016 Clinical Practice Guidelines by the Infectious Diseases Society of America and the American Thoracic Society. Clin Infect Dis. 2016;63:1–51.

3 Kollef M, Shorr A, Tabak Y, et al. Epidemiology and outcomes of healthcare associated pneumonia: results from a large US database of culture-positive pneumonia. Chest. 2005;128:3854–62.

4 Carratala J, Mykietiuk A, Fernandez-Sabe N, et al. Health care-associated pneumonia requiring hospital admission. Arch Intern Med. 2007;167:1393–99.

5 Venditti M, Falcone M, Corrao S, et al. Outcomes of patients hospitalized with community-acquired, healthcare-associated and hospital-acquired pneumonia. Ann Intern Med. 2009;150:19–26.

6 Valles J, Martin-Loeches I, Torres A, et al. Epidemiology, antibiotic therapy and clinical outcomes of healthcare-associated pneumonia in critically ill patients: a Spanish cohort study. Intensive Care Med. 2014;40:572–81.

7 Micek S, Kollef K, Reichely R, et al. Health care-associated: pneumonia and community-acquired pneumonia: a single center experience. Antimicrob Agents Chemother. 2007;51:3568–73.

8 Chalmers J, Taylor J, Singanayagam A, et al. Epidemiology, antibiotic therapy, and clinical outcomes in health care-associated pneumonia: a UK cohort study. Clin Infect Dis. 2011;53:107–13.

9 Chalmers JD, Rother C, Salih W, Ewig S. Healthcare-associated pneumonia does not accurately identify potentially resistant pathogens: a systematic review and meta-analysis. Clin Infect Dis. 2014;58:330–9.

10 Kalil A, Klompas M, Haynatzki G, et al. Treatment of hospital-acquired pneumonia with linezolid or vancomycin; a systematic review and meta-analysis: BMJ Open. 2013;3:e00912.

11 Walkey A, O'Donnell M, Wiener R. Linezolid vs. glycopeptide antibiotics for the treatment of suspected methicillin-resistant Staphylococcus aureus nosocomial pneumonia. Chest. 2011;139:1148–55.

12 Dimopoulos G, Poulakou G, Pneumatikos I, et al. Short- vs. long-duration antibiotic regimens for ventilator-associated pneumonia: a systematic review and meta-analysis. Chest. 2013;144:1759–67.

13 Attridge R, Frei C, Pugh M, et al. Health care-associated pneumonia in the intensive care unit: guideline-concordant antibiotics and outcomes. J Crit Care. 2016;36:265–71.

14 Rothberg M, Zilberberg M, Pekow P, et al. Association of guideline-based antimicrobial therapy and outcomes in healthcare-associated pneumonia. J Antimicrob Chemother. 2015;70:1573–9.

15 Jones BE, Jones MM, Huttner B, et al. Trends in antibiotic use and nosocomial pathogens in hospitalized veterans with pneumonia at 128 medical centers, 2006–2010. Clin Infect Dis. 2015;61:1403–10.

16 Kollef M, Morrow L, Baughman R, et al. Health care-associated pneumonia (HCAP): a critical appraisal to improve identification, management, and outcomes—proceedings of the HCAP summit. 2008;46:S296–334.

17 Ewig S, Welte T, Chastre J, Torres A. Rethinking the concepts of community-acquired and health-care associated pneumonia. Lancet Infect Dis. 2010;10:279–87.

Chapter 8

Tuberculosis

Peter Daley and Marek Smieja

Case Presentation 1

A 40-year-old man, who emigrated from India to Canada two years previously, presents with fever and cough for several weeks. He is coughing up thick sputum, sometimes streaked with blood. He had hemoptysis on one occasion. Fever is more marked in the evenings and he has sweats at night. He has lost 10 kg in the past two months.

On examination, the patient is thin, almost to the point of emaciation; the trachea is deviated to the right side. There is dullness to percussion over the apex of the lung. Auscultation reveals moist crepitations and bronchial breathing over the same area.

A chest radiograph reveals a dense opacity in the right apical region with a small cavity. You admit him to hospital into a negative pressure isolation room and order sputum examination for acid-fast bacilli (AFB) and mycobacterial culture. His first sputum examination is negative for AFB. You wonder whether a more sensitive molecular test for *Mycobacterium tuberculosis* would help to rapidly diagnose this man's suspected pulmonary tuberculosis.

8.1 Epidemiology

Tuberculosis (TB) is an infectious disease caused by the bacterium *Mycobacterium tuberculosis complex*, and remains a major cause of poverty and mortality throughout the world. An estimated 1.7 billion people, or nearly one-third of the world's population, have latent TB infection (LTBI) [1], and in 2015, there were an estimated 10.4 million new active TB cases and 1.8 million deaths [2].

The year 2015 represented the deadline for the Global Plan to Stop TB, which intended to reverse the rising incidence of TB and to half the prevalence and mortality compared to 1990. Mortality and prevalence estimates are on target to achieve this goal. The End TB Strategy now targets a reduction in deaths by 95%, and incidence by 90%, between 2015 and 2035; however, the current rate of decline in incidence of 1.5% per year will need to be accelerated to 4–5% per year if this is to be achieved. TB remains in the top 10 causes of death in the world, causing more deaths than infection with the human immunodeficiency virus (HIV) or malaria. Six countries account for 60% of incident TB cases (India, Indonesia, China, Nigeria, Pakistan, and South Africa), and three countries account for 45% of incident multi-drug resistant (MDR) TB cases (India, China, and the Russian Federation).

Significant gaps still exist in key TB control indicators [2], and 4.3 million annual incident cases are not reported. MDR treatment success is only 52%. Only 20% of patients eligible for MDR treatment are receiving it.

Evidence-Based Infectious Diseases, Third Edition. Edited by Dominik Mertz, Fiona Smaill, and Nick Daneman.

Only 55% of notified TB cases are tested for HIV. TB control programs in high incidence countries rely heavily on international donors, with a U.S.$2 billion annual shortfall in required funding. Many TB patients pay for their own care, reducing access and adherence.

8.2 Risk Factors for Infection and Disease

The principal mode of transmission for *M. tuberculosis* is by airborne droplets, and consequently, the primary infective focus is in the lungs. Infection generally does not manifest as disease, and progression to disease depends on a number of contributing factors. The risk factors for developing TB can be divided into factors that increase the probability of exposure to infection, and factors that increase the probability of disease among those who become infected.

Given the low incidence of TB in industrialized countries, the major risk factor for exposure is previous habitation in endemic areas. Refugees and immigrants from TB-endemic areas of the world are at high risk of developing TB because of previous exposure, particularly in their first 5–10 years after arrival. Other groups at risk of TB exposure are household or institutional contacts of active TB cases, aboriginal people, the homeless, injection drug users, and people in long-term care institutions.

Among those with LTBI, the strongest risk factor for progression to disease is concurrent HIV infection, associated with a 50–200-fold increase. Other risk factors include increasing age, malignancy, silicosis, liver or kidney disease, transplantation and other immuno-suppression, chronic use of corticosteroids, alcoholism, malnutrition, gastrectomy, jejunoileal bypass, and diabetes mellitus. The increased risk associated with biologic immunosuppressive therapy varies from quite low to a relative risk (RR) of 29.3 [3]. Indoor air pollution may be associated with developing active disease, although meta-analyses disagree [4,5]. Smoking, alcohol consumption, diabetes, and low body mass index are independent and synergistic risk factors [6]. Second-hand smoke exposure is significantly associated with risk of active disease (RR 1.59, 95% confidence interval [CI] 1.11–2.27) [7].

Among newly acquired LTBI, 5% develop active TB within two years, and a further 5% are estimated to develop TB life-long [8]. Among patients with untreated HIV, the risk following exposure to *M. tuberculosis* may be as high as 8% per year, or a cumulative 50% or higher risk of developing active TB [9].

8.3 Diagnosis of Active TB

8.3.1 Clinical Presentation

The classic clinical features of active pulmonary TB include chronic cough, hemoptysis, expectoration of thick sputum, and constitutional symptoms such as fatigue or night sweats, anorexia, and weight loss. We could find no data indicating a contribution of physical examination findings to diagnosis.

8.3.2 Microbiologic Testing

Diagnosis of active TB requires demonstration of the pathogen by acid-fast stained smears, culture of the organism, or amplification of specific DNA. Respiratory specimens (expectorated sputum, induced sputum, bronchoalveolar lavage, gastric lavage, pleural biopsy) are the most commonly examined. Because a single day collection may be more convenient for patients, a meta-analysis of eight studies concluded that same-day collection is equally accurate as two-day collection [10]. Among patients with scant sputum, sputum induction detects more cases, but was not associated with an increase in early treatment in a randomized, non-blinded trial in South Africa [11]. A variety of other specimens such as urine, cerebrospinal fluid, pleural fluid, pus, or tissue biopsy specimens can be collected in suspected cases of extrapulmonary TB, but the sensitivity is lower than respiratory specimens. Histopathologic examination may reveal granulomatous inflammation. Fresh or frozen tissue can be cultured for mycobacteria.

8.3.3 Nucleic Acid Amplification Tests (NAAT)

The Cepheid Xpert MTB/RIF test has been strongly recommended by the World Health Organization (WHO) as the initial test for active TB among adults and children with HIV or at risk of MDR, and given a conditional recommendation as the initial sputum test among all adults and children with suspected TB [12]. Xpert MTB/RIF may be used as an add-on test following sputum collection for smear and culture among adults at low risk of HIV or MDR. Xpert MTB/RIF should be used as the initial test for cerebrospinal fluid and may be used for nonrespiratory specimens [13]. Although Xpert MTB/RIF is more expensive than microscopy, Xpert MTB/RIF costs less when it replaces conventional culture and susceptibility testing [13]. The test detects *M. tuberculosis* and drug resistance to rifampin, and does not require laboratory facilities or advanced training since the automated DNA extraction and detection occur in the same tube. This is the first time that NAAT has been recommended to replace conventional testing for active TB diagnosis in developing countries. Xpert MTB/RIF has been rolled out to 21 countries, including 1.4 million test cartridges, in a project funded by UNITAID, assisted by a reduced price provided by the manufacturer. Novel applications of NAAT include testing easily available specimens such as urine [14].

8.3.4 Smear Examination

Mycobacteria are acid-fast bacilli (AFB), which can be demonstrated in appropriately prepared specimens by Ziehl–Neelsen (ZN) or related stains. At least 100 fields, which examine only 1% of the entire smear, must be examined under the oil immersion objective before a specimen is declared negative. To find one AFB per field, there must be a minimum of 10^6 bacilli/mL of sputum. In surveys, the smear detects only about 50% of all culture-positive cases. Sensitivity of smear is increased using fluorescent stains as compared to conventional ZN method, with similar specificity [15]. Using light-emitting diode bulbs can allow conversion of conventional light microscopes to fluorescence capacity, without loss of specificity [16]. Pre-treatment of sputum by physical or chemical means is associated with an increase in smear sensitivity compared to direct examination [17].

Whereas a positive AFB smear may be diagnostic in an endemic country, fewer than 50% of AFB-positive sputa in industrialized countries may be due to *M. tuberculosis*. The remainder are due to non-tuberculous mycobacteria.

8.3.5 Mycobacterial Culture

As sputum AFB stain is insensitive, culture for mycobacteria will markedly improve detection. Results of culture by the conventional solid egg media take a mean of 32 days, whereas liquid culture using Mycobacterium Growth Indicator Tube (Becton-Dickinson, USA) requires a mean of 14.2 days [18]. Culture has an analytic sensitivity many times greater than sputum examination, and can detect as few as 10–100 bacilli/mL. Newer rapid liquid culture techniques such as Microscopic Observation Drug Susceptibility (MODS) are faster and less costly than liquid culture, with similar performance for detection [19] and susceptibility [20]. Culture techniques require expensive biosafety level 3 laboratories, due to risk of laboratory-acquired TB infection.

Drug susceptibility testing (DST) is performed on growth in culture. Colorimetric redox indicator methods are rapid and simple and have 89–100% sensitivity and specificity for rifampin and isoniazid [21]. Molecular DST for first line drugs is accurate and may be cost effective due to earlier results compared to conventional DST [22]. Molecular testing now offers high accuracy second-line DST from culture or direct from smear-positive sputum [23]. Rapid DST may also be possible using proteomic methods [24].

8.3.6 Chest Radiograph

Although compatible changes on the chest x-ray may contribute to the diagnosis of active TB, these are not alone adequate because of low specificity and poor inter-rater reliability.

8.3.7 Serological Tests

Commercial antibody tests from blood demonstrate inadequate and variable performance for the diagnosis of TB, and are not recommended [25]. In contrast, adenosine deaminase testing of sterile fluids has excellent performance for the diagnosis of extrapulmonary TB [26].

8.3.8 Antigen Testing

Novel applications for detection include urine lipo-arabinomannan, a cell wall protein in mycobacteria. Although sensitivity is low, in late-stage HIV when TB diagnosis is difficult, the test may add some diagnostic benefit in combination with conventional tests [27].

8.3.9 Whole Genome Sequencing (WGS)

The increasing access to rapid WGS and bioinformatics analysis has provided superior resolution for molecular epidemiology compared to conventional molecular typing techniques, including the definition of transmission events not detected by traditional epidemiology [28,29]. WGS is also being used for rapid susceptibility testing, including the detection of novel resistance mutations, and amplification directly from sputum [30].

8.3.10 Interferon Gamma Release Assays (IGRAs)

The role of IGRAs for the diagnosis of active TB is controversial since they cannot distinguish active TB from latent TB infection (LTBI). The WHO has discouraged their use for active TB.

Case Presentation 1 (continued)

The Xpert MTB/RIF is positive for TB and negative for rifampin resistance and small numbers of acid-fast bacilli are seen. You start him on isoniazid (INH), rifampicin (rifampin), pyrazinamide, and ethambutol. He consents to HIV antibody testing and tests negative. Two weeks later, his culture confirms *M. tuberculosis*. One week later, his isolate is found to be fully susceptible to all first-line antituberculosis drugs, and you discontinue his ethambutol. You plan to treat him with three drugs for a total of two months, followed by a further four months of isoniazid and rifampicin. You warn him about potential drug side effects, and prescribe vitamin B6 to minimize his chance of neuropathy. You notify the local public health department to arrange contact tracing. You ask the department about the availability of directly observed therapy (DOT), and wonder about the need for DOT in this man.

8.4 Treatment

8.4.1 Drug-susceptible Active TB Treatment

The aim of treatment is to prevent transmission, cure patients, prevent relapses, and avert deaths. The treatment of pulmonary TB has been subjected to numerous randomized clinical trials, primarily in high-prevalence countries, although no systematic review of such trials was identified. A number of studies conducted by the British Medical Research Council in Singapore,

Hong Kong, India, and East Africa compared various durations and regimens [31], and found that a combination of isoniazid (INH), rifampicin (RIF), and pyrazinamide (PZA) for two months, followed by INH and RIF for a further four months, resulted in high (>96%) cure rates. The WHO guidelines [32] (currently under revision) strongly recommend these three drugs, together with ethambutol (ETH), for initial treatment of drug-susceptible active TB, for a total duration of treatment of six months. Some experts recommend extended duration among TB patients with HIV. In patients with cavitary disease and culture positivity at two months, CDC recommends seven months' total duration [33].

Daily doses are strongly recommended, with an alternative of thrice weekly doses where treatment is directly observed, but not in HIV prevalent areas. Sputum smear monitoring should be done at two months, and at three months if still positive. Drug susceptibility testing (DST) is recommended if smears fail to clear at three months, although developed countries will perform initial DST on all cases. Generally, empirical treatment pending microbiological diagnosis is discouraged, although when risk of progression or transmission is high, and indirect evidence supports the diagnosis, empirical treatment may be considered [33].

Evidence to support shortened duration of treatment is urgently needed in order to improve completion rate. Trials to shorten treatment without increasing relapse are limited by duration of post-trial follow-up, and the definition of the appropriate biomarker for relapse [34].

The benefits of directly observed treatment, short course (DOTS) to improve completion rate remains unclear. Eleven trials from Tanzania, Pakistan, Nepal, Taiwan, Thailand, South Africa, Swaziland, Australia, and the United States were included in a meta-analysis, which demonstrated no increase in completion rate when DOTS programs were compared to other methods of treatment delivery [35]. There may be other benefits due to integrated DOTS programs besides completion rate, however, such as access to diagnosis and record keeping. Even with DOTS, high completion rates are not assured, because patients are often transient or challenged by social or psychiatric problems. Material incentives in developed countries do not improve adherence [36], but reminder systems may assist [37].

There is insufficient evidence of benefit for adjunctive corticosteroid treatment in pulmonary TB [38], although it reduces mortality due to TB meningitis [39]. Nutritional or vitamin supplementation is not associated with benefit [40].

The treatment of TB in the setting of HIV consists of standard therapies with the duration of treatment at least as long as in HIV negative persons. HIV-coinfected patients tend to do equally well clinically and microbiologically, but they have an increased case fatality rate and TB recurrence rate. Early initiation of antiretroviral therapy after TB therapy reduces overall mortality, but increases Immune Reconstitution Inflammatory Syndrome-associated mortality [41].

Secondary prophylaxis with INH given to HIV/TB-co-infected patients was more effective than placebo in preventing recurrent TB [42]. Trimethoprim/sulfamethoxazole for prophylaxis of *Pneumocystis jiroveci* should be given to all HIV patients with TB, and is associated with a reduction in mortality compared to placebo in HIV/TB coinfection (Hazard Ratio [HR] 0.79, 95% CI 0.63–0.99) [43].

8.4.2 Drug-resistant Active TB Treatment

In settings with high rates of primary INH resistance, INH, RIF, and ETH may be used for continuation phase (weak recommendation, further research urgently needed) [32]. In 2016, the WHO recommended that TB resistant to RIF (RIF resistant) should be treated in the same way as TB resistant to RIF and INH (multi-drug resistant [MDR]). In 2015, the global proportion of RIF resistant/MDR-TB among new cases was 3.9% (95% CI 2.7–5.1) and 21% (95% CI 15–28) among previously treated cases. MDR-TB is concentrated in Russia, China, and India. Among MDR-TB, 9.5% are also extensively drug resistant (XDR), meaning resistant to INH, RIF, one injectable and one fluoroquinolone. The global treatment success rate (defined as cure [bacteriologically confirmed cases that are smear or culture negative in the last month of treatment, and on at least one previous occasion] or completed treatment without proof of smear or culture negative status) for HIV negative susceptible TB is 83%; for HIV positive susceptible, 75%; for MDR, 52%; and for XDR, 28% [2]. Global death rates for HIV negative susceptible TB is 3%; for HIV positive susceptible, 11%; for MDR, 17%; and for XDR, 27% [2].

Randomized trials are not available to guide the treatment of drug-resistant TB, and previous WHO guidelines suggested at least 18 months of treatment. Recent guidelines conditionally recommend that low-risk patients (not previously treated with second-line drugs, and susceptible to fluoroquinolones and injectable drugs) may be treated for 9–12 months [44]. At least five effective drugs should be used in the intensive phase, and high-dose INH and ETH should be considered (conditional recommendations). A meta-analysis of 14 observational studies demonstrated better MDR treatment outcomes with individualized treatment compared to standardized treatment [45].

Two novel drugs for MDR treatment have been recently developed. Bedaquiline added to standard MDR treatment in an open-label, uncontrolled trial of highly drug resistant TB was associated with culture conversion rates between 62.2% and 73.1% at 120 weeks [46]. Delaminid was reported in three industry-sponsored trials in extensively drug-resistant (XDR) TB, in addition to optimized backbone treatment [47]. Two-month culture conversion was non-significantly higher, and mortality was non-significantly lower in patients receiving six months of delamanid compared to two months. Delamanid has been recommended by the WHO for treatment of MDR-TB among children [48].

Case Presentation 1 (continued)

You treat your patient for a total of six months. At two months, his sputum smears and culture are negative. At four weeks, his transaminase levels rise to three times baseline, but as he is asymptomatic, you continue his therapy and these normalize by week 8. He completes therapy and is asked to present one year later for X-ray follow-up. Contact tracing reveals no immediate family or fellow workers with symptoms or a positive TB skin test. You reassure him that the chances of a future recurrence are very low and quite treatable if recurrence does occur.

8.5   Prevention of TB

Case Presentation 2

You are asked to see a 25-year-old asymptomatic woman who recently immigrated to Canada from the Philippines. Her screening intradermal 5-unit PPD test is positive at 13 mm of induration. She does not recall any previous skin testing. She received BCG vaccine as a young child and has had no known exposure to active TB among family, friends, or occupational contacts. She denies respiratory symptoms, has an unremarkable clinical examination, and has a normal chest radiograph. You diagnose latent TB infection (LTBI) and recommend INH treatment for nine months, although you wonder whether the BCG vaccine is responsible for her TB skin test reactivity. She also asks whether a blood test she has heard about for TB would be better than the skin test.

8.6   Diagnosis of Latent TB Infection

8.6.1   Tuberculin Skin Test (TST)

The tuberculin skin test consists of injecting five units of purified protein derivative S (PPD-S) intradermally into the volar aspect of the forearm, and measuring the millimeters of induration in the transverse diameter 48–72 hours later. The test measures delayed-type hypersensitivity to mycobacterial antigen. Conversion of the skin test may take three months after exposure to infection, and an increase of 10 mm or more identifies patients who are at high risk for developing active TB [8].

8.6.2 Interferon Gamma Release Assays (IGRA)

Gamma-interferon release by lymphocytes stimulated with mycobacterial antigen can detect infection with *M. tuberculosis* based on memory immune response. IGRA has been shown to be more specific than the tuberculin skin test, correlate better with TB exposure, be less confounded by BCG vaccination and non-tuberculous mycobacterial infections, be less complex to administer and interpret, and only require one patient visit [49]. Performance is difficult to assess due to the lack of a reference standard for the diagnosis of LTBI, but IGRA better predicts progression to active TB compared to tuberculin skin test (TST) [49]. Unfortunately, neither test works well in advanced HIV disease, due to anergy [50]. Many jurisdictions have discontinued the TST in favor of the IGRA.

8.7 Treatment of LTBI

Treatment of LTBI is the strategy of treating asymptomatic infected patients to prevent future active TB. In the United States, screening for LTBI is recommended for populations with previous residence in high incidence countries, and populations living in high-risk congregate settings [51]. Many treatment regimens have been compared to placebo in clinical trials, and in a meta-analysis of 53 studies, INH for six months (Odds Ratio [OR] 0.64), INH for nine months (OR 0.52), RIF for three to four months (OR 0.41), and INH/RIF for three to four months (OR 0.52) are effective [52]. Shorter RIF regimens may be less toxic than longer INH regimens [53].

In cases exposed to known MDR-TB, the role of prophylaxis is unclear as no randomized studies have been completed [54].

Case Presentation 2 (continued)

Your patient is treated with daily INH and vitamin B6. She increasingly complains of tiredness and headaches, and difficulty concentrating on her studies. After five months, she decides not to continue treatment. You convince her to complete six months of therapy, which you know is an acceptable alternative. You emphasize that treatment for latent TB infection is imperfect and that a small chance of future TB remains. You recommend that should she develop symptoms compatible with TB, she will need to be investigated for this. You estimate that her baseline lifetime risk of TB reactivation was up to 5%, and following treatment, you have reduced this risk to 2% or less.

8.8 TB Prophylaxis in HIV

In HIV, where risk of activation of LTBI is high and diagnosis of LTBI is difficult, continuous INH prophylaxis has been recommended. Among 2,056 HIV infected patients in the Ivory Coast, a randomized trial of INH prophylaxis for six months reported reduced mortality (adjusted HR 0.65, 95% CI 0.48–0.88) [55]. INH prophylaxis for 36 months was superior to 6 months [56]. In a meta-analysis, INH prophylaxis was associated with a reduction in relative risk of TB of 35% [57]. Empirical TB treatment was not superior to INH prophylaxis in preventing mortality in a randomized trial [58].

8.9 Vaccination

Childhood immunization with BCG has been studied in three meta-analyses, which pooled both randomized controlled trials and case-control studies. BCG was shown to reduce miliary and meningeal TB by 75 to 86%, and pulmonary TB in children only by 50%.

Several novel TB vaccines are in early phase trials. MVA85A-IMX313 has undergone a Phase 1 trial in 30 previously BCG vaccinated adults. It was well tolerated and created an immune response [59]. M72/AS01 was tested among 240 HIV negative and HIV positive adults in India, and found to be well tolerated and immunogenic [60]. A large randomized trial of MVA85A in infants

in South Africa, however, was not shown to be protective [61].

8.10   Conclusion

Although TB continues to cause a very large number of deaths and contribute to poverty in many countries, new investment, new tools, and new technologies are reversing incidence and mortality, and contributing very hopeful targets to the End TB Strategy for 2035.

References

1 Dye C, Scheele S, Dolin P, Pathania V, Raviglione MC. Consensus statement. Global burden of tuberculosis: estimated incidence, prevalence, and mortality by country. WHO Global Surveillance and Monitoring Project. JAMA. 1999 Aug 18;282(7):677–86.

2 Global tuberculosis report 2016. Geneva: World Health Organization, 2016.

3 Dobler CC. Biologic Agents and Tuberculosis. Microbiol Spectr. 2016 Dec;4(6).

4 Kurmi OP, Sadhra CS, Ayres JG, Sadhra SS. Tuberculosis risk from exposure to solid fuel smoke: a systematic review and meta-analysis. J Epidemiol Community Health. 2014 Dec;68(12):1112–8.

5 Lin HH, Suk CW, Lo HL, Huang RY, Enarson DA, Chiang CY. Indoor air pollution from solid fuel and tuberculosis: a systematic review and meta-analysis. Int J Tuberc Lung Dis. 2014 May;18(5):613–21.

6 Patra J, Jha P, Rehm J, Suraweera W. Tobacco smoking, alcohol drinking, diabetes, low body mass index and the risk of self-reported symptoms of active tuberculosis: individual participant data (IPD) meta-analyses of 72,684 individuals in 14 high tuberculosis burden countries. PLoS One. 2014;9(5):e96433.

7 Dogar OF, Pillai N, Safdar N, Shah SK, Zahid R, Siddiqi K. Second-hand smoke and

the risk of tuberculosis: a systematic review and a meta-analysis. Epidemiol Infect. 2015 Nov;143(15):3158–72.

8 Ferebee SH. Controlled chemoprophylaxis trials in tuberculosis: a general review. Bibl Tuberc. 1970;26:28–106.

9 Selwyn PA, Hartel D, Lewis VA, et al. A prospective study of the risk of tuberculosis among intravenous drug users with human immunodeficiency virus infection. NEnglJMed. 1989;320(9):545–50.

10 Davis JL, Cattamanchi A, Cuevas LE, Hopewell PC, Steingart KR. Diagnostic accuracy of same-day microscopy versus standard microscopy for pulmonary tuberculosis: a systematic review and meta-analysis. Lancet Infect Dis. 2013 Feb;13(2):147–54.

11 Peter JG, Theron G, Pooran A, Thomas J, Pascoe M, Dheda K. Comparison of two methods for acquisition of sputum samples for diagnosis of suspected tuberculosis in smear-negative or sputum-scarce people: a randomised controlled trial. Lancet Respir Med. 2013 Aug;1(6):471–8.

12 Steingart KR, Schiller I, Horne DJ, Pai M, Boehme CC, Dendukuri N. Xpert(R) MTB/RIF assay for pulmonary tuberculosis and rifampicin resistance in adults. Cochrane Database Syst Rev. 2014 Jan 21(1):CD009593.

13 Automated Real-Time Nucleic Acid Amplification Technology for Rapid and Simultaneous Detection of Tuberculosis and Rifampicin Resistance: Xpert MTB/RIF Assay for the Diagnosis of Pulmonary and Extrapulmonary TB in Adults and Children: Policy Update. WHO Guidelines Approved by the Guidelines Review Committee. Geneva2013.

14 Marangu D, Devine B, John-Stewart G. Diagnostic accuracy of nucleic acid amplification tests in urine for pulmonary tuberculosis: a meta-analysis. Int J Tuberc Lung Dis. 2015 Nov;19(11):1339–47.

15 Steingart KR, Henry M, Ng V, et al. Fluorescence versus conventional sputum smear microscopy for tuberculosis: a systematic review. Lancet Infect Dis. 2006 Sep;6(9):570–81.

16 Chang EW, Page AL, Bonnet M. Light-emitting diode fluorescence microscopy for tuberculosis diagnosis: a meta-analysis. Eur Respir J. 2016 Mar;47(3):929–37.

17 Steingart KR, Ng V, Henry M, et al. Sputum processing methods to improve the sensitivity of smear microscopy for tuberculosis: a systematic review. Lancet Infect Dis. 2006 Oct;6(10):664–74.

18 Rageade F, Picot N, Blanc-Michaud A, et al. Performance of solid and liquid culture media for the detection of Mycobacterium tuberculosis in clinical materials: meta-analysis of recent studies. Eur J Clin Microbiol Infect Dis. 2014 Jun;33(6):867–70.

19 Leung E, Minion J, Benedetti A, Pai M, Menzies D. Microcolony culture techniques for tuberculosis diagnosis: a systematic review. Int J Tuberc Lung Dis. 2012 Jan;16(1):16–23, i–iii.

20 Minion J, Leung E, Menzies D, Pai M. Microscopic-observation drug susceptibility and thin layer agar assays for the detection of drug resistant tuberculosis: a systematic review and meta-analysis. Lancet Infect Dis. 2010 Oct;10(10):688–98.

21 Coban AY, Deveci A, Sunter AT, Martin A. Nitrate reductase assay for rapid detection of isoniazid, rifampin, ethambutol, and streptomycin resistance in Mycobacterium tuberculosis: a systematic review and meta-analysis. J Clin Microbiol. 2014 Jan;52(1):15–9.

22 Drobniewski F, Cooke M, Jordan J, et al. Systematic review, meta-analysis and economic modelling of molecular diagnostic tests for antibiotic resistance in tuberculosis. Health Technol Assess. 2015 May;19(34):1–188, vii–viii.

23 Theron G, Peter J, Richardson M, Warren R, Dheda K, Steingart KR. GenoType(R) MTBDRsl assay for resistance to second-line anti-tuberculosis drugs. Cochrane Database Syst Rev. 2016 Sep 08;9:CD010705.

24 Ceyssens PJ, Soetaert K, Timke M, et al. Matrix-assisted laser fesorption ionization-time of flight mass dpectrometry for combined species identification and drug sensitivity testing in mycobacteria. J Clin Microbiol. 2017 Feb;55(2):624–34.

25 Steingart KR, Flores LL, Dendukuri N, et al. Commercial serological tests for the diagnosis of active pulmonary and extrapulmonary tuberculosis: an updated systematic review and meta-analysis. PLoS Med. 2011 Aug;8(8):e1001062.

26 Gui X, Xiao H. Diagnosis of tuberculosis pleurisy with adenosine deaminase (ADA): a systematic review and meta-analysis. Int J Clin Exp Med. 2014;7(10):3126–35.

27 Shah M, Hanrahan C, Wang ZY, et al. Lateral flow urine lipoarabinomannan assay for detecting active tuberculosis in HIV-positive adults. Cochrane Database Syst Rev. 2016 May 10(5):CD011420.

28 Cannas A, Mazzarelli A, Di Caro A, Delogu G, Girardi E. Molecular typing of mycobacterium tuberculosis strains: a fundamental tool for tuberculosis control and elimination. Infect Dis Rep. 2016 Jun 24;8(2):6567.

29 Nikolayevskyy V, Kranzer K, Niemann S, Drobniewski F. Whole genome sequencing of Mycobacterium tuberculosis for detection of recent transmission and

tracing outbreaks: a systematic review. Tuberculosis (Edinb). 2016 May;98:77–85.

30 Swaminathan S, Sundaramurthi JC, Palaniappan AN, Narayanan S. Recent developments in genomics, bioinformatics and drug discovery to combat emerging drug-resistant tuberculosis. Tuberculosis (Edinb). 2016 Dec;101:31–40.

31 Fox W, Ellard GA, Mitchison DA. Studies on the treatment of tuberculosis undertaken by the British Medical Research Council tuberculosis units, 1946–1986, with relevant subsequent publications. Int J Tuberc Lung Dis. 1999;3(10 Suppl 2) S231–S79.

32 Treatment of Tuberculosis: Guidelines. WHO Guidelines Approved by the Guidelines Review Committee. 4th ed. Geneva2010.

33 Nahid P, Dorman SE, Alipanah N, et al. Official American Thoracic Society/ Centers for Disease Control and Prevention/Infectious Diseases Society of America Clinical Practice Guidelines: Treatment of Drug-Susceptible Tuberculosis. Clin Infect Dis. 2016 Oct 01;63(7):e147–95.

34 Phillips PP, Mendel CM, Burger DA, et al. Limited role of culture conversion for decision-making in individual patient care and for advancing novel regimens to confirmatory clinical trials. BMC Med. 2016 Feb 04;14:19.

35 Karumbi J, Garner P. Directly observed therapy for treating tuberculosis. Cochrane Database Syst Rev. 2015 May 29(5):CD003343.

36 Lutge EE, Wiysonge CS, Knight SE, Sinclair D, Volmink J. Incentives and enablers to improve adherence in tuberculosis. Cochrane Database Syst Rev. 2015 Sep 03(9):CD007952.

37 Liu Q, Abba K, Alejandria MM, Sinclair D, Balanag VM, Lansang MA. Reminder systems to improve patient adherence to tuberculosis clinic appointments for diagnosis and treatment. Cochrane Database Syst Rev. 2014 Nov 18(11):CD006594.

38 Critchley JA, Orton LC, Pearson F. Adjunctive steroid therapy for managing pulmonary tuberculosis. Cochrane Database Syst Rev. 2014 Nov 12(11):CD011370.

39 Prasad K, Singh MB, Ryan H. Corticosteroids for managing tuberculous meningitis. Cochrane Database Syst Rev. 2016 Apr 28;4:CD002244.

40 Grobler L, Nagpal S, Sudarsanam TD, Sinclair D. Nutritional supplements for people being treated for active tuberculosis. Cochrane Database Syst Rev. 2016 Jun 29(6):CD006086.

41 Abay SM, Deribe K, Reda AA, et al. The effect of early initiation of antiretroviral therapy in TB/HIV-coinfected Patients: a systematic review and meta-analysis. J Int Assoc Provid AIDS Care. 2015 Nov-Dec; 14(6):560–70.

42 Fitzgerald DW, Desvarieux M, Severe P, et al. Effect of post-treatment isoniazid on prevention of recurrent tuberculosis in HIV-1infected individuals: a randomised trial. Lancet. 2000;356 1470–4.

43 Nunn AJ, Mwaba P, Chintu C, et al. Role of co-trimoxazole prophylaxis in reducing mortality in HIV infected adults being treated for tuberculosis: randomised clinical trial. BMJ. 2008 Jul 10;337:a257.

44 WHO Treatment Guidelines for Drug-Resistant Tuberculosis, 2016 Update. WHO Guidelines Approved by the Guidelines Review Committee. Geneva2016.

45 Kibret KT, Moges Y, Memiah P, Biadgilign S. Treatment outcomes for multidrug-resistant tuberculosis under DOTS-Plus: a systematic review and meta-analysis of published studies. Infect Dis Poverty. 2017 Jan 17;6(1):7.

46 Pym AS, Diacon AH, Tang SJ, et al. Bedaquiline in the treatment of multidrug- and extensively drug-resistant tuberculosis. Eur Respir J. 2016 Feb;47(2):564–74.

47 Gupta R, Geiter LJ, Wells CD, Gao M, Cirule A, Xiao H. Delamanid for extensively drug-resistant tuberculosis. N Engl J Med. 2015 Jul 16;373(3):291–2.

48 The Use of Delamanid in the Treatment of Multidrug-Resistant Tuberculosis in Children and Adolescents: Interim Policy Guidance. WHO Guidelines Approved by the Guidelines Review Committee. Geneva 2016.

49 Diel R, Goletti D, Ferrara G, et al. Interferon-gamma release assays for the diagnosis of latent Mycobacterium tuberculosis infection: a systematic review and meta-analysis. Eur Respir J. 2011 Jan;37(1):88–99.

50 Cattamanchi A, Smith R, Steingart KR, et al. Interferon-gamma release assays for the diagnosis of latent tuberculosis infection in HIV-infected individuals: a systematic review and meta-analysis. J Acquir Immune Defic Syndr. 2011 Mar 01;56(3):230–8.

51 Force USPST, Bibbins-Domingo K, Grossman DC, et al. Screening for latent tuberculosis infection in adults: US Preventive Services Task Force Recommendation Statement. JAMA. 2016 Sep 06;316(9):962–9.

52 Stagg HR, Zenner D, Harris RJ, Munoz L, Lipman MC, Abubakar I. Treatment of latent tuberculosis infection: a network meta-analysis. Ann Intern Med. 2014 Sep 16;161(6):419–28.

53 Sharma SK, Sharma A, Kadhiravan T, Tharyan P. Rifamycins (rifampicin, rifabutin and rifapentine) compared to isoniazid for preventing tuberculosis in HIV-negative people at risk of active TB. Cochrane Database Syst Rev. 2013 Jul 05(7):CD007545.

54 Fraser A, Paul M, Attamna A, Leibovici L. Drugs for preventing tuberculosis in people at risk of multiple-drug-resistant pulmonary tuberculosis. Cochrane Database Syst Rev. 2006 (2):CD005435.

55 Group TAS, Danel C, Moh R, et al. A trial of early antiretrovirals and isoniazid preventive therapy in Africa. N Engl J Med. 2015 Aug 27;373(9):808–22.

56 Den Boon S, Matteelli A, Ford N, Getahun H. Continuous isoniazid for the treatment of latent tuberculosis infection in people living with HIV. AIDS. 2016 Mar 13;30(5):797–801.

57 Ayele HT, Mourik MS, Debray TP, Bonten MJ. Isoniazid prophylactic therapy for the prevention of tuberculosis in HIV infected adults: a systematic review and meta-analysis of randomized trials. PLoS One. 2015;10(11):e0142290.

58 Hosseinipour MC, Bisson GP, Miyahara S, et al. Empirical tuberculosis therapy versus isoniazid in adult outpatients with advanced HIV initiating antiretroviral therapy (REMEMBER): a multicountry open-label randomised controlled trial. Lancet. 2016 Mar 19;387(10024):1198–209.

59 Minhinnick A, Satti I, Harris S, et al. A first-in-human phase 1 trial to evaluate the safety and immunogenicity of the candidate tuberculosis vaccine MVA85A-IMX313, administered to BCG-vaccinated adults. Vaccine. 2016 Mar 08;34(11):1412–21.

60 Kumarasamy N, Poongulali S, Bollaerts A, et al. A Randomized, Controlled Safety, and Immunogenicity Trial of the M72/AS01 Candidate Tuberculosis Vaccine in HIV-Positive Indian Adults. Medicine (Baltimore). 2016 Jan;95(3):e2459.

61 Tameris MD, Hatherill M, Landry BS, et al. Safety and efficacy of MVA85A, a new tuberculosis vaccine, in infants previously vaccinated with BCG: a randomised, placebo-controlled phase 2b trial. Lancet. 2013 Mar 23;381(9871):1021–8.

Chapter 9

Clostridium Difficile Infection in Adults
Louis Valiquette

Clostridium difficile (C. difficile) is a globally emergent enteric pathogen and is the leading cause of health-associated infectious diarrhea. In 2011, it was responsible for almost 500,000 infections and 29,000 deaths in the United States alone [1]. Clinical presentation of a *C. difficile* infection (CDI) varies from asymptomatic carriage to fulminant colitis. Most patients will present with mild to moderate non-bloody diarrhea, but on average, 18% of patients will suffer from severe CDI [2]. Severe or complicated CDI (cCDI) definitions vary according to sources but usually include: laboratory parameters (leukocytosis, increased in serum creatinine, low serum albumin etc.), imaging/endoscopy findings (toxic megacolon, pancolitis, pseudomembranes, etc.), and significant clinical outcomes (shock, need for ICU admission, colon perforation, need for colectomy or death) [3,4]. Recurrence (rCDI) is present when CDI re-occurs within eight weeks of the onset of a prior episode, after completion of initial treatment [4]. In the last decade, the frequency and severity of CDI have increased significantly worldwide due to the emergence of a hypervirulent strain designated as NAP1/BI/027 [5,6]. A deletion in the negative regulatory gene *tcdC* may allow to increased toxin production, although the exact mechanisms is not clearly understood [7].

Case Presentation 1

An 84-year-old male patient with chronic obstructive pulmonary disease and severe congestive heart disease is presenting to the emergency room after having had watery diarrhea, fevers, and abdominal cramps for three days. He was not aware of any sick contacts. His family doctor is treating him for an acute exacerbation of his respiratory condition with ciprofloxacin, and he is currently on treatment day 7. You are considering *C. difficile* and want to order the appropriate test.

9.1 Diagnosis

CDI is defined by the presence of clinical symptoms and the identification of *C. difficile* toxin or toxin-producing *C. difficile* in stools or colonoscopic or histopathological findings demonstrating pseudomembranous colitis [3,8].

The most frequent clinical presentation is diarrhea associated with prior antibiotic exposure. It must be kept in mind that diarrhea is a common symptom in hospitalized patients and is associated with several infectious and non-infectious causes like viral gastroenteritis, antibiotic-associated diarrhea, enteral feeding, drug-induced diarrhea, and so on.

Evidence-Based Infectious Diseases, Third Edition. Edited by Dominik Mertz, Fiona Smaill, and Nick Daneman.
© 2018 John Wiley & Sons Ltd. Published 2018 by John Wiley & Sons Ltd.

Fever, leukocytosis, and abdominal pain in the lower quadrants are other frequently associated symptoms. Stools are usually watery or mucoid with a characteristic foul odor. Detection of pseudomembranes by endoscopy is specific as other pathogens have only been rarely associated with their presence, but is poorly sensitive. Since pseudomembranous colitis involves only the right colon in approximately 30% of patients, total colonoscopy is preferred. Endoscopy is still useful to obtain a rapid diagnosis and in patients in ileus, but must be used with caution in patients with fulminant colitis as it has been associated with perforation. Imaging studies such as radiography and CT are useful to identify complications (perforation, toxic megacolon, etc.), but have low sensitivity and specificity to diagnose CDI [3,8].

CDI diagnosis is made in the laboratory by detecting the presence of two enterotoxins: toxin A and toxin B. They are encoded by *tcdA* and *tcdB* genes, located in the pathogenicity locus (PaLoc). Non-toxigenic *C. difficile* strains do not possess the PaLoc, and hence, the ability to produce toxins and disease. Consequently, CDI diagnosis cannot be based on *C. difficile* culture alone. On the other hand, identifying the toxin alone does not define CDI, as individuals might also be colonized by toxigenic strains.

Tests with low sensitivity might lead to patients not being treated and suffering of CDI complications, but also to sustained transmission due to the lack of appropriate isolation. On the other side, false-positives may lead to overlooking another serious disease process, and unnecessary treatments and isolation [8]. For this reason, it is recommended to only test loose or unformed stools and not to repeat testing during the same episode of diarrhea. Testing after treatment completion is not recommended as cured patients might continue to excrete toxigenic *C. difficile* asymptomatically during weeks [3,8–10].

Reference tests for CDI are the cell cytotoxin assay (CCTA) and the toxigenic culture (TC), but they are rarely used in a clinical setting because of long turnaround time and the need for specialized expertise [10]. They have been replaced by more rapid and convenient tests like toxin A and B immunoassays (EIA), glutamate dehydrogenase (GDH, a highly conserved enzyme in toxigenic and non-toxigenic *C. difficile* strains) detection, and nucleic acid amplification tests (NAATs). Highly specific (99%), toxin A and B EIA are not sensitive enough to be used as stand-alone tests (65–80%). To compensate for this lack of sensitivity, a multi-step approach consisting of the detection of GDH followed by EIA and/or NAAT confirmation has been proposed [3]. A two-step approach using GDH testing followed by toxin A and B EIA had reported sensitivity and specificity rates of 85% and 99%, respectively [11]. NAATs are frequently used as stand-alone tests because of their capacity to accommodate large volumes and provide rapid results. However, due to their very high sensitivity, they will also detect patients colonized with toxigenic *C. difficile* strains. Because asymptomatic carriage of toxigenic *C. difficile* is prevalent in hospitalized patients, there is a clear risk of overestimation of the true incidence of CDI [8].

Case Presentation 1 (continued)

On the same day as the GDH was reported positive, a toxin A and B EIA was completed and also found positive. Neither leukocytosis nor an increase in the serum creatinine was observed. You want to select the best first-line treatment to limit the consequences in your very frail patient. Considering his age and comorbidities, you are wondering if fidaxomicin would be an appropriate first-line treatment.

9.2 Treatment

Before starting antibiotics directly targeted at *C. difficile*, we suggest stopping any other concomitant antibiotic, antimotility drug, and proton pump inhibitor, if possible, and to administer adequate replacement of fluid and electrolytes.

For non-severe initial CDI, metronidazole is still an acceptable option considering its low cost and the potential of oral vancomycin to promote the acquisition of vancomycin-resistant enterococci [3]. However, metronidazole is not an interesting option for rCDI because prolonged treatments have been associated with persistent peripheral neuropathy, and colon concentrations decrease rapidly as inflammation subsides. Additionally, the recent analysis of pooled data from two Phase 3 randomized-controlled trials (RCTs) comparing tolevamer (a toxin-binding drug, proven inferior to metronidazole), vancomycin, and metronidazole, demonstrated that vancomycin was associated with higher clinical success than metronidazole (OR = 1.58, 95% CI 1.04–2.40,

$p = .034$). In a small RCT, vancomycin has also been shown to be superior to metronidazole in patients with severe CDI, with clinical cure rates of 97% versus 76% ($p = .02$) [12]. Vancomycin given at doses of 125 mg four times daily reaches fecal concentrations ranging between 200 and 1,000 ug/ml [13]. This clearly exceeds the reported minimal inhibitory concentration (MIC) for *C. difficile* (MIC90 between 1 and 2 ug/ml). Higher dosages of vancomycin are recommended in clinical guidelines for patients with cCDI, but there are no data available to support this practice [3]. In cCDI, recommended regimen consists of intravenous metronidazole and oral vancomycin, and consideration for administrating vancomycin by rectal enemas, if a severe ileus is present (Table 9.1).

Fidaxomicin, a novel unabsorbed macrocyclic antibiotic, is the first agent approved by

Table 9.1 Treatment options of the initial CDI episode.

Severity of the disease	Agent	Comments
Mild to moderate	• Metronidazole 500 mg orally 3 times daily for 10–14 days • Vancomycin 125 mg orally 3 times daily for 10–14 days • Fidaxomicin 200 mg orally twice daily for 10–4 days	• The most recent guidelines from the Infectious Disease Society of America (IDSA) recommend vancomycin and fidaxomicin as first-line agents. Metronidazole is an accepted alternative for nonsevere CDI when access to vancomycin and fidaxomicin is limited [3]. • Fidaxomicin has been shown to decrease the risk of further recurrence, but initial cure is comparable to vancomycin [15,16]. Its high cost and the equipoise regarding its efficacy against NAP1/BI/027 strains limit its use.
Severe	• Vancomycin 125 mg orally 4 times daily for 10–14 days • Fidaxomicin 200 mg orally twice daily for 10–14 days	• Pharmacokinetic data does not support an increased dosage of vancomycin unless the patient has severe diarrhea, especially for the first 48 hours of treatment [13]. • Fidaxomicin was not inferior to vancomycin in the subgroup analysis restricted to patients with severe CDI, same limitation and benefits as above [15,16].
Complicated	• Metronidazole 500 mg 3 times daily intravenously PLUS • Vancomycin 500 mg orally/nasogastric tube 4 times daily. If complete ileus, vancomycin can be instilled via a rectal tube (500 mg in 100 mL of normal saline 4 times daily) • Tigecycline 50 mg twice daily intravenously	• The risk of colon perforation must be considered while administering vancomycin in retention enema. • Very limited data to support tigecycline use in CDI treatment, but could be an interesting option to provide broader antimicrobial coverage in patients with concomitant sepsis.

the FDA for CDI. A meta-analysis of two phase III RCTs has demonstrated non-inferiority between vancomycin and fidaxomicin for initial clinical cure and superiority of fidaxomicin over vancomycin in the prevention of further recurrences [14]. Overall, fidaxomicin reduced persistent diarrhea, recurrence, or death by 40% (95% CI, 26%–51%; $p < .001$) corresponding to a number needed to treat of 7.9. Individually, each study demonstrated a significant reduction in rCDI [15,16]. Limited effect on fecal flora, inhibition of spore production, and longer post-antibiotic effect might explain fidaxomicin's superiority over vancomycin. However, considering its higher cost and the absence of a significant effect in patients infected with NAP1/BI/027 strains on rCDI, fidaxomicin has not replaced vancomycin in guidelines.

For a first episode of non-severe CDI, oral metronidazole remains an adequate first-line treatment if the accessiblity to other options is limited. We recommend the use of oral vancomycin for patients with severe or complicated CDI, and/or patients at higher risk for recurrences. The best available agent to decrease the risk of rCDI after a first episode appear to be fidaxomicin.

Case Presentation 1 (continued)

You have selected a 10-day course of oral metronidazole (500 mg, 3 times daily). The patient's symptoms subsided and he was well for two weeks. But now he is presenting again with 7–8 loose stools per day, and his *C. difficile* test is positive. What would be the best therapeutic option in this patient, at this stage? What would you do if this recurrence was his fifth?

Recurrent CDI has an important clinical burden, as up to one-third of patients will need readmission or develop severe CDI [17]. The most important factor linked to rCDI is the disruption of the colon indigenous flora, hence, treatment strategies for rCDI are different. Patients with a first rCDI episode might benefit from fidaxomicin as the lower

rCDI rate was similar in that subpopulation [18]. Tapering and sequential ("chaser") regimen have been used to allow the indigenous flora to recover while *C. difficile* growth is controlled. Vancomycin tapering regimens usually involve a standard treatment of 14 days, followed by six to eight weeks of decreasing dosage. Rifaximin and fidaxomicin have both been studied as sequential treatments after standard or tapering regimens of vancomycin, and have shown promise [19].

For years, fecal microbiota transplantation (FMT) was only supported by case series and systematic reviews of case series with all the inherent limitations of non-randomized study designs. However, more recently, an open-label randomized clinical trial was stopped before completion due to superiority of the FMT arm [20]. Indeed, 13 FMT patients (81%) were cured after a first treatment compared to 7 (27%) in the control arm. Three patients, who did not respond initially to their first treatment, received a second administration of which two were cured for a combined efficacy of 94% in favor of FMT (Table 9.2).

This large treatment effect was probably overestimated by the use of a non-standard comparator (i.e., high dose oral vancomycin). Of interest, a recent small open-label trial did not find a significant difference between FMT administered by fecal enema and tapering oral vancomycin treatment (rCDI rate, respectively: 56% and 42%) [21]. With these contradictory results and given the potential risk of transmission of infectious and non-infectious conditions, we cannot make a recommendation for routine use of FMT, and it should only be considered in patients with multiple rCDI and failure to conventional therapy.

Case Presentation 1 (continued)

Finally, the patient receives a course of 14 days of vancomycin without further recurrences. One month later, he again needs a course of antibiotics for another respiratory superinfection. His family physician calls you to ask if he can do something to decrease the risk of CDI?

Table 9.2 Treatment options of recurrent CDI.

	Agent	Comments
First episode of rCDI	• Vancomycin 125 mg orally 3 times daily for 10–14 days • Fidaxomicin 200 mg orally twice daily for 10 days	• Fewer secondary recurrences with fidaxomicin in a *post hoc* subgroup analysis [18]. In the most recent IDSA's guidelines, tapered oral vancomycin is suggested for a first rCDI episode (weak recommendation/low quality of evidence) [3].
Multiple recurrence (more than one rCDI episode)	• Vancomycin 125 mg orally 4 times daily for 14 days followed by tapered regimen (125 mg orally 3 times daily for 7 days, 125 mg orally twice daily for 7 days, 125 mg orally once daily for 7 days, 125 mg orally once every two days for two weeks)* • Fidaxomicin 200 mg orally twice daily for 10 days • Vancomycin 125 mg orally 4 times daily for 14 days followed by rifaximin 400 mg 3 times daily for 14 days. • Vancomycin 125 mg orally 4 times daily for 14 days followed by fidaxomicin 200 mg orally twice daily for 10 days. • Fecal microbiota transplantation (FMT) via rectal enema or nasoduodenal infusion.	• All the suggested treatments for multiple rCDI, apart for FMT, are based on retrospective cohort studies, case-series and expert opinions. • One pilot RCT showed a significant reduction in recurrent diarrhea in patients with CDI receiving rifaximin after a standard treatment, but did not shown a significant decrease in rCDI [19]. • FMT is the most efficient treatment for multiple rCDI (clinical cure >90%), as supported by two recent RCTs [20,22]. However, risk of transmission of infectious and non-infectious conditions must be considered.

*Several dosage variations exist; no superiority have been demonstrated for one option in particular.

9.3 Primary Prophylaxis

Probiotics are preparations of living, low pathogenicity organisms which when administered in adequate amounts might confer a health benefit to the host. A great variety of commercial probiotic formulations are available, including different bacterial and yeast strains. The effect of one type of strain, or a combination of specific strains, cannot be generalized to other species or strains. Probiotics are generally regarded as safe. Despite a broad utilization in children and adults, very rare cases of infections have been reported and mostly in immunosuppressed patients. If these rare complications occur, however, they can be associated with significant morbidity and mortality.

In a meta-analysis evaluating different probiotic formulations in the primary prevention of CDI, probiotics were found to reduce markedly and significantly the incidence of CDI (RR 0.36, 95% CI, 0.26–0.49) [23]. These results need to be interpreted with caution as only three individual trials were significant, with two of these having an unusually high CDI rate in the control group, and the majority of the included studies had a very small sample size. Since the release of the aforementioned meta-analysis, a large—albeit underpowered due to a lower than expected event rate of 1%—multi-center study did not demonstrate a significant effect of a probiotic formulation (two strains of *Lactobacillus* sp. and two strains of *Bifidobacteria sp.*) in adults older than 65 years exposed to antibiotics (RR 0.71, 95% CI, 0.34–1.47) [24]. Finally, a very recent meta-analysis using a Bayesian hierarchical model concluded that there was considerable uncertainty regarding the efficacy of *Lactobacillus* probiotic treatments to prevent CDI due to between-study heterogeneity [25]. Therefore, there is conflicting evidence to support the use of probiotics for primary prevention of CDI and evidence is not sufficient to recommend their routine use [3].

9.4 Secondary Prophylaxis

In some situations, a patient currently or recently treated for CDI might require additional antimicrobial therapy for a concomitant infection, which potentially increases the risk of rCDI. Vancomycin, probiotics, and monoclonal antibodies targeting specifically toxins have all been studied in this context.

Two recent retrospective cohort studies have specifically addressed the use of vancomycin to prevent rCDI in patients treated with systemic antimicrobials for another infection. In the first study, oral vancomycin prophylaxis decreased the risk of further recurrences in patients with rCDI receiving systemic antimicrobials (adjusted hazard ratio: 0.47, 95%CI, 0.32–0.69), but not in patients treated for an initial episode [26]. In the second, the incidence was significantly lower in patients on vancomycin prophylaxis during the follow-up period (4.2% vs. 26.6%, OR 0.12, 95% CI, 0.04–0.4) [27]. The most important hurdles to bring these results into practice are the variable dosage regimens used, the different follow-up periods and eligibility criteria, and the risk of bias due to the lack of RCT data. However, awaiting the results of more supportive data from RCTs, vancomycin could be considered during the course of systemic antibiotic therapy in patients at risk for rCDI.

Data are insufficient to support the use of probiotics alone or as an adjunct to antibiotics in CDI therapy to prevent further rCDI [28].

Passive immunization with the infusion of monoclonal antibodies directed at toxin A (actoxumab) and B (bezlotoxumab) have been studied in two large phase 3 RCTs. In both trials, the rate of rCDI was significantly lower with bezlotoxumab (MODIFY I: 17% and MODIFY II 16%) compared with the groups receiving the placebo (MODIFY I: 28%; MODIFY II: 26%) [29]. The number needed to treat to prevent one episode of rCDI was 10, but was 6 in older patients (≥65 years of age) and those with previous CDI. The actoxumab arm was discontinued in MODIFY I after an interim analysis because of a rate of rCDI similar to placebo and more serious adverse events. Bezlotoxumab has been recently approved by the U.S. Food and Drug Administration (FDA); however, the high cost of monoclonal antibodies will probably limit their use.

References

1 Lessa FC, Mu Y, Bamberg WM, Beldavs ZG, Dumyati GK, Dunn JR, et al. Burden of Clostridium difficile infection in the United States. N Engl J Med. 2015;372(9):825–34.

2 Abou Chakra CN, Pepin J, Sirard S, Valiquette L. Risk factors for recurrence, complications and mortality in Clostridium difficile infection: a systematic review. PLoS One. 2014;9(6):e98400.

3 McDonald LC, Gerding DN, Johnson S, Bakken JS, Carroll KC, Coffin SE, et al. Clinical Practice Guidelines for Clostridium difficile Infection in Adults and Children: 2017 Update by the Infectious Diseases Society of America (IDSA) and Society for Healthcare Epidemiology of America (SHEA). Clin Infect Dis. 2018 Feb 15. doi: 10.1093/cid/cix1085. [Epub ahead of print] PubMed PMID: 29462280.

4 Debast SB, Bauer MP, Kuijper EJ. European Society of Clinical Microbiology and Infectious Diseases: update of the treatment guidance document for Clostridium difficile infection. Clin Microbiol Infect. 2014 Mar;20 Suppl 2:1–26. doi:10.1111/1469-0691.12418. PubMed PMID: 24118601.

5 Loo VG, Poirier L, Miller MA, Oughton M, Libman MD, Michaud S, et al. A predominantly clonal multi-institutional

outbreak of Clostridium difficile-associated diarrhea with high morbidity and mortality. N Engl J Med. 2005;353(23):2442–9.

6 Pepin J, Valiquette L, Alary ME, Villemure P, Pelletier A, Forget K, et al. Clostridium difficile-associated diarrhea in a region of Quebec from 1991 to 2003: a changing pattern of disease severity. CMAJ. 2004;171(5):466–72.

7 Abt MC, McKenney PT, Pamer EG. Clostridium difficile colitis: pathogenesis and host defence. Nat Rev Microbiol. 2016;14(10):60920.

8 Crobach MJ, Planche T, Eckert C, Barbut F, Terveer EM, Dekkers OM, et al. European Society of Clinical Microbiology and Infectious Diseases: update of the diagnostic guidance document for Clostridium difficile infection. Clin Microbiol Infect. 2016;22 Suppl 4: S63–81.

9 Martin JS, Monaghan TM, Wilcox MH. Clostridium difficile infection: epidemiology, diagnosis and understanding transmission. Nat Rev Gastroenterol Hepatol. 2016;13(4):206–16.

10 Planche T, Wilcox MH. Diagnostic pitfalls in Clostridium difficile infection. Infect Dis Clin North Am. 2015;29(1):63–82.

11 Planche T, Aghaizu A, Holliman R, Riley P, Poloniecki J, Breathnach A, et al. Diagnosis of Clostridium difficile infection by toxin detection kits: a systematic review. Lancet Infect Dis. 2008;8(12):777–84.

12 Zar FA, Bakkanagari SR, Moorthi KM, Davis MB. A comparison of vancomycin and metronidazole for the treatment of Clostridium difficile-associated diarrhea, stratified by disease severity. Clin Infect Dis. 2007;45(3):302–7.

13 Gonzales M, Pepin J, Frost EH, Carrier JC, Sirard S, Fortier LC, et al. Faecal pharmacokinetics of orally administered vancomycin in patients with suspected Clostridium difficile infection. BMC Infect Dis. 2010;10:363.

14 Crook DW, Walker AS, Kean Y, Weiss K, Cornely OA, Miller MA, et al. Fidaxomicin versus vancomycin for Clostridium difficile infection: meta-analysis of pivotal randomized controlled trials. Clin Infect Dis. 2012;55 Suppl 2:S93–103.

15 Louie TJ, Miller MA, Mullane KM, Weiss K, Lentnek A, Golan Y, et al. Fidaxomicin versus vancomycin for Clostridium difficile infection. N Engl J Med. 2011;364(5):422–31.

16 Cornely OA, Crook DW, Esposito R, Poirier A, Somero MS, Weiss K, et al. Fidaxomicin versus vancomycin for infection with Clostridium difficile in Europe, Canada, and the USA: a double-blind, non-inferiority, randomised controlled trial. Lancet Infect Dis. 2012;12(4):281–9.

17 Sheitoyan-Pesant C, Abou Chakra CN, Pepin J, Marcil-Heguy A, Nault V, Valiquette L. Clinical and healthcare burden of multiple recurrences of Clostridium difficile infection. Clin Infect Dis. 2016;62(5):574–80.

18 Cornely OA, Miller MA, Louie TJ, Crook DW, Gorbach SL. Treatment of first recurrence of Clostridium difficile infection: fidaxomicin versus vancomycin. Clin Infect Dis. 2012;55 Suppl 2:S154–61.

19 Garey KW, Ghantoji SS, Shah DN, Habib M, Arora V, Jiang ZD, et al. A randomized, double-blind, placebo-controlled pilot study to assess the ability of rifaximin to prevent recurrent diarrhoea in patients with Clostridium difficile infection. J Antimicrob Chemother. 2011;66(12):2850–5.

20 van Nood E, Vrieze A, Nieuwdorp M, Fuentes S, Zoetendal EG, de Vos WM, et al. Duodenal infusion of donor feces for recurrent Clostridium difficile. N Engl J Med. 2013;368(5):407–15.

21 Hota SS, Sales V, Tomlinson G, Salpeter MJ, McGeer A, Coburn B, et al. Oral Vancomycin Followed by Fecal Transplantation Versus Tapering Oral Vancomycin Treatment for Recurrent Clostridium difficile Infection: An Open-Label, Randomized Controlled Trial. Clin Infect Dis. 2017;64(3):265–71.

22 Kelly CR, Khoruts A, Staley C, Sadowsky MJ, Abd M, Alani M, et al. Effect of fecal microbiota transplantation on recurrence

in multiply recurrent Clostridium difficile infection: a randomized trial. Ann Intern Med. 2016;165(9):609–16.

23 Goldenberg JZ, Ma SS, Saxton JD, Martzen MR, Vandvik PO, Thorlund K, et al. Probiotics for the prevention of Clostridium difficile-associated diarrhea in adults and children. Cochrane Database Syst Rev. 2013(5):CD006095.

24 Allen SJ, Wareham K, Wang D, Bradley C, Hutchings H, Harris W, et al. Lactobacilli and bifidobacteria in the prevention of antibiotic-associated diarrhoea and Clostridium difficile diarrhoea in older inpatients (PLACIDE): a randomised, double-blind, placebo-controlled, multicentre trial. Lancet. 2013;382(9900):1249–57.

25 Sinclair A, Xie X, Saab L, Dendukuri N. Lactobacillus probiotics in the prevention of diarrhea associated with Clostridium difficile: a systematic review and Bayesian hierarchical meta-analysis. CMAJ Open. 2016;4(4):E706–E18.

26 Carignan A, Poulin S, Martin P, Labbe AC, Valiquette L, Al-Bachari H, et al. Efficacy of secondary prophylaxis with vancomycin for preventing recurrent Clostridium difficile infections. Am J Gastroenterol. 2016;111(12):1834–40.

27 Van Hise NW, Bryant AM, Hennessey EK, Crannage AJ, Khoury JA, Manian FA. Efficacy of oral vancomycin in preventing recurrent Clostridium difficile infection in patients treated with systemic antimicrobial agents. Clin Infect Dis. 2016;63(5):651–3.

28 Pillai A, Nelson R. Probiotics for treatment of Clostridium difficile-associated colitis in adults. Cochrane Database Syst Rev. 2008(1):CD004611.

29 Wilcox MH, Gerding DN, Poxton IR, Kelly C, Nathan R, Birch T, et al. Bezlotoxumab for Prevention of Recurrent Clostridium difficile Infection. N Engl J Med. 2017;376(4):305–17.

Chapter 10

Urinary Tract Infections

Thomas Fekete

10.1 Urinary Tract Infections in Women

Case Presentation 1

An otherwise healthy 35-year-old woman is seen in the outpatient clinic for a two-day history of worsening urinary burning and frequency. She has two children at home and is currently using oral contraceptives. She recalls a urinary tract infection (UTI) from about six years earlier that responded to a three-day course of antibiotics, and she has had no sequelae of UTI since. She has no symptoms of vaginal itching or discharge. On examination she looks mildly uncomfortable but otherwise in no distress. She is afebrile and has normal vital signs. There is no costovertebral angle tenderness. There is slight discomfort with deep palpation over the pubis, but the bladder is not enlarged. The patient refuses a pelvic examination since she has just seen her gynecologist two weeks earlier for a routine check-up and was told everything was normal.

UTIs are a common medical problem, with U.S. costs estimated at more than US$1.6 billion in 1995 [1]. Estimates of the incidence of UTIs range from 100–200/100,000 women per year, but even if the data are inconclusive, UTIs are so common that 40% of adult women report having had at least one lifetime UTI. In young, sexually active women, the rate of UTIs has been reported to be as high as 0.5 episodes per woman year [2].

Case Presentation 1 (continued)

Urine dipstick testing is done in the office. It is strongly positive for leukocyte esterase and nitrites, but negative for blood, protein, and glucose. Is there sufficient evidence to make a clinical diagnosis of UTI and initiate antibiotic treatment in this patient?

10.1.1 Diagnosis

The pretest probability of UTI in an otherwise healthy woman with one or more UTI symptoms is about 50%, and a systematic review revealed that dysuria and frequency without vaginal discharge or irritation as in our patient raised the probability to more than 90% [3]. While a positive urine dipstick can further raise this probability, a negative result will still leave a high post-test probability of UTI. It is a fair question to ask how low a probability would argue against further workup or initiation of therapy. The systematic review above made a formal evaluation of clinical features of UTI. The authors identified nine individual studies that allowed an assessment of individual features such as

Evidence-Based Infectious Diseases, Third Edition. Edited by Dominik Mertz, Fiona Smaill, and Nick Daneman.
© 2018 John Wiley & Sons Ltd. Published 2018 by John Wiley & Sons Ltd.

Table 10.1 Likelihood ratios (LR) for some important UTI clinical features.

Clinical features	Positive LR	Negative LR
Dysuria	1.5	0.5
Frequency	1.8	–
Hematuria	2.0	–
Vaginal discharge	0.3	–
Vaginal irritation	0.2	–
Back pain	1.6	0.8
Vaginal discharge on examination	0.7	–
Costovertebral angle tenderness	1.7	–

dysuria or vaginal irritation so that each symptom could be given a likelihood ratio for the presence of a UTI. This likelihood ratio could be applied to a prior probability of UTI (as determined by the patient or the physician) so that a reasonable clinical diagnosis could be made. The likelihood ratios for some of the most important clinical features (where the 95% confidence interval did not include 1.0) are in Table 10.1.

The two most common tests used on the commercial dipstick to assess possible bacteriuria and pyuria (though not necessarily true infection) are the nitrite (nitrate reductase) and the leukocyte esterase tests. The nitrite test measures the presence of the enzyme nitrate reductase—a bacterial enzyme present in many Gram-negative bacteria. False positives are rare, but false negatives rates range from 10% to 30%, especially when infections are caused by nitrite-negative organisms, when the urine has a low pH or there is urobilinogen or ascorbic acid in the urine. Leukocyte esterase measures the presence of white blood cells in the urine. While other conditions can cause pyuria, the clinical setting is usually sufficiently clear to rule out other conditions. False-negative results can be found with low concentrations of urinary leukocytes, the presence of ascorbic acid, phenazopyridine, or large amounts of protein. The clinical benefit of treatment for women with typical symptoms in the absence of a positive dipstick and cultures

has been evaluated in a double-blind randomized controlled trial in which women were randomized to a three-day course of trimethoprim versus placebo [4]. The speed and degree of improved dysuria strongly favored the treatment arm suggesting an infectious entity despite negative screening tests. A systematic review of dipstick testing indicates negative dipstick results have the capacity to rule out even low levels (about 10^2) of bacteriuria [5], but this may illustrate the weakness of bacteriuria as a marker for people with dysuria destined to respond clinically to antibiotics.

In terms of non-invasive diagnostic tests that can be done in the ambulatory setting, there are two options: microscopic analysis of the urinary sediment and urine culture. Urine microscopy (semi-quantitative measurement of urine leukocytes) is done as a routine part of the urinalysis in many hospital laboratories, but the urine dipstick is almost as reliable in confirming UTI as the microscopic analysis [6] and is quicker and less expensive than microscopy. Both tests are imperfect but, in an Emergency Room study, each test had roughly the same number of false negatives and false positives when compared with the results of urine culture [7]. In pregnancy, the urine culture is the test of choice since management decisions are culture based. Less is known about the usefulness of dipstick testing in hospitalized patients, who experience higher rates of pyuria and UTI than ambulatory patients. Zaman and colleagues found high specificity using >10 WBC/μL and >5 WBC/μL (94% and 90%), but lower sensitivity with these values (57% and 84%, respectively) [8]. The positive predictive values were 91% and 77%, and the negative predictive values were 68% and 93%, respectively.

A management strategy that does not include any kind of urine testing might be appealing as a way of reducing costs, but could result in overtreatment. In a cohort of 231 Canadian women presenting with dysuria, about 80% thought that they had a UTI [9]. Physician diagnosis of a UTI occurred in 92% of cases; however, urine cultures were positive in only 53% of patients. As a result, unnecessary antibiotics were frequently prescribed. Combining clinical features and urine testing for pyuria and nitrates could have reduced the number of unnecessary treatment courses considerably. Unfortunately, it would have delayed the treatment of infection in a number of women with true cystitis (positive urine culture but negative dipstick test). The careful clinician might interpret this as a choice between overtreatment and delayed diagnosis. Luckily, the consequences of either approach are modest both economically (since the drugs and the diagnostic tests are fairly inexpensive) and in toxicity (since the medications are well tolerated and a short delay in the treatment of UTI almost never leads to serious sequelae). McIsaac et al. reported that by using an algorithm of requiring a positive urine dipstick before treatment would lead to a reduction in unnecessary antibiotic use from 40% of all drugs used to 27%, and a reduction in total urine cultures obtained from 87% to 40%; however, it also led to a reduction in the sensitivity for UTI from 92% to 81%. This algorithm would result in one delay of therapy in every 13 women with UTI [9].

The threshold concentration of organisms in the urine distinguishing contamination from infection has been the source of disagreement. While quantitative cultures usually show a large number of organisms present ($>10^5$/mL), about 25–30% of UTIs will have fewer organisms ($>10^3$/mL) with indistinguishable clinical presentations and responses to treatment [10]. By strict definition, a UTI should have $>10^3$ colony forming units of microbe per mL of urine (as opposed to the frequently noted cutoff of 10^5) [11]. Urine cultures demand time for processing and growth (at least 18 hours) and further time for identification of the microbe and determination of antimicrobial susceptibility. A treatment delay while these results are awaited can increase the morbidity of UTI, and the culture itself modestly increases the cost of diagnosis. However, there are no RCTs that have randomized patients with presenting UTI symptoms to urine culture versus no culture.

The common recommendations to obtain urine cultures in patients who require hospitalization, who are allergic to first-line antibiotics, or who fail therapy is done in anticipation of possible changes in treatment based on resistance or drug intolerance. Severely ill patients may also benefit from a urine culture insofar as it might guide appropriate changes in treatment if there is a failure to respond to initial therapy. Withholding treatment until a culture report is available is reasonable only for those patients with a low suspicion of infection or significant drug allergy. The benefit of obtaining a culture when there is a plan to initiate treatment immediately is to help interpret potential treatment failure. In earlier studies of healthy ambulatory women, treatment failures had been rare (<5%), but changing resistance rates to popular treatments such as fluoroquinolones or trimethoprim/sulfamethoxazole (TMP/SMX) with resistance rates of 20% or higher may increase this rate significantly. We recommend that women who come to the clinic with symptoms of cystitis have a point of care dipstick test before antibiotics are initiated. We suggest that women who have had prior cystitis and call with recurrent symptoms can be offered empirical treatment without an office visit, but should come in for testing if they have previously failed therapy, have had resistant organisms, or have multiple allergies.

10.1.2 Other Diagnostic Testing

UTI can be defined as simple or complicated based on the respective absence or presence of documented or suspected structural or physiologic abnormalities of the urinary tract. There is no information in Case 1 to suggest abnormal urinary anatomy and physiology.

Case Presentation 1 (continued)

After confirming the patient's sulfa allergy, the physician prescribed a five-day course of nitrofurantoin (100 mg orally twice a day). A phone call to the patient two days after the completion of therapy showed that her symptoms were totally resolved and that she had experienced only mild nausea on antimicrobial therapy.

10.1.3 Therapy
for the Ambulatory Patient

In ambulatory patients with UTIs, cultures show a great preponderance of *Escherichia coli* (*E. coli*). It is a common commensal of the gastrointestinal tract, and UTI strains are a subset of gastrointestinal-adapted strains that are also able to adhere to the periurethral area and to the cells lining the urinary tract. Similarly, other uropathogenic Gram-negative bacteria (such as *Klebsiella* spp., *Proteus* spp.) can cause UTIs in otherwise healthy people.

There are two important Gram-positive uropathogens of ambulatory women. The first is *Staphylococcus saprophyticus*, a coagulase-negative staphylococcus present in young women especially during the summer months. The second is *Enterococcus*. This is the third most common genus after *Escherichia* and *Klebsiella*, and because of its high degree of intrinsic antibiotic resistance, it understandably tends to cause infection in people who have previously received antibiotics. As an example of emerging uropathogens, consider

E. coli strain ST131 (sequence type represents an analysis of several *E. coli* genes that are highly preserved but have small mutational changes over time). ST131 *E. coli* is pandemic and has a combination of virulence genes (including adherence to the colon and uroepithelium) and plasmid-based resistance genes [12]. This includes beta-lactamases conferring the extended-spectrum beta-lactamase (ESBL) phenotype as well as genes for resistance to multiple classes of antibiotic. Eradication will be nearly impossible because of ST131's adaptation to human mucosal surfaces, thus permitting prolonged asymptomatic carriage. More recently, a variant of this strain that acquired carbapenemase genes has been making its way around the world [13].

Many studies on UTI outcomes including mostly older studies have used a microbiologic outcome rather than a clinical one for several reasons. First, studies in which symptoms were absent or minimal (such as asymptomatic bacteriuria or infections in catheterized patients) do not have a clear clinical metric. Second, symptoms may recede on their own or even with ineffective treatment. Third, some researchers prefer a more objective outcome than hard-to-corroborate symptoms. Fourth, recurrent (especially late) bacteriuria may be a matter of concern. Asymptomatic bacteriuria is a minor concern (except in pregnancy), and our treatment goals are now symptom-directed to provide maximum relief from morbidity rather than to chase cultures. Thus, it can be difficult to correlate results from older, microbiologic studies to patient experience. Ongoing studies will include both measures when feasible though patients and providers are likely to be much more interested in clinical metrics.

There are many choices of antimicrobials for the treatment of UTIs and a number of potential treatment durations. The patient in Case 1 had resolution of symptoms of her first UTI after a five-day course of therapy. A systematic review of the relative efficacy of single-dose versus three-day or longer therapy shows better outcomes with the three-day or longer therapy [14]. Unsurprisingly, in the management of uncomplicated cystitis in women, three-day courses have fewer side effects (relative risk [RR] 0.83, 95% CI 0.79–0.91) and similar failure rates as compared to prolonged courses (RR 1.16, 95% CI 0.96–1.41 at early and 1.17, 95% CI 0.99–1.38 at later follow-up). Therefore, there is no compelling reason to use more expensive and potentially toxic durations of antibiotic treatment for uncomplicated cystitis

Nitrofurantoin has been recommended as first-line therapy. It requires a five-day course and is generally well tolerated. It has little impact on the gastrointestinal flora and has reasonable activity against some drug-resistant strains. It is not a good choice for serious infection. The only drug still given in a single dose is fosfomycin, which has a long half-life (5.7 hours) and high urinary levels (a single 3 g dose is given as a sachet dissolved in liquid) [15]. The use of single-dose fosfomycin gives a lower cure rate than TMP/SMX or fluoroquinolones [16]. Generic TMX/SMX and ciprofloxacin are still the least expensive options in most settings.

Numerous studies have demonstrated the inferiority of β-lactams for UTI [17]. That is not to say that some patients do not respond well to inexpensive β-lactams such as amoxicillin, but that the overall rates of response and relapse are disappointing as compared with other drugs even in the absence of β-lactam resistance. Expanding the spectrum by using amoxicillin/clavulanate does not provide robust initial improvement or prevention of recurrence. A randomized trial of three-day regimens of amoxicillin/clavulanate or ciprofloxacin showed a clinical cure rate of 58% for the β-lactam and 77% for ciprofloxacin ($p < 0.001$) [18]. Surprisingly, the durability of response seemed equal regardless of the initial susceptibility of the organism to amoxicillin/clavulanate. The authors speculate that a large share of failure is attributable to a failure to eradicate the organism from the urogenital tract (45% vs. 10% persistent colonization, respectively). However,

β-lactams are recommended for the treatment of UTI during pregnancy given their favorable safety profile and the concerns about toxicity for the alternative agents. The increasing resistance rates to fluoroquinolones, however, may make beta-lactam more comparable in terms of efficacy for empiric treatment.

A Cochrane review about fluoroquinolones for uncomplicated cystitis in women indicates that, although as a class fluoroquinolones have shown good clinical outcomes in the published literature, there might be clinically important differences in efficacy and tolerability within the class or compared with other agents [19]. In July 2016, the FDA issued an advisory that fluoroquinolones no longer be used for uncomplicated UTI because of concerns about rare but serious toxicity including tendon, muscle, joint, nerve, and central nervous system problems [20].

A potential limitation of guidelines is that they may not keep up with changes in microbial resistance. Failure to follow guidelines has been documented, but the consequences are unclear. In a large primary care setting, of the 30% of patients with UTIs who would have met criteria for guideline directed therapy, only 25% were treated in a manner compatible with the 1999 IDSA guideline [21]. A national survey of prescribing practices showed that fluoroquinolone use steadily increased. In fact, fluoroquinolones have surpassed TMP/SMX as the most utilized treatment for uncomplicated UTIs in ambulatory women [22]. While there are regional differences, the overall trend appears to be an increase in the use of fluoroquinolones to treat older women. A more nuanced approach of using TMP/SMX and nitrofurantoin is as first-line therapy for uncomplicated cystitis. Both of these drugs as well as fosfomycin have been proposed as fluoroquinolone sparing agents, but head-to-head comparisons are scarce [23]. Regardless of this lack of evidence, we suggest following these current recommendations given the safety and resistance concerns with fluoroquinolones.

The use of non-antibiotic treatments for UTI is appealing, but the evidence basis for most of these interventions is lacking. A Cochrane review of alkalization of urine for treatment of UTI showed that of 172 potential studies flagged for review, none of them met the inclusion criteria, and thus, there was no quantitative conclusion possible regarding either safety or efficacy of this approach [24].

10.1.4 Prognosis

Response to treatment is usually fast although it may take days for all symptoms to resolve. There is even some clinical success with organisms that are reported to be resistant to the drug chosen for treatment. This might result from spontaneous cure or from achieving high enough a concentration of antimicrobial in the urine to result in cure despite apparent resistance. In an Israeli study [25], all patients received a five-day course of TMP/SMX, and in the patients with strains that were susceptible, the success rate was 82% as compared with 42% in whom the organism was resistant. In a large British study showing a relatively low incidence of trimethoprim resistance (14%), half the patients with in vitro resistance to trimethoprim receiving a three-day course of trimethoprim were symptomatically resolved in one week [26]. The time to resolution of symptoms was longer (when it occurred), but given the rate of resistance and the fairly good clinical response even in patients with resistant strains, the authors calculated that they would need to treat 23 patients to find one who returned for retreatment. Thus, they make the case for continued empiric therapy with TMP/ SMX without the need for a pretreatment urine culture.

Case Presentation 2

A 63-year-old woman is seen in the office for a two-day history of dysuria. She had recently retired from her secretarial job because of complications of her diabetes (early cataracts and mild, painful neuropathy) that had made it difficult for her to travel to work. She had recently completed a course of cephalexin for cellulitis of the left foot with clinical improvement. Her current voiding symptoms were moderately severe. She thought she might have had a fever and some mild sweats but at the time of the clinic visit she was afebrile. The remainder of the examination was unremarkable except for mild left costovertebral angle tenderness and diminished sensation in both feet. A pelvic examination was normal. A urine specimen was obtained: The dipstick test was positive for leukocyte esterase and glucose, and negative for all other tests including nitrite.

Like the previous patient, this woman also has a short history of irritative voiding symptoms, but there are some important distinctions. In addition to being older, this patient has long-standing diabetes with complications. The presence of significant diabetic peripheral neuropathy might portend autonomic neuropathy and incomplete bladder emptying. Significant residual bladder urine increases the risk of upper tract infection and treatment failure as well as the intrinsic risk for cystitis [27]. Furthermore, this patient's previous course of antibiotics (a cephalosporin) raises a concern of a more antibiotic-resistant organism. There are two potential strategies with respect to obtaining urine cultures for this patient:

- Obtain a culture before initiating antibiotics (early culture).
- Obtain a culture only if there is a clinical failure of empiric therapy (late culture).

Early culture is reasonable when urine can be obtained in the office and if culture reports are promptly and reliably available. A late-culture strategy makes sense if cultures are difficult to obtain and if adherence with medication and follow-up is likely to be excellent. These strategies have not been formally compared in clinical trials, but the low cost of urine cultures and the increasing rate of antibiotic resistance in uropathogens has tilted the equation in favor of testing in this situation.

Duration of treatment for complicated UTI without sepsis or clear kidney involvement is not as straightforward as that for other UTIs. The uncertainty is driven by the disparity of reasons why these infections occur. We suggest that a range of 5–14 days be considered. Patients with minor complications, quick clinical response, and known susceptible organisms would be at the shorter end and those with slower clinical responses or more significant risk factors should be at the upper end. For the average patient, we suggest a seven-day course.

Case Presentation 2 (continued)

A urine culture was requested, and while culture results were awaited, the patient began a course of antibiotics with TMP/SMX (160/800 mg orally twice a day) with the intention of giving a seven-day course of treatment. The laboratory report on the culture showed that she had an *E. coli* that was resistant to ampicillin but susceptible to all the other agents tested. The patient responded clinically within two days of starting treatment. At the conclusion of her seven-day course of therapy, she was asymptomatic, and at the time of follow-up clinic visit, had no symptoms or physical findings of UTI.

10.1.5   Follow-up

Follow-up for the woman with a symptomatic UTI is simple. If symptoms have resolved, the treatment is considered successful and no further visit or diagnostic testing is needed. Both of the cases presented had good responses and would not need follow-up. It would be sufficient to have telephone contact to assure that the treatment was successful.

10.1.6   Asymptomatic Bacteriuria

Asymptomatic bacteriuria refers to the presence of significant numbers of bacteria in the urine in the absence of symptoms such as urinary burning, frequency, or urgency. In young, healthy women, the prevalence of asymptomatic bacteriuria is 5–6% [28]. In the vast majority of cases of asymptomatic bacteriuria, the bacteriuria resolves spontaneously or persists without clinical symptoms or sequelae. However, the likelihood of developing cystitis within a week of the detection of asymptomatic bacteriuria is eight times higher than the risk within a week of having a sterile urine culture. Underlying conditions known to be associated with higher rates of asymptomatic bacteriuria are pregnancy, indwelling urinary catheter or post-removal, advanced age (>65 years), and diabetes mellitus. Treatment of asymptomatic bacteriuria does not correlate with better clinical outcomes in most cases [29]. Until recently, there was little evidence of harm in treating asymptomatic bacteriuria, but an Italian paper showed a higher rate of symptomatic UTI with more resistant bacteria for at least a year after treatment with antibiotics for asymptomatic bacteriuria [30].

There is evidence favoring treatment of asymptomatic bacteriuria during pregnancy [31]. This Cochrane review showed substantial benefits of treatment for asymptomatic bacteriuria during pregnancy. The elimination of bacteriuria was greater with antibiotics than with placebo or no treatment, the reduction of pyelonephritis was impressive (RR 0.23, 95% CI 0.13–0.41), and the pregnancy outcome (fewer preterm RR 0.27 or low birthweight babies RR 0.64) was enhanced. However the studies referenced were older and of low quality. A recent Dutch study showed that asymptomatic bacteriuria was associated with more pyelonephritis but not with poor birth outcomes [32]. This does not change current recommendations to screen and treat, but it bears watching in other developed countries, especially if there are limited treatment options. Asymptomatic bacteriuria is recommended to be treated before invasive procedures when bleeding is anticipated (including surgery and cystoscopy). There is evidence that prophylaxis with a single dose of pre-procedure ciprofloxacin can appreciably reduce the risk of post-cystoscopy bacteriuria in women with negative urine cultures undergoing diagnostic cystoscopy [33], but it may be time to reconsider this approach as fluoroquinolone resistance increases.

Case Presentation 2 (continued)

Three months later, the patient noted the onset of dysuria and urinary frequency over a period of two days. At the time of the office visit, she was uncomfortable, but had no fever or constitutional symptoms. Her urinalysis again showed a positive leukocyte esterase on the dipstick and a large number of white blood cells on microscopic analysis. She was given another course of TMP/SMX after a urine culture was sent. This time, the culture showed >100,000 colony-forming units of *Klebsiella pneumoniae*. This organism was resistant to ampicillin but susceptible to all other antibiotics tested.

In this situation, the patient had a new infection after cure of the previous UTI. Recurrence of UTI is a common problem with rates reported as high as 44% at one year [34]. Recurrent symptoms following apparent cure of a UTI can represent a relapse of the previous infection or a reinfection. In this case, the patient clearly had a reinfection since the organism isolated was a different species from that of the prior infection.

Case Presentation 2 (continued)

Although she felt completely well at the conclusion of her second course of antibiotics, the patient is frustrated and asks, "Why does this keep happening to me? Can't something be done to prevent another one of these infections?"

10.1.7 Prevention

The timing and frequency of recurrent UTI is unpredictable. Most of the known risk factors for UTI are difficult to control. Efforts to reduce UTIs by the ingestion of cranberry juice have been, at best, mildly effective while the use of a lactobacillus GG beverage was not helpful in preventing UTI [35]. Cranberry juice prophylaxis for ambulatory women was studied in a Cochrane systematic review and found to be somewhat helpful for those who can tolerate it [36]. A more recent RCT of cranberry capsules (more convenient than juice) for prevention of UTI showed no measurable benefit in women who resided in nursing homes [37]. Change in vaginal pH, in particular, the use of spermicide (often accompanying diaphragms), has been associated with an increased risk of UTI in several studies [2]. Sexual activity can predispose to UTIs [2] and this may be especially problematic with newer sex partners. In postmenopausal women, not taking estrogen replacement therapy is a risk factor for recurrent UTI [27]. Topical or systemic estrogens will reduce the rate of recurrent UTI in these women [38]. Clearly, the use of systemic estrogens should be informed by their risk/benefit for medical problems other than UTI.

The controversy over seeking an anatomic explanation for recurrent UTI is not fully resolved, but in adults, it is rare to identify correctable lesions [39]. In this study, 104 adult women referred to Urology for UTI consultation showed that only 4% had a potentially treatable problem (urethral diverticula).

Evidence exists to support antimicrobial prevention of recurrent infections. Women with frequent, uncomplicated recurrences (usually two or more infections in a six-month period) may benefit from one of three antibiotic use strategies:

- continuous low-dose prophylaxis [40].
- postcoital prophylaxis [41].
- pre-emptive short course treatment (without medical consultation) at first sign of infection [42].

Each of these strategies reduces the frequency and morbidity of UTI, but there are no controlled trials comparing them. A study of postcoital prophylaxis with TMP/SMX was shown to reduce UTIs by 12-fold (from 3.6 per patient year to 0.3 per patient year) [41]. Self-directed therapy appeals to many women. In one study, 172 women were given the opportunity to initiate levofloxacin therapy at the first indication of a UTI [43]. Roughly 50% of the women studied had one or more UTIs (on average, two per woman for those who had UTI), and 95% of suspected UTIs had positive urinalysis and/or urine culture with clinical and microbiologic cures >92%. A prevention study showed that 3 g of fosfomycin taken orally every 10 days for six months lowered significantly the infection rate to 0.14 infections per patient compared to 2.97 infections per patient year of placebo recipients [44]. The benefits of these approaches may diminish as the number of women with colonization/infection by resistant bacteria rises.

Whether prophylaxis is offered or not, there tends to be a slow trend toward cessation of recurrent infections in women without anatomic or physiologic reasons to have recurrent UTI. For women on continuing prophylaxis or postcoital prophylaxis, it might make sense to stop this treatment every year or so to see if the propensity to recurrent infections has faded. The patient in Case 2 will need to be aware of her urinary infection pattern and attend to her possible bladder dysfunction. This may entail consultation with a urologist who can assess her urodynamics and help determine the best way to maintain good voiding patterns. If she asks about the potential benefit of probiotics, she can be told that a Cochrane analysis of probiotics in adults and children failed to show any benefit [45].

The problem of UTI in people with spinal cord injury has also led to a study of preventive measures. The U.S. Agency for Health Care Policy initiated a meta-analysis of the role of prophylactic antibiotics in adults and adolescents with neurogenic bladder secondary to spinal cord injury [46].

They showed a reduction in the number of episodes of asymptomatic bacteriuria, but not in the number of symptomatic UTIs. This calls into question the practice of aggressive prophylaxis, especially in an environment of rising rates of *Clostridium difficile* infection. Patients with spinal cord injuries are also a target population for a new concept in infection prevention: bacterial interference. *E. coli* strain 83972 isolated from a child with persistent, symptom-free bacteriuria has been shown to reduce both bacteriuria and UTI in a placebo-controlled trial where it was instilled into the bladder and established colonization [47]. Other trials are under way, and this may be an attractive option in other patient groups with a risk for recurrent UTI.

10.2 Urinary Tract Infections in Men

Case Presentation 3

A 40-year-old man presented to his physician with a three-day history of dysuria. The pain was moderately severe but only present during voiding. He had no urethral discharge and he had no pelvic pain. He had not been sexually active for over one month prior to his dysuria. On examination, his temperature was 37.4 °C and the general physical examination was normal. The rectal examination showed a mildly enlarged but non-tender prostate. Urine analysis showed pyuria and bacteriuria. Urine culture was obtained and he was given ciprofloxacin 750 mg every 12 hours pending culture results. The culture eventually showed 10^5 colony forming units per mL of *E. coli* susceptible to ciprofloxacin.

10.2.1 Clinical Presentation

The presentation in this case is comparable to UTIs that are seen in women. However, in men it is important to consider involvement of the prostate gland as well as the bladder, ureters, and kidneys. The literature on UTI in men is limited and groups together urinary infections, such as cystitis and pyelonephritis, with prostatitis. It is easy to "rule in" prostatitis with a variety of clinical features (prostate tenderness, post-prostate examination urethral discharge) because acute prostatitis is often defined as a UTI in a man with additional features supporting prostate inflammation [48]. However, in men with features of UTI, it can be impossible to rule out some degree of prostatitis at the time of initial diagnosis since there may be only subtle or subclinical features of prostate involvement, which would only be revealed by prostate biopsy or culture of prostatic secretions. Thus, the absence of prostate tenderness or post-prostate examination urethral discharge does not exclude the possibility of prostatitis in a man with dysuria and positive urine cultures [48]. Because of this overlap, acute prostatitis and UTI can be considered to form a continuum in men.

10.2.2　Diagnosis

The diagnosis of UTI in men is made in a similar fashion to that in women. Urine collection is less likely to be compromised by contamination from skin flora. Pyuria and bacteriuria are both highly predictive of significant positive cultures. The lower limit of a positive quantitative culture is 10^3 colony-forming units per mL [49]. The sensitivity and specificity of this cut-off were both 97%, and it was unimportant as to whether a clean-catch midstream specimen or an uncleansed first void specimen was used. Importantly, although less common than in women, the prevalence of asymptomatic bacteriuria in men ranges from less than 1% in healthy young men to up to 40% in men in long-term care facilities, thus a positive urine culture does not necessarily imply the presence of a UTI [50].

10.2.3　Other Investigations

The evaluation of the cause of UTI in men differs from that in women since it is believed that there should be some diagnosable anatomic or physiologic factor to account for the UTI in men. Recent studies in this area may suffer from referral bias, though. Furthermore, in no case do they mention whether corrective procedures were done or whether they improved outcomes. A Scandinavian study of 83 men with UTI showed that 19 had some upper tract finding and 35 had lower tract problems [51]. Using cystourethroscopy, uroflowmetry, digital rectal examination, and measurement of post-void residual by abdominal ultrasound, the investigators identified a correctable defect in only one man with an upper tract lesion, but 41% of the men had a lower tract abnormality, most of which were already known. Another study designed to compare intravenous urography with ultrasound and plain film showed that half of the men studied had some abnormality (most of which were not correctable) [52]. The most common problem found was bladder outflow obstruction that was actually diagnosed by urodynamics (which was not part of the formal study protocol but was available for many but not all of the patients). A community-based study from Australia showed that of gay men with UTI (one-third of whom were HIV positive), clinical management was satisfactory, and of the men who underwent further investigation, only 14% had detectable abnormalities [53]. One thing lacking in all these studies is a sense of the rate of baseline abnormalities in similar populations of men without UTIs. Given the high rate of prostate symptoms recorded in community-based surveys [54], UTIs might simply coexist with some of the voiding problems and other prostate complaints seen in so many men. Therefore, no recommendations to routinely screen men with UTIs for underlying anatomic abnormalities can be made.

10.2.4　Treatment Strategies for Men

The organisms that cause urinary tract infections in men (including acute and chronic prostatitis) are the same as those found in women [55]. The same virulence factors (P fimbriae, adhesins, hemolysins) that make bacteria successful uropathogens in women (particularly as a cause of pyelonephritis) also make them uropathogenic in men [56]. Thus, *E. coli*, *Klebsiella* spp., *Enterococcus* spp., *Proteus* spp., and various other Gram-negative bacteria comprise the vast majority of uropathogens in men.

There are few randomized controlled trials comparing treatment strategies for male urinary tract infection or prostatitis, and no systematic reviews. Because of the possibility of concurrent prostatitis in men, the drugs selected for initial therapy are often those that penetrate well into the prostate gland. These include TMP+/-SMX and the fluoroquinolones. Clinical trials of TMP/SMX for UTI in men have been disappointing. In an effort to compare a short course (10 days) to a long course (12 weeks) for recurrent UTI, the investigators of a multicenter U.S. Veterans Administration study [57] found only 306 patients to screen; 38 were randomized and 30 were available for analysis at the end of the study. Notably, fewer than half of the men studied were symptomatic from their UTI, and two did not even have pyuria. Of interest, the long course of therapy was superior—60% microbiologic success for 12 weeks and only 20% for 10 days (RR 3, 95% CI 1.01–8.95). Recurrent infections were from the same organism in the majority of cases. Another study of 42 men with recurrent UTI showed that a longer course of treatment (6 weeks vs. 2 weeks) had a lower failure rate at a six-week post-treatment follow-up visit (68% vs. 32%; RR 2.2, 95% CI 1.05–4.49) [58]. This contrasts with a study of male veterans showing that short courses of a quinolone or TMP/SMX had comparable or better outcomes than longer courses and there were fewer antibiotic associated complications [59]. While a retrospective database review is considered a weak study design, the large number of subjects (>33,000) does suggest that shorter courses could be studied safely, and points toward no benefit in the absence

of recurrence of UTI of longer treatment durations.

The clinical response to fluoroquinolones in men with UTI appear to be better than with other antibiotics. Fluoroquinolones have good prostate penetration in animal models, and agents studied appear comparable in the treatment of male UTI/prostatitis. When norfloxacin was compared with TMP/SMX in 109 men with UTI recurrence in a randomized controlled trial, the clinical cure rate was similar; however, the bacterial eradication rate was 93% with norfloxacin and 67% with TMP/SMX ($p < 0.05$) [60].

In another study [61], ciprofloxacin was compared with TMP/SMX in men with UTI and early bacterial eradication rate (days 5–9 following antibiotics) favored ciprofloxacin (82% vs. 52%; $p = 0.035$). Of note, the drug doses used in the study were low (ciprofloxacin 250 mg orally every 12 hours, and TMP/SMX 160/800 mg orally every 12 hours) and the duration was brief (mean of 7 days). An open-label study of ciprofloxacin for chronic bacterial prostatitis showed a good outcome with a four-week course [62]. The bacteriologic cure rate was 92% at three months after the end of therapy and 70% at two years post-therapy. A randomized controlled trial comparing two versus four weeks of ciprofloxacin for men with febrile UTIs showed no significant difference in either early response or at one-year follow-up [63].

How does this evidence apply to the example of the patient in Case 3 above? The treatment with ciprofloxacin or TMP/SMX is rational and should be of one to two weeks' duration. Assuming that he has no further symptoms, he does not need investigative studies, but incomplete resolution or relapse should occasion a work-up. An ultrasound and plain abdominal radiograph can look for structural lesions such as kidney stones or hydronephrosis. A urologic evaluation could find problems with bladder emptying or structural disease of the lower urinary tract (including the prostate gland). While his prognosis is good, he may require a longer course of antibiotics for subsequent UTI while suspecting persisting prostatitis. Treatment benefit is lower for men with chronic prostatitis/chronic pelvic pain syndrome. A multicenter six-week trial of levofloxacin versus placebo in 80 men showed some improvement in both groups, but no benefit of the antibiotic over the placebo [64]. A double-blind, randomized trial of nearly 200 men compared ciprofloxacin plus tamsulosin, ciprofloxacin plus placebo, tamsulosin plus placebo, and two placebos [65]. The four groups were indistinguishable in terms of clinical response or measurement of disease using the NIH scoring system, thus antibiotics can currently not be recommended for the treatment of chronic prostatitis.

10.3 Severe and Complex Urinary Tract Infections

Case Presentation 4

A 59-year-old diabetic woman with no other prior medical problems was seen in the Emergency Department with a 36-hour history of fever, chills, and flank pain. She attempted to go to work that day, but after two hours at the office, her co-workers became alarmed when she nearly fainted on the way to the copier. In the ED, she was slightly confused and sweaty. Her oral temperature was 38.9°C, pulse 110, and respiratory rate 24. Her blood pressure was 92/60 mmHg. She had right flank tenderness on palpation. Urine obtained by bladder catheterization was cloudy and had numerous WBC and bacteria on microscopic examination. She had a WBC of 22,000 with 80% neutrophils, 14% band forms, and 6% lymphocytes. Her finger stick blood glucose was 21 mmol/L and her creatinine was 100 μmol/L.

This patient has a severe urinary tract infection requiring hospital admission [3]. In addition to fever and flank tenderness, she has sepsis with hypotension, rapid heart and

respiratory rates, confusion, and the clinical diagnosis of pyelonephritis. Furthermore, her diabetes is out of control and she is dehydrated.

Because this woman is diabetic, she could be presenting with a complicated UTI. This is defined as either a disruption of the normal anatomy or physiology (as in this patient) of the urinary tract. Obstructions to urine flow such as stones, tumors, or strictures can lead to more clinically severe infections. Alterations to barriers that normally maintain the unidirectional flow of urine such as vesicoureteral reflux and external bladder catheters can also predispose to complicated infections. The presence of stones or catheters can also contribute a surface for the growth of microbes as well as some protection from host defenses such as complement and phagocytosis. Physiologic problems such as incomplete bladder emptying with residual urine or poor ureteral muscular function can contribute to UTI complexity. Risk factors for pyelonephritis are similar to those of cystitis: sexual activity, family history, diabetes, and incontinence [66].

10.3.1 Diagnosis of Severe Urinary Tract Infections

The work-up for patients with severe UTI starts with urine collection for urinalysis and culture. Quantitation of pyuria or bacteriuria cannot distinguish mild from severe UTI. A review of quantitative pyuria in 1983 showed a sensitivity of 97% and a specificity of 98% for the finding of concomitant bacteriuria [67]. Pyuria and UTI in the setting of an indwelling bladder catheter is still a topic of interest, but a recent study has shown that the high specificity of pyuria for bacteriuria (90%) is offset by a low sensitivity (37%) [68]. In a British hospital study, urine dipstick testing on hospitalized patients was highly sensitive (98.3%) for bacteriuria; negative results on leukocyte esterase, nitrite, blood, and protein had a 98.3% negative predictive value for a positive culture result [69].

Blood cultures are commonly performed in patients with severe UTI, but blood culture positivity is rarely in excess of 20–25%, even in the most severe hospitalized cases [70]. Positive blood cultures have the same organism that is found in the urine, and thus, may add little to the determination of the specific etiology of the UTI [71]. Whether positive blood cultures are associated with worse outcomes, such as prolonged hospitalization, has not been determined [72]. There is some evidence from a retrospective chart review that young women with severe UTI and positive blood cultures do have higher rates of genitourinary abnormality, persistent fever, and abnormal heart rate than women without bacteremia [73]. A study of pregnant women with severe UTI showed that those who were bacteremic had a longer hospital stay than those who were not [74]. The management implications for patients with positive blood cultures is hard to assess since they often have other markers of severity that call for more intensive treatment [75]. Positive blood cultures rarely surprise the clinician or independently change the therapeutic approach [76].

10.3.2   Site of Care

The initial management of severe UTI includes a decision about hospitalization, which is based on the need for intravenous fluids, vasopressors, close nursing care, and adherence to a medical regimen. The patient in Case 4 might be stabilized in the Emergency Department, but would likely require hospital admission for assessment and treatment of her hemodynamic instability.

For patients with otherwise uncomplicated severe UTI, the choice of hospital admission increases the cost of treatment, however it is difficult to ascertain whether it improves outcome. This topic has not been studied in a controlled fashion except to show that for patients who can be managed in the ambulatory environment with oral therapy, there is no advantage to parenteral medications [77]. A retrospective survey of women evaluated in an Emergency Department showed that patients who were admitted (28 out of a total of 111) were older, had higher degrees of fever, were more likely to be diabetic or to have some genitourinary abnormality, or to be vomiting than women who were managed as outpatients [78]. It is notable that 12% of the patients initially discharged from the Emergency Department returned. A large population-based study of pyelonephritis in the Seattle area showed that the majority were managed in the ambulatory environment [79]. However the outpatient site of care was much more commonly chosen for women between 15–54 as compared to children, older women, or men of any age.

10.3.3   Treatment

After obtaining cultures and other laboratory tests, antibiotics are given empirically until susceptibility results are available.

The bacterial species that cause serious UTIs are similar to those that cause cystitis. There is a preponderance of *E. coli* and other Gram-negative rods. There are different phylogenetic characteristics and excess virulence factors in uropathogens causing pyelonephritis as compared to those causing cystitis or just found in normal fecal flora [80]. These bacteria usually have the same adherence properties, but may have additional virulence attributes that permit ascent of the ureter and in some cases deeper invasion such as bacteremia. For the critically ill, septic patient in whom even a short delay in treatment could be significant, broad therapy is appropriate until culture results permit a narrowing. Empiric choice of antibiotics should be based on the local epidemiology to best address the changing resistance patterns in patients with severe pyelonephritis. Empiric choices include broad-spectrum β-lactam, cephalosporins, carbapenems, and aminoglycoside. TMP/SMX and fluoroquinolones are discouraged due to resistance rates >10% in many settings. De-escalation can be done when cultures are back.

So long as there is no contraindication such as vomiting or hypotension, oral antibiotics are effective. In one study, route of administration of ciprofloxacin was randomized to intravenous or oral therapy with about 70 patients per arm [77]. Over one-third of the patients were bacteremic. There was no discernable difference in any of the outcome measures between oral and intravenous therapy, although the study was not powered to show modest superiority of either regimen. Because of the good bioavailability of oral ciprofloxacin, this outcome was not surprising. The presence of enterococci required a change in regimen in both groups, although the patients were doing well clinically at the time of the change. Among specific fluoroquinolones, there is no clear evidence as to which is most effective. This is largely because the comparative clinical trials have been powered for equivalence. Duration of therapy is longer than the 3-d regimen for cystitis, but when treating susceptible organisms, 7-d regimens seem to be equivalent to 14-d courses [81]. This Swedish study was well designed with placebo for the second 7-d in the short treatment group. Success was >96% in both arms.

There is evidence to suggest that for severe UTI, fluoroquinolones are superior to TMP/SMX, but this is largely based on higher rates of TMP/SMX resistance. Aminoglycosides are another therapeutic option for severe UTIs. Most uropathogens from ambulatory patients are still susceptible to aminoglycosides (with the exception of *Enterococcus* spp.). However, careful monitoring is required because of the possibility for nephrotoxicity and ototoxicity. Once-a-day dosing schedules for aminoglycosides can reduce the risk of nephrotoxicity of a seven-day treatment course without sacrificing efficacy [82].

Other classes of drugs have been studied in equivalence trials for the treatment of severe UTI. In one study, piperacillin/tazobactam and imipenem were equivalent for severe UTI with a microbiologic success rate of about 50% and clinical success of about 80% for each [83]. In another study, patients were randomized to a single dose of intravenous ceftriaxone followed by oral cefixime versus daily intravenous ceftriaxone. Both groups of patients received a 10-day course of therapy and their outcomes were nearly identical. This cohort of patients was well enough to tolerate oral therapy after the first day, and had about 75% bacteriologic and 90% clinical cure for each arm. Our patient in Case 4 might well be able to be discharged home after one or just a few doses of parenteral antibiotics.

Durability of response is a concern with severe UTI. In a comparison of hospitalized patients with severe UTI who received a short course of intravenous cefuroxime (for 2–3 days), patients who had follow-up with norfloxacin (a fluoroquinolone) did better microbiologically than those who had ceftibuten (a cephalosporin) [84]. The relative probability of bacterial eradication at 7- to 14-day follow-up after the conclusion of therapy was 0.84 (95% CI 0.74–0.97) with ceftibuten being less effective. This study did not explain why the responses were shorter lived for the cephalosporin, but it would be logical to assume that failure to eradicate the organism in other gastrointestinal and urogenital sites might have led to recurrence despite the 10-day course of therapy and the initial use of a parenteral cephalosporin. In some patients, duration alone may account for differences in outcomes. Patients with spinal cord injuries are prone to developing UTIs, but there may be difficulty in correlating clinical response with microbial response since the bacteriuria associated with relapse can be variably symptomatic. Nevertheless, a randomized trial comparing 3 versus 14 days of ciprofloxacin therapy for adults with symptomatic UTI in the presence of spinal cord injury showed a much higher rate of relapse in those who got the shorter course (RR 2.5 for early relapse and 2.1 for late relapse) [85].

As is the case with less severe UTIs, the prospect of more resistance can influence choices of initial therapy and may limit alternatives in the face of drug allergy [86]. Between 1992 and 1996, there was a doubling in the prevalence of TMP/SMX resistance in the Seattle area [87]. In a review of resistance rates in the 1990s outside the USA, percentage of *E. coli* isolates resistant to TMP/SMX varied from 12% in Holland to 60% in Bangladesh, and resistance to fluoroquinolones varied from 0% to 13% in Spain and 18% in Bangladesh [88]. The emergence of resistance has been dramatic. For example, between 2000 and 2010, the resistance of *E. coli* obtained from outpatient urine samples went from 3% to 17% to fluoroquinolones and from 18% to 24% for TMP/SMX [89]. It was stable for nitrofurantoin (0.8 to 1.6%), but it rose for ceftriaxone from 0.2 to 2.3%. In the same vein, another large network analysis showed similar changes in samples obtained in 2003 and 2012 [90]. Bacteria with resistance patterns typical of hospital-acquired strains now threaten women with community-acquired UTIs. In addition to fluoroquinolone resistance, community-acquired strains show extended-spectrum β-lactamase (ESBL) resistance. In a Spanish study, there was a threefold increase between 2000 and 2003 in the isolation of ESBL-producing *E. coli* among ambulatory women with UTIs [91]. The strains were from several different clones, but shared a CTX-M ESBL gene, suggesting that carrying this gene does not interfere with colonization of the healthy gastrointestinal and genitourinary tracts. The only antibiotic exposure risk factor in this case–control study was exposure to a second-generation cephalosporin, cefuroxime (OR = 21, CI 95%, 5.38–85.22; $p < 0.05$). In this study and others, the presence of ESBL genes was strongly associated with co-resistance including those for fluoroquinolones and trimethoprim. The rate of resistance to fluoroquinolones and cephalosporins continues to increase around the world [86].

10.3.4 How Quickly Should a Severe UTI Respond to Therapy?

Duration of fever is easily measured, and there is a wide range of rates of improvement. A retrospective survey of patients admitted with fever and UTI showed that the mean duration of fever (T > 37.5 °C at some point during a 12-hour interval) was 39 hours with a median of 34 hours [92]. At 48 hours, about one-quarter of the patients were still febrile. Elements associated with longer fever were increased serum creatinine, younger age, higher initial white blood cell counts, and the presence of *E. coli* as the causative agent. The interpretation of this data is difficult since the choice of hospital admission and initial antibiotics were uncontrolled, but it shows that temperature elevations can persist in people doing well and having no underlying medical problems. The presence of persistent fever in a patient making a good clinical response is a poor reason to initiate a detailed work-up for complicated UTI since fever was weakly correlated with abnormal results of imaging studies of the urinary tract that were done at the physician's request in some patients in this study.

References

1 Foxman B, Barlow R, D'Arcy H, Gillespie B, Sobel JD. Urinary tract infection: self-reported incidence and associated costs. Ann Epidemiol. 2000;10(8):509–15.
2 Hooton TM, Scholes D, Hughes JP, Winter C, Roberts PL, Stapleton AE, et al. A prospective study of risk factors for symptomatic urinary tract infection in young women. N Engl J Med. 1996;335(7):468–74.
3 Bent S, Nallamothu BK, Simel DL, Fihn SD, Saint S. Does this woman have an acute uncomplicated urinary tract infection? JAMA. 2002;287(20):2701–10.
4 Richards D, Toop L, Chambers S, Fletcher L. Response to antibiotics of women with symptoms of urinary tract infection but negative dipstick urine test results: double blind randomised controlled trial. BMJ. 2005;331(7509):143.

5 St John A, Boyd JC, Lowes AJ, Price CP. The use of urinary dipstick tests to exclude urinary tract infection: a systematic review of the literature. Am J Clin Pathol. 2006;126(3):428–36.

6 Komaroff AL. Urinalysis and urine culture in women with dysuria. Ann Intern Med. 1986;104(2):212–8.

7 Lammers RL, Gibson S, Kovacs D, Sears W, Strachan G. Comparison of test characteristics of urine dipstick and urinalysis at various test cutoff points. Ann Emerg Med. 2001;38(5):505–12.

8 Zaman Z, Borremans A, Verhaegen J, Verbist L, Blanckaert N. Disappointing dipstick screening for urinary tract infection in hospital inpatients. J Clin Pathol. 1998;51(6):471–2.

9 McIsaac WJ, Low DE, Biringer A, Pimlott N, Evans M, Glazier R. The impact of empirical management of acute cystitis on unnecessary antibiotic use. Arch Intern Med. 2002;162(5):600–5.

10 Stamm WE. Quantitative urine cultures revisited. Eur J Clin Microbiol. 1984;3(4):279–81.

11 Rubin RH, Shapiro ED, Andriole VT, Davis RJ, Stamm WE. Evaluation of new anti-infective drugs for the treatment of urinary tract infection. Infectious Diseases Society of America and the Food and Drug Administration. Clin Infect Dis. 1992;15 Suppl 1:S216–27.

12 Rogers BA, Sidjabat HE, Paterson DL. Escherichia coli O25b-ST131: a pandemic, multiresistant, community-associated strain. J Antimicrob Chemother. 2011;66(1):1–14.

13 Peirano G, Bradford PA, Kazmierczak KM, Badal RE, Hackel M, Hoban DJ, et al. Global incidence of carbapenemase-producing Escherichia coli ST131. Emerg Infect Dis. 2014;20(11):1928–31.

14 Katchman EA, Milo G, Paul M, Christiaens T, Baerheim A, Leibovici L. Three-day vs longer duration of antibiotic treatment for cystitis in women: systematic review and meta-analysis. Am J Med. 2005;118(11):1196–207.

15 Patel SS, Balfour JA, Bryson HM. Fosfomycin tromethamine. A review of its antibacterial activity, pharmacokinetic properties and therapeutic efficacy as a single-dose oral treatment for acute uncomplicated lower urinary tract infections. Drugs. 1997;53(4):637–56.

16 Gupta K, Hooton TM, Roberts PL, Stamm WE. Short-course nitrofurantoin for the treatment of acute uncomplicated cystitis in women. Arch Intern Med. 2007;167(20):2207–12.

17 Hooton TM, Winter C, Tiu F, Stamm WE. Randomized comparative trial and cost analysis of 3-day antimicrobial regimens for treatment of acute cystitis in women. JAMA. 1995;273(1):41–5.

18 Hooton TM, Scholes D, Gupta K, Stapleton AE, Roberts PL, Stamm WE. Amoxicillin-clavulanate vs ciprofloxacin for the treatment of uncomplicated cystitis in women: a randomized trial. JAMA. 2005;293(8):949–55.

19 Rafalsky V, Andreeva I, Rjabkova E. Quinolones for uncomplicated acute cystitis in women. Cochrane Database Syst Rev. 2006;(3):CD003597.

20 U.S. Food & Drug Administration (FDA) Drug Safety Communication: FDA updates warnings for oral and injectable fluoroquinolone antibiotics due to disabling side effects: (http://www.fda.gov/Drugs/DrugSafety/ucm511530.htm).

21 Grover ML, Bracamonte JD, Kanodia AK, Bryan MJ, Donahue SP, Warner AM, et al. Assessing adherence to evidence-based guidelines for the diagnosis and management of uncomplicated urinary tract infection. Mayo Clin Proc. 2007;82(2):181–5.

22 Kallen AJ, Welch HG, Sirovich BE. Current antibiotic therapy for isolated urinary tract infections in women. Arch Intern Med. 2006;166(6):635–9.

23 Hooton TM, Besser R, Foxman B, Fritsche TR, Nicolle LE. Acute uncomplicated cystitis in an era of increasing antibiotic resistance: a proposed approach to empirical therapy. Clin Infect Dis. 2004;39(1):75–80.

24 O'Kane DB, Dave SK, Gore N, Patel F, Hoffmann TC, Trill JL, et al. Urinary alkalisation for symptomatic uncomplicated urinary tract infection in women. Cochrane Database Syst Rev. 2016;4:CD010745.

25 Raz R, Chazan B, Kennes Y, Colodner R, Rottensterich E, Dan M, et al. Empiric use of trimethoprim-sulfamethoxazole (TMP-SMX) in the treatment of women with uncomplicated urinary tract infections, in a geographical area with a high prevalence of TMP-SMX-resistant uropathogens. Clin Infect Dis. 2002;34(9):1165–9.

26 McNulty CA, Richards J, Livermore DM, Little P, Charlett A, Freeman E, et al. Clinical relevance of laboratory-reported antibiotic resistance in acute uncomplicated urinary tract infection in primary care. J Antimicrob Chemother. 2006;58(5):1000–8.

27 Stamm WE, Raz R. Factors contributing to susceptibility of postmenopausal women to recurrent urinary tract infections. Clin Infect Dis. 1999;28(4):723–5.

28 Hooton TM, Scholes D, Stapleton AE, Roberts PL, Winter C, Gupta K, et al. A prospective study of asymptomatic bacteriuria in sexually active young women. N Engl J Med. 2000;343(14):992–7.

29 Trautner BW. Asymptomatic bacteriuria: when the treatment is worse than the disease. Nat Rev Urol. 2011;9(2):85–93.

30 Cai T, Nesi G, Mazzoli S, Meacci F, Lanzafame P, Caciagli P, et al. Asymptomatic bacteriuria treatment is associated with a higher prevalence of antibiotic resistant strains in women with urinary tract infections. Clin Infect Dis. 2015;61(11):1655–61.

31 Smaill FM, Vazquez JC. Antibiotics for asymptomatic bacteriuria in pregnancy. Cochrane Database Syst Rev. 2015(8):CD000490.

32 Kazemier BM, Koningstein FN, Schneeberger C, Ott A, Bossuyt PM, de Miranda E, et al. Maternal and neonatal consequences of treated and untreated asymptomatic bacteriuria in pregnancy: a prospective cohort study with an embedded randomised controlled trial. Lancet Infect Dis. 2015;15(11):1324–33.

33 Kartal ED, Yenilmez A, Kiremitci A, Meric H, Kale M, Usluer G. Effectiveness of ciprofloxacin prophylaxis in preventing bacteriuria caused by urodynamic study: a blind, randomized study of 192 patients. Urology. 2006;67(6):1149–53.

34 Ikaheimo R, Siitonen A, Heiskanen T, Karkkainen U, Kuosmanen P, Lipponen P, et al. Recurrence of urinary tract infection in a primary care setting: analysis of a 1-year follow-up of 179 women. Clin Infect Dis. 1996;22(1):91–9.

35 Kontiokari T, Sundqvist K, Nuutinen M, Pokka T, Koskela M, Uhari M. Randomised trial of cranberry-lingonberry juice and Lactobacillus GG drink for the prevention of urinary tract infections in women. BMJ. 2001;322(7302):1571.

36 Jepson RG, Williams G, Craig JC. Cranberries for preventing urinary tract infections. Cochrane Database Syst Rev. 2012;10:CD001321.

37 Juthani-Mehta M, Van Ness PH, Bianco L, Rink A, Rubeck S, Ginter S, et al. Effect of cranberry capsules on bacteriuria plus pyuria among older women in nursing homes: a randomized clinical trial. JAMA. 2016;316(18):1879–87.

38 Raz R, Stamm WE. A controlled trial of intravaginal estriol in postmenopausal women with recurrent urinary tract infections. N Engl J Med. 1993;329(11):753–6.

39 Fowler JE, Jr., Pulaski ET. Excretory urography, cystography, and cystoscopy in the evaluation of women with urinary-tract infection: a prospective study. N Engl J Med. 1981;304(8):462–5.

40 Nicolle LE. Prophylaxis: recurrent urinary tract infection in women. Infection. 1992;20 Suppl 3:S203–5; discussion S6–10.

41 Stapleton A, Latham RH, Johnson C, Stamm WE. Postcoital antimicrobial prophylaxis for recurrent urinary tract infection. A randomized, double-blind,

placebo-controlled trial. JAMA. 1990;264(6):703–6.

42 Chew LD, Fihn SD. Recurrent cystitis in nonpregnant women. West J Med. 1999;170(5):274–7.

43 Gupta K, Hooton TM, Roberts PL, Stamm WE. Patient-initiated treatment of uncomplicated recurrent urinary tract infections in young women. Ann Intern Med. 2001;135(1):9–16.

44 Rudenko N, Dorofeyev A. Prevention of recurrent lower urinary tract infections by long-term administration of fosfomycin trometamol. Double blind, randomized, parallel group, placebo controlled study. Arzneimittelforschung. 2005;55(7):420–7.

45 Schwenger EM, Tejani AM, Loewen PS. Probiotics for preventing urinary tract infections in adults and children. Cochrane Database Syst Rev. 2015;12):CD008772.

46 Vickrey BG, Shekelle P, Morton S, Clark K, Pathak M, Kamberg C. Prevention and management of urinary tract infections in paralyzed persons. Evid Rep Technol Assess (Summ). 1999(6):1–3.

47 Darouiche RO, Thornby JI, Cerra-Stewart C, Donovan WH, Hull RA. Bacterial interference for prevention of urinary tract infection: a prospective, randomized, placebo-controlled, double-blind pilot trial. Clin Infect Dis. 2005;41(10):1531–4.

48 Lipsky BA. Prostatitis and urinary tract infection in men: what's new; what's true? Am J Med. 1999;106(3):327–34.

49 Lipsky BA, Ireton RC, Fihn SD, Hackett R, Berger RE. Diagnosis of bacteriuria in men: specimen collection and culture interpretation. J Infect Dis. 1987;155(5):847–54.

50 Nicolle LE. Asymptomatic bacteriuria: when to screen and when to treat. Infect Dis Clin North Am. 2003;17(2):367–94.

51 Ulleryd P, Zackrisson B, Aus G, Bergdahl S, Hugosson J, Sandberg T. Selective urological evaluation in men with febrile urinary tract infection. BJU Int. 2001;88(1):15–20.

52 Andrews SJ, Brooks PT, Hanbury DC, King CM, Prendergast CM, Boustead GB, et al. Ultrasonography and abdominal radiography versus intravenous urography in investigation of urinary tract infection in men: prospective incident cohort study. BMJ. 2002;324(7335):454–6.

53 Russell DB, Roth NJ. Urinary tract infections in men in a primary care population. Aust Fam Physician. 2001;30(2):177–9.

54 Nickel JC, Downey J, Hunter D, Clark J. Prevalence of prostatitis-like symptoms in a population based study using the National Institutes of Health chronic prostatitis symptom index. J Urol. 2001;165(3):842–5.

55 Cornia PB, Takahashi TA, Lipsky BA. The microbiology of bacteriuria in men: a 5-year study at a Veterans' Affairs hospital. Diagn Microbiol Infect Dis. 2006;56(1):25–30.

56 Ulleryd P, Lincoln K, Scheutz F, Sandberg T. Virulence characteristics of Escherichia coli in relation to host response in men with symptomatic urinary tract infection. Clin Infect Dis. 1994;18(4):579–84.

57 Smith JW, Jones SR, Reed WP, Tice AD, Deupree RH, Kaijser B. Recurrent urinary tract infections in men. Characteristics and response to therapy. Ann Intern Med. 1979;91(4):544–8.

58 Gleckman R, Crowley M, Natsios GA. Therapy of recurrent invasive urinary-tract infections of men. N Engl J Med. 1979;301(16):878–80.

59 Drekonja DM, Rector TS, Cutting A, Johnson JR. Urinary tract infection in male veterans: treatment patterns and outcomes. JAMA Intern Med. 2013;173(1):62–8.

60 Sabbaj J, Hoagland VL, Cook T. Norfloxacin versus co-trimoxazole in the treatment of recurring urinary tract infections in men. Scand J Infect Dis Suppl. 1986;48:48–53.

61 Allais JM, Preheim LC, Cuevas TA, Roccaforte JS, Mellencamp MA, Bittner MJ. Randomized, double-blind comparison of ciprofloxacin and trimethoprim-

sulfamethoxazole for complicated urinary tract infections. Antimicrob Agents Chemother. 1988;32(9):1327–30.

62 Weidner W, Ludwig M, Brahler E, Schiefer HG. Outcome of antibiotic therapy with ciprofloxacin in chronic bacterial prostatitis. Drugs. 1999;58 Suppl 2: 103–6.

63 Ulleryd P, Sandberg T. Ciprofloxacin for 2 or 4 weeks in the treatment of febrile urinary tract infection in men: a randomized trial with a 1 year follow-up. Scand J Infect Dis. 2003;35(1):34–9.

64 Nickel JC, Downey J, Clark J, Casey RW, Pommerville PJ, Barkin J, et al. Levofloxacin for chronic prostatitis/chronic pelvic pain syndrome in men: a randomized placebo-controlled multicenter trial. Urology. 2003;62(4):614–7.

65 Alexander RB, Propert KJ, Schaeffer AJ, Landis JR, Nickel JC, O'Leary MP, et al. Ciprofloxacin or tamsulosin in men with chronic prostatitis/chronic pelvic pain syndrome: a randomized, double-blind trial. Ann Intern Med. 2004;141(8):581–9.

66 Scholes D, Hooton TM, Roberts PL, Gupta K, Stapleton AE, Stamm WE. Risk factors associated with acute pyelonephritis in healthy women. Ann Intern Med. 2005;142(1):20–7.

67 Stamm WE. Measurement of pyuria and its relation to bacteriuria. Am J Med. 1983;75(1B):53–8.

68 Tambyah PA, Maki DG. The relationship between pyuria and infection in patients with indwelling urinary catheters: a prospective study of 761 patients. Arch Intern Med. 2000;160(5):673–7.

69 Patel HD, Livsey SA, Swann RA, Bukhari SS. Can urine dipstick testing for urinary tract infection at point of care reduce laboratory workload? J Clin Pathol. 2005;58(9):951–4.

70 McMurray BR, Wrenn KD, Wright SW. Usefulness of blood cultures in pyelonephritis. Am J Emerg Med. 1997;15(2):137–40.

71 Thanassi M. Utility of urine and blood cultures in pyelonephritis. Acad Emerg Med. 1997;4(8):797–800.

72 Grover SA, Komaroff AL, Weisberg M, Cook EF, Goldman L. The characteristics and hospital course of patients admitted for presumed acute pyelonephritis. J Gen Intern Med. 1987;2(1):5–10.

73 Smith WR, McClish DK, Poses RM, Pinson AG, Miller ST, Bobo-Moseley L, et al. Bacteremia in young urban women admitted with pyelonephritis. Am J Med Sci. 1997;313(1):50–7.

74 Wing DA, Park AS, Debuque L, Millar LK. Limited clinical utility of blood and urine cultures in the treatment of acute pyelonephritis during pregnancy. Am J Obstet Gynecol. 2000;182(6):1437–40.

75 Hsu CY, Fang HC, Chou KJ, Chen CL, Lee PT, Chung HM. The clinical impact of bacteremia in complicated acute pyelonephritis. Am J Med Sci. 2006;332(4):175–80.

76 Chen Y, Nitzan O, Saliba W, Chazan B, Colodner R, Raz R. Are blood cultures necessary in the management of women with complicated pyelonephritis? J Infect. 2006;53(4):235–40.

77 Mombelli G, Pezzoli R, Pinoja-Lutz G, Monotti R, Marone C, Franciolli M. Oral vs intravenous ciprofloxacin in the initial empirical management of severe pyelonephritis or complicated urinary tract infections: a prospective randomized clinical trial. Arch Intern Med. 1999;159(1):53–8.

78 Pinson AG, Philbrick JT, Lindbeck GH, Schorling JB. ED management of acute pyelonephritis in women: a cohort study. Am J Emerg Med. 1994;12(3): 271–8.

79 Czaja CA, Scholes D, Hooton TM, Stamm WE. Population-based epidemiologic analysis of acute pyelonephritis. Clin Infect Dis. 2007;45(3):273–80.

80 Johnson JR, Owens K, Gajewski A, Kuskowski MA. Bacterial characteristics in relation to clinical source of Escherichia coli isolates from women with acute cystitis

or pyelonephritis and uninfected women. J Clin Microbiol. 2005;43(12):6064–72.

81 Sandberg T, Skoog G, Hermansson AB, Kahlmeter G, Kuylenstierna N, Lannergard A, et al. Ciprofloxacin for 7 days versus 14 days in women with acute pyelonephritis: a randomised, open-label and double-blind, placebo-controlled, non-inferiority trial. Lancet. 2012;380(9840):484–90.

82 Drusano GL, Ambrose PG, Bhavnani SM, Bertino JS, Nafziger AN, Louie A. Back to the future: using aminoglycosides again and how to dose them optimally. Clin Infect Dis. 2007;45(6):753–60.

83 Naber KG, Savov O, Salmen HC. Piperacillin 2 g/tazobactam 0.5 g is as effective as imipenem 0.5 g/cilastatin 0.5 g for the treatment of acute uncomplicated pyelonephritis and complicated urinary tract infections. Int J Antimicrob Agents. 2002;19(2):95–103.

84 Cronberg S, Banke S, Bergman B, Boman H, Eilard T, Elbel E, et al. Fewer bacterial relapses after oral treatment with norfloxacin than with ceftibuten in acute pyelonephritis initially treated with intravenous cefuroxime. Scand J Infect Dis. 2001;33(5):339–43.

85 Dow G, Rao P, Harding G, Brunka J, Kennedy J, Alfa M, et al. A prospective, randomized trial of 3 or 14 days of ciprofloxacin treatment for acute urinary tract infection in patients with spinal cord injury. Clin Infect Dis. 2004;39(5):658–64.

86 Walker E, Lyman A, Gupta K, Mahoney MV, Snyder GM, Hirsch EB. Clinical management of an increasing threat: outpatient urinary yract infections due to multidrug-resistant uropathogens. Clin Infect Dis. 2016;63(7):960–5.

87 Gupta K, Scholes D, Stamm WE. Increasing prevalence of antimicrobial resistance among uropathogens causing acute uncomplicated cystitis in women. JAMA. 1999;281(8):736–8.

88 Gupta K, Hooton TM, Stamm WE. Increasing antimicrobial resistance and the management of uncomplicated community-acquired urinary tract infections. Ann Intern Med. 2001;135(1):41–50.

89 Sanchez GV, Master RN, Karlowsky JA, Bordon JM. In vitro antimicrobial resistance of urinary Escherichia coli isolates among U.S. outpatients from 2000 to 2010. Antimicrob Agents Chemother. 2012;56(4):2181–3.

90 Sanchez GV, Babiker A, Master RN, Luu T, Mathur A, Bordon J. Antibiotic resistance among urinary isolates from female outpatients in the United States in 2003 and 2012. Antimicrob Agents Chemother. 2016;60(5):2680–3.

91 Calbo E, Romani V, Xercavins M, Gomez L, Vidal CG, Quintana S, et al. Risk factors for community-onset urinary tract infections due to Escherichia coli harbouring extended-spectrum beta-lactamases. J Antimicrob Chemother. 2006;57(4):780–3.

92 Behr MA, Drummond R, Libman MD, Delaney JS, Dylewski JS. Fever duration in hospitalized acute pyelonephritis patients. Am J Med. 1996;101(3):277–80.

Chapter 11

Sexually Transmitted Infections

Courtney A. Thompson, Darrell H. S. Tan, and Kaede Sullivan

Case Presentation 1

A 17-year-old girl presents to the city sexual health clinic with vaginal discharge. She has a new boyfriend and is "on the pill"; she and her partner do not use condoms as their relationship "is monogamous." On examination, she has mild lower abdominal tenderness to palpation, cervicitis, and cervical discharge. There is cervical motion tenderness and left adnexal tenderness on bimanual examination. Her 17-year-old boyfriend has accompanied her to the clinic and is assessed separately; he reports a small amount of urethral discharge and mild dysuria. Examination reveals copious urethral discharge with meatal edema. A Gram stain of the discharge reveals Gram-negative intracellular diplococci.

- How accurate is the clinical diagnosis of sexually transmitted infections (STI)?
- Do laboratory test results change the range of diagnostic possibilities in an individual with a possible STI?
- How helpful are historical and clinical findings in the diagnosis of pelvic inflammatory disease?

Sexually transmitted infections (STI) are caused by a large and heterogeneous group of pathogens. Many can be transmitted by both nonsexual and sexual routes; for example,

enteric pathogens can be transmitted through food and water as well as via sexual intercourse. This chapter focuses on infectious agents that are principally transmitted via sexual contact, although the general principles described in later sections can be applied to the larger group of STIs. Human immunodeficiency virus (HIV) infection is discussed in Chapter 12.

A notable feature of STIs is their high incidence and prevalence (notwithstanding likely under-diagnosis). *Chlamydia trachomatis* infection is the most common reportable infectious disease in the United States and Canada [1,2]. Approximately 15.7% of adults in the United States have serologic evidence of herpes simplex virus type 2 (HSV-2) infection [3]. Transient human papillomavirus (HPV) infection is acquired through sexual activity by 33–55% of young adults in the United States and Europe [4–6]. Worldwide, there were an estimated 131 million new cases of chlamydia (100–166 million), 78 million of gonorrhoea (53–110 million), 143 million of trichomoniasis (98–202 million), and 6 million of syphilis (4–8 million) in 2012 [7].

STIs are also associated with significant morbidity as well as large economic costs.

Genital chlamydia infection is associated with tubal infertility [8], ectopic pregnancies [9], and chronic pelvic pain [10,11]. Certain HPV genotypes (most notably 16 and 18 as well as

Evidence-Based Infectious Diseases, Third Edition. Edited by Dominik Mertz, Fiona Smaill, and Nick Daneman.
© 2018 John Wiley & Sons Ltd. Published 2018 by John Wiley & Sons Ltd.

31, 33, 35, 39, 45, 51, 52, 56, 58, 59, and 68) are strongly associated with cervical and anal cancers [12,13]. Infection of pregnant women with sexually transmitted pathogens may increase the risk of premature delivery and may cause severe illness in the newborn [14–17].

The burden of disease associated with these infections is further augmented by the synergistic relationship between STI and HIV infection, owing to physical disruption of host mucosa, recruitment of immunologically active cells to the genital tract, and increases in HIV viral burden in genital secretions. A meta-analysis of observational studies estimated the relative risk of HIV acquisition in the context of another STI to be 3.7 (95% CI 2.7–5.0) [18].

This chapter reviews the evidence for the clinical and microbiologic diagnosis and syndromic management (i.e., the use of more broadly targeted therapy in response to a clinical constellation of symptoms or signs) of these infections. Evidence related to the interaction between contraceptive choice and STI is also reviewed. The second part of the chapter focuses on empiric and targeted management of STI, including some issues related to management in pregnancy. Finally, evidence of effectiveness for population-based STI prevention strategies is discussed.

11.1 Diagnosis of STI

11.1.1 Clinical and Syndromic Diagnosis

Sexually transmitted pathogens cause several common syndromes. Infection with *Neisseria gonorrhoeae*, *Chlamydia trachomatis*, and *Mycoplasma genitalium* frequently results in urethritis, cervicitis, or pelvic inflammatory disease, while vaginal discharge is commonly caused by infection with *Trichomonas vaginalis*, *Candida* species, or by bacterial vaginosis. HSV, *Treponema pallidum*, and *Haemophilus ducreyi* are common agents of ulcerative genital disease.

Although specific sexually transmitted causes of urethritis, cervicitis, and vaginitis are challenging to diagnose clinically, empiric management can be initiated based on a syndromic approach. The World Health Organization (WHO) developed syndromic algorithms for the management of STI in 2003 [19]. In a meta-analysis evaluating the algorithm for vaginal discharge [20], flowcharts limited to basic history and risk assessment alone yielded poor sensitivity (27.4%), but moderate specificity (84.9%) for identifying cervicitis caused by *N. gonorrhoeae* or *C. trachomatis*, compared with improved sensitivity (90.1%), but reduced specificity (35.5%) with the addition of speculum exam and basic laboratory investigations, such as Gram stain [21]. The poor diagnostic performance of these algorithms resulted in frequent over or under-treatment [21]. However, meta-analysis assessment of the WHO algorithm for vaginitis caused by trichomoniasis or bacterial vaginosis demonstrated improved diagnostic yield compared with that for cervicitis. Algorithms including history and risk assessment with speculum examination and vaginal discharge microscopy resulted in 91.7% sensitivity, 99.9% specificity, 99.9% positive predictive value (PPV), and only 0.02% missed treatments [19]. There are no randomized controlled trials (RCTs) assessing the clinical diagnosis of pelvic inflammatory disease (PID). A Swedish cohort study found three clinical and laboratory features: erythrocyte sedimentation rate (ESR), fever, and adnexal tenderness to identify 65% of cases compared to laparoscopy [22].

Sexually transmitted causes of genital ulcer disease (GUD) can be categorized according to the presence of tenderness, the number of lesions, and ulcer characteristics, although clinicians' ability to accurately identify causative organisms based on these features is limited [23]. Genital herpes, caused by herpes simplex virus types 1 and 2 (HSV-1 and HSV-2) typically presents as multiple vesicles on an erythematous base, and is the most common cause of painful ulcers in industrialized world settings. Chancroid, caused by *Haemophilus ducreyi*, typically causes purulent, moderately tender ulcers with an undermined border. The primary chancre of syphilis is typically a solitary, painless, indurated but non-purulent ulcer, teeming with *Treponema pallidum* spirochetes. The primary lesion of lymphogranuloma venereum (LGV) is classically a small painless papule, pustule, nodule, or erosion. However, among men who have sex with men (MSM), the most common presentation is acute proctitis, characterized by rectal bleeding, pain, tenesmus, mucoid discharge, and constipation; friable colonic ulcers have also been described. Finally, donovanosis, caused by *Klebsiella granulomatis* usually begins as a papule or nodule that rapidly progresses to a "beefy red" non-tender ulcer.

11.1.2 Asymptomatic Screening

Population-based screening may be useful for preventing both the complications and transmission of STI, but in non-pregnant populations, there is limited evidence to guide policy for most pathogens. An exception is *C. trachomatis*, which would be markedly under-diagnosed if testing were limited to symptomatic individuals, especially in women [24,25]. There is moderate evidence that screening for chlamydia in asymptomatic young women may prevent pelvic inflammatory disease. Three RCTs have assessed this question, but only one study was of good quality and demonstrated a statistically significant benefit of asymptomatic screening versus routine practice (RR 0.44, 95% CI 0.20–0.90) [26]. Although routine screening of heterosexual men is not currently recommended, mathematical models that account for transmissibility do suggest that including males in screening programs would likely provide additional gains in women's health at reasonable cost [24]. Asymptomatic screening likely has the greatest yield in specific populations, such as MSM and pregnant women. Evidence for

routine screening of STI in MSM is limited, but is recommended based on the higher rates of disease in this population [2].

11.1.3 Laboratory Testing

11.1.3.1 *Neisseria gonorrhoeae* and *Chlamydia trachomatis*

In experienced hands, the use of urethral Gram stain for the identification of Gram-negative diplococci appears very sensitive and specific for the detection of *N. gonorrhoeae* in men [27]. It can be performed on-site in STI clinic settings, and facilitates rapid diagnosis and treatment in high-risk patients.

For definitive diagnosis, culture was long considered the gold standard test for both *N. gonorrhoeae* and *C. trachomatis*. However, the sensitivity of *N. gonorrhoeae* culture is low in genital specimens compared to nucleic acid amplification tests (NAAT) [28]. The poor sensitivity is largely due to loss of organism viability associated with transport delay [29]. However, due to emerging multidrug resistance in *N. gonorrhoeae*, culture of this organism, which is required for antimicrobial susceptibility testing, remains a valuable technique for surveillance and management of refractory cases. Sensitivity of *C. trachomatis* culture is equally poor and is labor-intensive as it requires a live cell culture. As a consequence, it is rarely performed outside of reference laboratories [30].

Due to the poor sensitivity of culture, NAATs have largely supplanted culture in the diagnosis of *N. gonorrhoeae* and *C. trachomatis*. Commonly used NAAT technologies include polymerase chain reaction (PCR), strand displacement amplification (SDA), and transmission-mediated amplification (TMA). NAATs have greatly improved detection of these pathogens in specimens acquired from the cervix, male urethra, and in male urine specimens. Female urine specimens have demonstrated variable sensitivity for both pathogens, but urine sampling is advantageous as it avoids discomfort associated with speculum examination. Additionally, NAATs performed on self-collected vaginal swab samples have been associated with satisfactory performance and may provide opportunities to increase screening uptake through home-, mail-, or Internet-based screening procedures. Although not FDA-approved, NAATs have also shown superior performance in samples collected from extra-genital sites such as the pharynx and rectum, and can be used following laboratory validation [28].

Lymphogranuloma venereum is a possible diagnosis when proctocolitis or unilateral inguinal or femoral lymphadenopathy is accompanied by a positive test for *C. trachomatis*. Genotyping using PCR and sequencing procedures is necessary to determine if a *C. trachomatis* serovar related to LGV (L1, L2, or L3) is present, and is available in various reference laboratories.

11.1.3.2 *Trichomonas Vaginalis*

Trichomonas vaginalis is a unicellular flagellated organism that causes vaginitis in women and urethritis in men. The wet mount is a test in which motile trichomonads are visualized from urethral or vaginal specimens under a microscope. While rapid and convenient, sensitivity may be <50% [5]. Culture can improve sensitivity but requires incubation and daily microscopy for up to seven days. Culture using special media has lower sensitivity than NAAT, but the exact sensitivity can vary depending on the gold standard definition used [31]. Available NAAT technologies for detection of *Trichomonas vaginalis* include polymerase chain reaction (PCR), and transmission-mediated amplification (TMA) and assays are now available for vaginal, endocervical, and urine samples in females and urine in males.

11.1.3.3 Chancroid

Direct Gram staining of purulent material from the ulcer base may reveal the characteristic "school of fish" or "railroad" arrangement of short, Gram-negative bacilli seen in chancroid. However, these can be difficult to visualize due to the presence of other organisms in a frequently polymicrobial setting [32]. Compared to PCR, *H. ducreyi* culture has a sensitivity of approximately 75% [33]. Because it does not grow readily on standard bacterial media, *H. ducreyi* culture is rarely performed outside of reference laboratories. The use of NAATs for the identification of *H. ducreyi* has improved sensitivity considerably [33]. These assays are not widely available, however, requiring laboratories to develop their own "laboratory-developed test" (LDT).

11.1.3.4 Herpes Simplex Virus

Viral culture, antigen tests, NAAT, and antibody tests are options for detecting HSV-1 and HSV-2. The sensitivity of visualizing multinucleated giant cells using a Tzanck smear is about 50% and is not considered an ideal detection method [34].

The gold standard test for diagnosis of genital herpes has traditionally been viral culture from genital lesions. However, viral culture is insensitive compared to NAAT, and requires considerable technician labor and skill to perform correctly. In addition, studies using PCR as the gold standard have shown that viral culture has lower sensitivity [35,36]. Currently, a number of highly sensitive molecular assays are available commercially for the detection of HSV-1 and HSV-2 from genital specimens and have been comprehensively reviewed elsewhere [37]. A PCR assay designed for use in cerebrospinal fluid in a rapid platform is commercially available, and may facilitate diagnosis of HSV meningitis and encephalitis [38].

11.1.3.5 Syphilis

Primary syphilis can be diagnosed by visualization of motile spirochetes from ulcer exudate using dark-field microscopy. However, this method requires both technical competence and experience, and has become rare in many settings.

Today, serologic testing is the mainstay of syphilis diagnosis in adults. These tests can be classified into two groups: non-treponemal tests and treponemal tests. Non-treponemal tests are based on reactivity of patient serum to antigen composed of cardiolipin, cholesterol, and lecithin. Examples include the rapid plasma reagin (RPR) and the Venereal Disease Research Laboratory (VDRL) tests. RPR is rapid and inexpensive, and was therefore used widely for syphilis screening despite lower sensitivity and specificity compared to the treponemal tests. Non-treponemal tests are less than 90% sensitive in primary syphilis. Sensitivity is higher in secondary and early latent syphilis. A small proportion of individuals with syphilis have a negative non-treponemal test for syphilis due to the "prozone" phenomenon, which occurs when extremely high titers of antibody disrupt the assay. This results in a false-negative test result, which becomes positive on dilution [39]. Non-treponemal tests revert to negative over time in approximately 30% of untreated individuals [40]. In addition, reports of falsely positive non-treponemal tests in the presence of other infectious diseases, rheumatologic diseases, and pregnancy are common [41].

By contrast, treponemal tests that identify antibodies directed against *Treponema* species components are highly specific, and are traditionally used for confirmation of positive non-treponemal tests. Examples include fluorescent treponemal antibody (FTA), *Treponema pallidum* particle agglutination (TP-PA), and enzyme immunoassay (EIA). When a rapid, automated, high throughput EIA assay became available, a reverse algorithm became widely used. Here, EIA is used first for screening, and when positive, RPR titers (1:2, 1:4, etc.) are used to assess disease stage and response to treatment. Because EIA is more sensitive than RPR, EIA-positive, RPR-negative cases emerged, causing concern about whether this represented latent disease or false positive EIA results. In the late 1990s, the Centers for Disease Control and Prevention (CDC) intervened and recommended that these cases undergo further confirmatory testing

by performing TP-PA and be accompanied by a detailed clinical and epidemiologic history as well as physical examination [42].

The diagnosis of neurosyphilis is challenging. While VDRL testing of cerebrospinal fluid (CSF) is well documented, the sensitivity of this test is poor. In a retrospective study performed in 38 individuals with positive CSF FTA-Abs (a test thought to be sensitive but non-specific for neurosyphilis), 15 had likely neurosyphilis on the basis of a compatible clinical history and other CSF abnormalities (e.g., leukocytosis or elevated protein), but only four of these 15 had a positive CSF VDRL (sensitivity 27%) [43].

Existing evidence does not support the routine use of PCR for the diagnosis of neurosyphilis in adults, and published studies have yielded poor sensitivity, particularly in non-primary disease [44].

11.1.3.6 *Mycoplasma genitalium*

M. genitalium is a slow-growing, fastidious organism that is very difficult to grow in culture [45]. As a result, NAAT is preferred for detecting this pathogen in urethral and endocervical specimens, although there are currently no commercially available tests routinely available. LDTs have been validated and are offered at various reference laboratories in North America.

11.1.3.7 Donovanosis

K. granulomatis is an obligate intracellular Gram-negative organism that typically resides within monocytes. Typically, diagnosis relies on Giemsa stains of biopsies or swabs from an ulcer surface showing large mononuclear cells containing deeply staining "Donovan bodies," some within intracytoplasmic cysts. PCR is not widely available [46].

11.1.4 Point-of-care Testing

Point-of-care (POC) tests allow rapid diagnosis outside of the laboratory with greater proximity to patient encounters. POC testing can be performed in medical clinics, emergency departments, urgent care facilities, or in some cases, at home. The goal of POC testing is to expedite diagnosis and treatment, and ideally limit the transmission and complications of STI.

POC tests have been described for detection of *C. trachomatis*, *N. gonorrhoeae*, *T. vaginalis*, *syphilis*, and HIV. Analysis of the myriad of assays currently in use globally is beyond the scope of this chapter. Overall, sensitivity is highly variable, and their impact on patient outcomes needs further research. Depending on the assay and the setting, cost and personnel requirements may be prohibitive [47]. Implementation of POC testing requires specialized training of clinical staff and adequate quality control measures.

11.2 Management of Sexually Transmitted Infections

Case Presentation 1 (continued)

The male teenager described above is treated syndromically for urethritis with 1 g of oral azithromycin, and 250 mg IM ceftriaxone. Because of the presence of abdominal discomfort, adnexal tenderness, and cervical motion tenderness, his female partner is treated for PID. Despite some uncertainty about her adherence, the treating physician manages her as an outpatient, with a two-week course of oral metronidazole and levofloxacin. Subsequent laboratory testing shows both to be infected with both *C. trachomatis* and *N. gonorrhoeae*.

- How effective is syndromic management of STI?
- How effective is directed treatment of STI?
- Does treatment of sexual partners reduce the risk of relapse or reinfection?
- Can behavioral interventions modify the future risk of sexually transmitted infection?

As previously discussed, the syndromic diagnosis of STI is substantially less accurate than laboratory-based diagnosis. Nonetheless, evidence exists to support management based on syndromic diagnoses, as this approach results in receipt of treatment by most infected individuals, and eliminates concerns related to non-treatment as a result of loss to follow-up.

11.2.1 *Neisseria gonorrhoeae*

A variety of drug regimens for the treatment of uncomplicated gonococcal urethritis and cervicitis have been assessed by RCTs, but the efficacy of many drugs has been compromised by the emergence of widespread antibiotic resistance in *N. gonorrhoeae*.

Although early RCTs of fluoroquinolones demonstrated good efficacy as single-dose therapy for uncomplicated gonococcal infections, emerging resistance has precluded their use in many regions [48]. The U.S. Centers for Disease Control and Prevention (CDC) issued an advisory in 2006 against empiric fluoroquinolone use for treatment of *N. gonorrhoeae* infection [49]. There is strong evidence linking in vitro resistance to fluoroquinolones to clinical treatment failure [50].

Treatment failure with use of oral cephalosporins emerged worldwide, prompting the CDC to issue updated guidelines, and currently, empiric treatment with dual therapy of intramuscular ceftriaxone plus oral azithromycin is recommended [51].

Because of the dynamic nature of antimicrobial resistance in *N. gonorrhoeae*, clinicians should remain abreast of changes in antimicrobial resistance patterns; in North America, an excellent resource in this regard is the Gonorrhea Isolate Surveillance Project (GISP) (http://www.cdc.gov/std/GISP/default.htm).

11.2.2 *Chlamydia trachomatis* Infections and Other Causes of Non-Gonococcal Urethritis or Cervicitis

The past three decades have seen an evolution in the understanding of so-called non-gonococcal urethritis, post-gonococcal urethritis, and mucopurulent cervicitis, with increasing recognition that these syndromes are most commonly caused by *C. trachomatis*. As such, early data on the treatment of chlamydial infections are derived from studies that did not explicitly identify this pathogen, or that grouped chlamydial infections with those caused by other non-gonococcal organisms.

The efficacy of tetracyclines in the treatment of chlamydial infections has been demonstrated in several RCTs. Minocycline (100 mg twice daily), doxycycline (100 mg twice daily), and tetracycline (250 mg four times daily) had equal efficacy in the treatment of non-gonococcal urethritis and mucopurulent cervicitis [52].

Macrolides are recommended as a valuable alternative to tetracyclines for the treatment of chlamydial infections, and the development of azithromycin has had a dramatic impact. An earlier systematic review and meta-analysis of 12 RCTs comparing azithromycin and doxycycline for the treatment of urethritis or cervicitis found no difference in microbiologic cure, or in the incidence of adverse drug events with efficacy of 97% and 98%, respectively [53]. More recently, concern has been raised for reduced efficacy of azithromycin in several randomized-controlled studies. A trial in the Los Angeles correctional system compared azithromycin (single dose 1 g) versus doxycycline (100 mg twice daily for 7 days) with direct-observed therapy (DOT) and microbiologic cure testing at 28 days. Overall efficacy was 97% for azithromycin and 100% for doxycycline, and did not demonstrate non-inferiority of azithromycin [54]. However, these results may not translate to routine practice where DOT is impractical. A double-blinded superiority trial of men comparing azithromycin to doxycycline demonstrated increased microbiological failure for *C. trachomatis* in men self-reporting suboptimal adherence (absolute RR 9.33, 95% CI 1.00–89.2) [55].

Fluoroquinolones have had variable efficacy in the treatment of chlamydial infections, and are alternative second-line treatment options. Two randomized trials comparing ciprofloxacin (750–1000 mg twice daily) to doxycycline found reduced eradication of chlamydia with ciprofloxacin (46–62%) compared to doxycycline (75–100%) [56,57]. In contrast, one week of ofloxacin at a dose of 300–400 mg twice daily appears to be equivalent to doxycycline, with both drugs reported to eradicate chlamydial infections in 97–100% of individuals with urethritis or cervicitis [58].

Untreated lower genital tract chlamydial infection is associated with adverse pregnancy outcomes, such as prematurity, low birth-weight, stillbirth, and postpartum endometritis [59,60]. A meta-analysis of trials comparing amoxicillin and erythromycin found the two drugs to have similar efficacy, although amoxicillin was associated with fewer adverse effects [61]. With increasing comfort related to the use of azithromycin in pregnancy, randomized trials have shown azithromycin to have equivalent efficacy but reduced adverse events compared to amoxicillin [62,63].

Although historically *M. genitalium* was not considered to be an independent cause of non-gonococcal urethritis and cervicitis, increasing evidence supports a role of *M. genitalium* in these infections. In a meta-analysis of 29 studies, *M. genitalium* was significantly associated with non-gonococcal and non-chlamydial urethritis in men (pooled OR 7.6, 95% CI 5.5–10.5]) with a prevalence of *M. genitalium* of about 10–35% [64]. In women, a meta-analysis showed *M. genitalium* was associated, albeit less strongly, with cervicitis (pooled OR 1.66, 95% CI 1.4–2.0) and PID (pooled OR 2.14, 95% CI 1.3–3.5) [65].

Unfortunately, *M. genitalium* is prone to the development of antimicrobial resistance and the only current agents with activity are tetracyclines, macrolides, and fluoroquinolones. Azithromycin has repeatedly demonstrated greater efficacy, but recent evidence suggests this is declining. Two small RCTs comparing azithromycin with doxycycline found *M. genitalium* clearance rates of 87% versus 45% ($p = 0.002$) [66], and 67% versus 31% ($p = 0.002$) [67], respectively. A more robust double-dummy RCT comparing these agents in 606 men found no significant difference in microbiological cure rates, but reduced efficacy of treatment overall [68]. Moxifloxacin is an alternative treatment option as demonstrated in a recent meta-analysis, but has declining efficacy for *M. genitalium* infection (100% prior to 2010 and 89% post-2010) [69].

11.2.3 Pelvic Inflammatory Disease (PID)

The agents of urethritis and cervicitis are strongly associated with PID, a syndrome characterized by lower abdominal pain, cervical motion tenderness, and uterine adnexal tenderness. However, while *N. gonorrhoeae*, *C. trachomatis*, or both organisms are identifiable in cervical culture specimens of 70% of individuals with clinically diagnosed PID, this infection is typically polymicrobial. Therapeutic regimens should include agents that are effective against these organisms, gram-negative bacilli and anaerobes. A Cochrane review of 37 RCTs found no increased efficacy of any one antibiotic regimen included in the current CDC guidelines. No difference in rate of cure was found for metronidazole-containing regimens compared to other anaerobic coverage [70].

A key clinical branch point in the management of PID involves determining whether individuals need hospital admission. The PEACH trial evaluated this question by randomizing 831 women to receive either inpatient treatment with intravenous cefoxitin and doxycycline, or outpatient treatment with a single intramuscular injection of cefoxitin and oral doxycycline. No significant differences were seen in short-term cure rates, nor in the development of longer-term sequelae [71].

11.2.4 Trichomoniasis

Metronidazole is recommended for the treatment of vaginal trichomoniasis. RCTs have found no significant difference in efficacy between a single 2 g dose of metronidazole and five- to seven-day courses of the drug dosed at 750–800 mg daily. Both regimens result in parasitologic cure in over 85% of individuals [72,73]. A single 2 g dose of tinidazole is equivalent in efficacy to 2 g of metronidazole for the treatment of vaginal trichomoniasis, and appears to be efficacious in individuals with prior failure of therapy associated with metronidazole-resistant trichomonads [74].

Topical therapies for trichomoniasis are not recommended. A multi-center, open-label RCT comparing single-dose oral metronidazole to intravaginal clotrimazole or sulfanilamide-allantoin-aminacrine hydrochloride suppositories found suppositories were associated with microbiologic failure in over 80% of participants [75].

11.2.5 Syphilis

Treatment recommendations for syphilis are dependent on the stage of infection. The presence of any neurologic, ocular, or otic signs or symptoms warrants a lumbar puncture to rule out neurosyphilis, which can complicate any stage. An area of controversy is whether neurologically asymptomatic HIV-positive patients with syphilis also require CSF examination. Mild CSF abnormalities are common in early stages of syphilis and of unknown clinical significance [76], but neurorelapse (symptomatic neurosyphilis despite prior adequate stage-specific treatment) has been well documented in HIV/syphilis co-infected individuals. A CD4 count ≤ 350 cells/mL and/or an RPR titer $\geq 1:32$ may be risk factors for the presence of CSF abnormalities in HIV/syphilis co-infection [77], but CSF examination has not been associated with improved clinical outcomes in the absence of neurologic symptoms.

Benzathine penicillin and aqueous penicillin G are recommended for the treatment of syphilis [78]. Although earlier studies on which these recommendations are based employed varying dosing regimens and outcome measures, more recently, randomized trials have demonstrated benzathine penicillin to have satisfactory rates of treatment success (generally defined as a ≥ fourfold decline in RPR titer) of 75%–95% depending on the time point assessed [78]. Few data are available on the treatment of late syphilis, with treatment recommendations based primarily on expert opinion. The recommendation that neurosyphilis be treated with 10–14 days of intravenous aqueous penicillin G is based on pharmacokinetic considerations, as treponemicidal drug concentrations are not reliably achieved in the CSF with benzathine penicillin [79].

Treponema pallidum remains universally susceptible to penicillin, with no recorded cases of drug resistance to date. However, alternative regimens are sometimes required for patients who are penicillin-allergic [78]. Small studies have evaluated ceftriaxone for early syphilis at doses of 1–2 g IM daily for 10 to 21 days, and shown response rates generally comparable to long-acting penicillin, but the need for repeated injections with this approach means it is seldom preferred. A 14-day course of doxycycline 100 mg twice daily (or tetracycline 500 mg 4 times daily) also produces response rates similar to benzathine penicillin in early syphilis, but may be limited by adherence challenges. RCTs have shown that azithromycin in a single oral dose of 1–2 g has similar or even better serological response rates compared with benzathine penicillin in early syphilis [80], but due to emerging drug resistance [81], azithromycin is not recommended unless all other therapies are not possible.

Importantly, penicillin remains the drug of choice in penicillin-allergic patients who are pregnant because of concerns about fetal toxicity with doxycycline and the failure of azithromycin to cross the placenta. While ceftriaxone may be a reasonable alternative, the evidence is restricted to case series [82,83].

Case reports published in the era before widespread antiretroviral therapy for HIV infection have raised concerns that HIV-infected individuals are more prone to relapse after syphilis treatment [84]. However, randomized trials have established that neither adding doses of benzathine penicillin [85] nor including additional oral antibiotics [86] is associated with improved serological response rates compared with a single dose of benzathine penicillin in co-infected patients.

Although definitive criteria for treatment success are lacking, response is usually defined as a fourfold decrease in non-treponemal titre. Nevertheless, a systematic review found that roughly 12.1% (interquartile range 4.9–25.6%) of patients will not reach this target, depending on the time point evaluated [87]. Moreover, roughly 20% of patients achieve a "serofast" state, defined as a persistent titer that is unchanged or ≤ twofold decreased [88]. The optimal management of such cases requires greater study. For patients with neurosyphilis, repeat lumbar puncture is advised every six months to ensure normalization of CSF pleocytosis, but normalization of the serum RPR may obviate the need for CSF examination in immunocompetent or antiretroviral-treated HIV-positive patients [89].

Syphilis treatment can be complicated by the Jarisch-Herxheimer reaction, an acute syndrome involving fever, chills, headache, myalgias, and intensification of skin rash within 24 hours of treatment, particularly in primary and secondary infections, in HIV-positive individuals, with RPR titers ≥1:32 and with penicillin therapy (reviewed in [90]). In pregnant women, the reaction can manifest as hemodynamic instability, uterine contractions and complications including preterm labor, prompting some experts to recommend 24 hours of continuous fetal monitoring if treatment is initiated during the second half of pregnancy [51].

11.2.6 Genital Herpes

Genital herpes, caused by both herpes simplex virus type 1 and 2 (HSV-1 or HSV-2), can have a wide range of clinical severity. First episode HSV infections can be classified according to whether pre-existing HSV antibody is present (non-primary infection) or not present (primary infection), with the latter being more severe [91]. In the year after a first clinical episode, recurrences occur in up to 90% of patients with HSV-2, and 20–50% for HSV-1; the median number of these recurrences in the first year is four for HSV-2 and one for HSV-1 [91,92]. This frequency is also greater with genital (as opposed to orolabial) infections, longer primary episodes, and the presence of immunosuppression. The frequency of symptomatic HSV reactivations generally decreases over time, by about 50% in year 2 after primary HSV-1 and by about 50% at years 3–5 after primary HSV-2, although some patients may experience similar or even higher rates of relapse over time [92].

Short courses of oral nucleoside analogues, including acyclovir and the prodrugs valacyclovir and famciclovir, can be used as episodic treatment in either first episodes or symptomatic recurrences of HSV, and reduce both the duration and severity of symptoms. Alternatively, for individuals with frequent HSV recurrences, chronic suppressive therapy with antiviral drugs is associated with 70–80% reductions in recurrences after four months [91], and improved health-related quality of life [93]. Clinical trials and systematic reviews have established the efficacy of a variety of regimens, as summarized in Table 11.1 [51,91,94,95]. Network meta-analysis has not shown the superiority of one oral antiviral drug over another for the prevention of genital herpes recurrences [95]. Of note, studies of topical antivirals for both genital and orolabial herpes have generally either shown no difference in efficacy compared with placebo, or been too poorly conducted to permit meaningful conclusions [94,96]. Despite decades of widespread use of these compounds, resistance rates remain low at <1% in immunocompetent versus 4–7% in immunocompromised populations, particularly those with chronic HSV ulcerations in the context of advanced AIDS [97].

Studies using highly sensitive PCR assays have shown that even in the absence of active herpes lesions, infected individuals exhibit frequent subclinical reactivations of HSV-1 and HSV-2 on mucosal surfaces [92]. This subclinical shedding is felt to be responsible for the vast majority of HSV transmission. Antiviral therapy has thus been studied as a strategy for preventing horizontal transmission. In a clinical trial of 1,484 heterosexual, monogamous, HSV-2 serodiscordant couples, use of valacyclovir 500 mg once daily by the HSV-2 seropositive partner was associated with a reduced probability of clinically symptomatic herpes infection (hazard ratio [HR] 0.25, 95% CI 0.08–0.75) and a reduced likelihood of HSV-2 seroconversion (HR 0.52, 95% CI 0.27–0.99) in the HSV-2 seronegative partner compared to placebo [98].

Table 11.1 Management strategies for genital herpes.

First episode	Recurrent HSV	Chronic suppression
Acyclovir 5 mg/kg iv q8h	Acyclovir 200 mg 5 times daily ×5d	Acyclovir 400 mg twice daily
Acyclovir 200 mg 5 times daily ×5–10d	Acyclovir 800 mg 3 times daily ×2d	Famciclovir 250 mg twice daily
Famciclovir 125–500mg 3 times daily ×5d	Famciclovir 125 mg twice daily ×5d	Valacyclovir 500–1,000 mg once daily
Valacyclovir 500–1,000 mg twice daily ×10d	Famciclovir 1,000 mg twice daily ×1d	
	Valacyclovir 500 mg twice daily ×3–5d	

Given the established safety record of acyclovir, valacyclovir, and famciclovir in pregnancy [99], antiviral therapy may also be used to prevent vertical HSV transmission. The risk of neonatal HSV infection is roughly 30–50% when primary infection occurs in the mother during the third trimester, 2–5% when recurrent vaginal lesions are present at the time of delivery, and roughly 1% for mothers with a history of recurrent genital herpes but only asymptomatic shedding at delivery [17,100,101]. In addition, there is a trend toward reduced transmission in women from whom HSV is isolated at the time of labor who undergo Caesarean delivery (OR 0.14, 95% CI 0.02–1.26) [17]. A systematic review found that acyclovir prophylaxis beginning at 36 weeks' gestation reduces both overall HSV detection at delivery (OR 0.11, 95% CI 0.04–0.31) and Caesarian deliveries for clinical recurrences (OR 0.25, 95% CI 0.15–0.40) [102]. Therefore, women with primary HSV in pregnancy should receive antiviral treatment for first episode infection, and offered Caesarian delivery if infection occurs in the third trimester. Women with recurrent HSV should be offered chronic suppressive therapy beginning at week 36, and any woman with lesions or prodromal symptoms at delivery should be offered Caesarian section.

HSV-2 is also a common co-infection in persons living with HIV, with a seroprevalence of up to 95% [91]. Having HSV-2 increases the risk of both HIV acquisition (RR = 1.7–3.1 depending on the population) [103] and transmission (roughly fourfold) [104], but randomized trials using acyclovir 400 mg twice daily have shown no impact on HIV prevention [105–107]. While meta-analyses suggest that HSV-2 is associated with increased HIV plasma viral load [108], HSV-2 seropositivity does not appear to accelerate HIV disease progression [109].

11.2.7 Chancroid

Clinical trials have established the efficacy of multiple antibiotic regimens for treating chancroid. Currently recommended options have cure rates of 88–100%, and include single-dose options such as azithromycin 1 g PO, ceftriaxone 250 mg IM, or ciprofloxacin 500 mg PO, as well as ciprofloxacin 500 mg PO twice daily for three days and erythromycin 500 mg PO qid for seven days [51]. A single 2 g dose of spectinomycin may be an alternative, but a randomized trial found a lower rate of cure with this regimen compared to erythromycin (48/55 = 87% vs. 61/61 = 100%, $p = 0.004$) [110]. Although penicillins, tetracyclines, and co-trimoxizole have previously been used, these agents are no longer suggested due to a high prevalence of drug resistance [111]. Concerns about intermediate resistance to ciprofloxacin and erythromycin have emerged more recently, but robust surveillance data are lacking.

Chancroid may be complicated by the development of fluctuant inguinal buboes. A small randomized trial compared aspiration to incision and drainage for the management of buboes during a chancroid outbreak in New Orleans [112]. Antimicrobial treatment regimens varied and follow-up was incomplete (85%), but 6/12 versus 0/11 evaluable participants required re-aspiration in the aspiration arm and incision and drainage arm, respectively ($p = 0.02$), suggesting the latter to be a more practical approach.

11.2.8 Lymphogranuloma Venereum

Treatment of LGV requires prolonged courses of antimicrobials that reach high intracellular concentrations, and options have historically included erythromycin, tetracycline, and doxycycline. Comparative trials are needed, but the strongest existing evidence is for doxycycline 100 mg twice daily for 21 days; a 2016 systematic review of nine observational studies found this regimen to have a pooled microbial cure rate of 98.5% (95% CI 96.3%–100%) for rectal LGV in MSM [113]. Azithromycin has also sometimes been used for LGV proctitis, based on its efficacy for non-LGV serovars of

C trachomatis, at a dose of 1g weekly for three weeks; however, the literature supporting this regimen is limited [114]. Moxifloxacin has been used successfully in rare cases of doxycycline failure [115]. In inguinal LGV, aspiration (as opposed to surgical excision) of fluctuant buboes is often recommended for symptomatic relief and to prevent chronic sinus formation [51], but published literature on this approach is lacking.

11.2.9 Donovanosis

Although published data on the management of granuloma inguinale are scant, azithromycin dosed either at 1 g weekly or 500 mg daily has been best studied and is most convenient. Treatment durations may vary, but most guidelines advise at least three weeks or until healing is complete [51,116]. Alternative regimens may include three weeks of ciprofloxacin 750 mg twice daily, doxycycline 100 mg twice daily, erythromycin 500 mg four times daily, or trimethoprim-sulfamethoxazole 160/800 mg twice daily [51,116].

11.2.10 Genital Warts

While genital warts are often said to involute spontaneously over time, there is little evidence to support this contention [117]. Fortunately, a large number of treatment modalities for genital warts have been evaluated in clinical trials.

In a systematic review of 18 clinical trials of self-administered therapies, imiquimod 3.75% and 5% cream, podophyllotoxin 0.5% solution and gel, as well as polyphenon E 10% and 15% ointment, were all superior to placebo at producing complete clearance in the short (2 weeks ± 2 weeks) and intermediate (16 weeks ± 8 weeks) term [118]. Although active therapies consistently caused more local adverse events (pain, erythema, inflammation, skin irritation, erosions, excoriations, and/or ulcerations) compared to placebo, there were no significant differences in dropouts related to adverse events, suggesting a high degree of acceptability overall. However, the limited number of trials comparing active therapies rendered it difficult to know which regimen should be preferred.

This limitation of the primary literature was addressed through network meta-analysis in a systematic review of 60 clinical trials and cost-effectiveness studies that included both self-administered and clinician-applied therapies. Consistent with the preceding review, all evaluated therapies (summarized in Table 11.2) were superior to placebo or to no treatment at producing complete clearance of lesions at the end of therapy, and few

Table 11.2 Management strategies for anogenital warts.

Self-administered	Provider-administered
Cidofovir 1% cream	Argon plasma coagulation
Imiquimod 3.75% or 5% cream	Cryotherapy (liquid nitrogen, cryoprobe)
Podofilox (podophyllotoxin) 0.5% solution or gel	Podophyllin resin 10–25%[a]

Sinecatechins 15% ointment	Surgical excision
	    Carbon dioxide laser
	    Curettage
	    Electrosurgery
	    Tangential scissor excision
	    Tangential shave excision

	Trichloroacetic acid or bichloroacetic acid 80–90% solution

[a] Safety concerns include neurologic toxicity, potential teratogenicity, fetal loss.

comparisons between active therapies found significant differences in this outcome [119]. However, those that did generally favored carbon dioxide (CO_2) laser therapy or podophyllotoxin 0.5% solution [119]. CO_2 laser therapy was the intervention most likely to produce clinical cure at the end of therapy overall at 97.1% (95% credible interval [CrI] 84.8%–99.9%) [119].

HIV infection is associated with an increased probability, frequency, and size of anogenital warts, but data are inadequate to suggest the need for different management strategies in HIV-positive individuals. However, the higher potential for squamous cell carcinomas in this population may warrant an increased index of suspicion for malignancy.

11.2.11 Treatment of Partners for Prevention of Reinfection

The importance of treating sex partners to prevent repeated infection has been demonstrated for several curable STI including trichomonal vaginitis, *C. trachomatis*, *N. gonorrhoeae*, and *M. genitalium* infection in women. In a study in which partners of women with trichomoniasis were randomized to either tinidazole or placebo, reinfection was strongly associated with the receipt of placebo (RR 4.7, 95% CI 1.3–25.3) [120]. A RCT of a behavioral intervention in women with a baseline STI found reinfection with gonorrhea or chlamydia to be strongly associated with sex with a partner who was not adequately treated (OR 5.6, 95% CI 3.0–10.5) [121]. Sexual contacts of persons with infectious syphilis may be incubating infection, and should be treated in the same way as patients with early syphilis. A randomized, open-label trial of single-dose azithromycin versus benzathine penicillin in 96 such individuals observed no cases of syphilis at three months among the 63 evaluable participants [122].

A practical challenge is ensuring partner receipt of medication. Expedited partner therapy (EPT) involves delivery of medications to sex partners via the patient without medical assessment, and might help improve partner treatment rates. A Cochrane review of EPT demonstrated a 29% lower risk of being re-infected for the EPT group compared with the simple patient referral group (RR = 0.71, 95% CI = 0.56–0.89), however, attrition rates were high in most studies [123]. Caution should be taken in implementing this approach in routine practice, as the partner receiving therapy does not receive medical assessment.

11.3 Prevention of STI

11.3.1 Condoms and Other Contraceptives

Evidence exists to support the effectiveness of latex male condoms in preventing transmission of several different STI. A prospective study of the impact of condom use on acquisition of either HIV or other STI in a community in Uganda found consistent condom use to be associated with a reduced risk of acquiring HIV infection (RR 0.4, 95% CI 0.2–0.9), syphilis (OR 0.7, 95% CI 0.5–0.9), and gonococcal or chlamydial infection (OR 0.5, 95% CI 0.3–1.0) [124]. In a review of 18 prospective studies published after June 2000, consistent condom use was associated with reduced acquisition of genital HSV-2, syphilis, and chlamydial infection by men and women; reduced acquisition of gonorrhoea by women, possibly reduced acquisition of trichomoniasis by women, and accelerated regression of cervical and penile HPV-associated lesions [125].

Other contraceptive practices, including the use of spermicides, oral contraceptive pills, and intrauterine contraceptive devices (IUD), may affect the risk of STI. Despite being bactericidal in vitro, there is no consistent evidence to suggest that the spermicide nonoxynol-9 reduces the risk of genital gonorrheal or chlamydia infection as demonstrated by three RCTs [126–128]. Further, nonoxynol-9 may increase the risk of GUD, which may enhance HIV transmission [127].

11.4   Strategies for Control of STI in the Community

11.4.1   Vaccination

Vaccination is becoming an increasingly important component of prevention strategies for viral STI. Conjugate virus-like particle (VLP) vaccines against both oncogenic (genotypes 16, 18, 31, 33, 45, 52, 58) and wart-associated (genotypes 6 and 11) HPV are now in clinical use in many countries. In published RCTs, these vaccines have been highly immunogenic [129–131], effective at preventing sexual acquisition of vaccine HPV strains [130,132,133], and consistent at reducing the risk of HPV-associated cervical dysplasia by >90% [133–135]. These vaccines are likely to reduce the risk of both future cervical cancer and need for invasive follow-up testing for women with abnormal Papanicolau smears. Furthermore, RCTs show that these vaccines prevent vulvar, vaginal, and perianal HPV-related lesions and neoplasia [136,137]. Unfortunately, effectiveness is limited to women without pre-existing HPV infection [138], necessitating vaccination before or shortly after initiation of coitarche. Vaccination has also been associated with reductions in external genital lesions in men and anal intraepithelial neoplasia in MSM [139,140].

Although VLP HPV vaccines are associated with a risk of anaphylaxis higher than other conjugate vaccines, severe adverse events are rare (rate of true anaphylaxis 2.6 per 100,000 vaccinations, 95% CI 1.0–5.3) [138]. Given the long latency of cervical cancer following HPV infection, data proving reductions in cervical cancer incidence as a result of vaccination are still pending.

11.4.2   Counseling and Behavioral Interventions

Several RCTs have evaluated behavioral interventions targeting groups perceived to be at increased risk of acquiring STI [141]. A recent systematic review identified marked between-study heterogeneity with respect to populations, interventions, and estimated effectiveness. However, behavioral and counseling interventions that are more intensive (e.g., multiple sessions, incorporate multiple modalities) do appear to have a moderate effect in reducing STI risk in adults and adolescents, with no increase in sexual risk-taking noted as a result of counseling [141]. Results, however, do not appear to be durable beyond six months post-intervention [141].

References

1 Public Health Agency of Canada. Report on Sexually Transmitted Infections in Canada 2012 Ottawa; Centre for Communicable Diseases and Infection Control2012. Available from: http://www.phac-aspc.gc.ca/sti-its-surv-epi/rep-rap-2012/tb-eng.php - toc

2 Centers for Disease Control and Prevention. Sexually Transmitted Disease Surveillance 2013. Atlanta: U.S. Department of Health and Human Services. 2014.

3 Bradley H, Markowitz LE, Gibson T, McQuillan GM. Seroprevalence of herpes simplex virus types 1 and 2—United States, 1999–2010. J Infectious Dis. 2014;209(3):325–33.

4 Wikstrom A, Popescu C, Forslund O. Asymptomatic penile HPV infection: a prospective study. Int J STD AIDS. 2000;11(2):80–4.

5 Winer RL, Lee SK, Hughes JP, Adam DE, Kiviat NB, Koutsky LA. Genital human papillomavirus infection: incidence and risk factors in a cohort of female university students. Am J Epidemiol. 2003;157(3):218–26.

6 Woodman CB, Collins S, Winter H, Bailey A, Ellis J, Prior P, et al. Natural history of cervical human papillomavirus infection in young women: a longitudinal cohort study. Lancet. 2001;357(9271):1831–6.

7 Newman L, Rowley J, Vander Hoorn S, Wijesooriya NS, Unemo M, Low N, et al. Global estimates of the prevalence and incidence of four curable sexually transmitted infections in 2012 based on systematic review and global reporting. PloS One. 2015;10(12):e0143304.

8 Tubal infertility: serologic relationship to past chlamydial and gonococcal infection. World Health Organization Task Force on the Prevention and Management of Infertility. Sex Transm Dis. 1995;22(2): 7–7.

9 Ankum WM, Mol BW, Van der Veen F, Bossuyt PM. Risk factors for ectopic pregnancy: a meta-analysis. Fertil Steril. 1996;65(6):1093–9.

10 Stacey CM, Munday PE, Taylor-Robinson D, Thomas BJ, Gilchrist C, Ruck F, et al. A longitudinal study of pelvic inflammatory disease. Brit J Obstet Gynaecol. 1992;99(12):994–9.

11 Safrin S, Schachter J, Dahrouge D, Sweet RL. Long-term sequelae of acute pelvic inflammatory disease. A retrospective cohort study. Am J Obstet Gynecol. 1992;166(4):1300–5.

12 Mitchell H, Drake M, Medley G. Prospective evaluation of risk of cervical cancer after cytological evidence of human papilloma virus infection. Lancet. 1986;1(8481): 573–5.

13 Palefsky JM, Holly EA, Ralston ML, Arthur SP, Hogeboom CJ, Darragh TM. Anal cytological abnormalities and anal HPV infection in men with Centers for Disease Control group IV HIV disease. Genitourinary Med. 1997;73(3):174–80.

14 Leitich H, Kiss H. Asymptomatic bacterial vaginosis and intermediate flora as risk factors for adverse pregnancy outcome. Best Prac Res Clin Obstet Gynaecol. 2007;21(3):375–90.

15 Rours GI, Duijts L, Moll HA, Arends LR, de Groot R, Jaddoe VW, et al. Chlamydia trachomatis infection during pregnancy associated with preterm delivery: a population-based prospective cohort study. Eur J Epidemiol. 2011;26(6):493–502.J

16 Hawkes S, Matin N, Broutet N, Low N. Effectiveness of interventions to improve screening for syphilis in pregnancy: a systematic review and meta-analysis. Lancet Infect Dis. 2011;11(9):684–91.

17 Brown ZA, Wald A, Morrow RA, Selke S, Zeh J, Corey L. Effect of serologic status and cesarean delivery on transmission rates of herpes simplex virus from mother to infant. JAMA. 2003;289(2):203–9.

18 Rottingen JA, Cameron DW, Garnett GP. A systematic review of the epidemiologic interactions between classic sexually transmitted diseases and HIV: how much really is known? Sex Transm Dis. 2001;28(10):579–97.

19 Bornstein J, Lakovsky Y, Lavi I, Bar-Am A, Abramovici H. The classic approach to diagnosis of vulvovaginitis: a critical analysis. Infectious Dis Obstet Gynecol. 2001;9(2):105–11.

20 Organization WH. Guidelines for the Management of Sexually Transmitted Infections Geneva2003. Available from: http://apps.who.int/iris/bitstream/10665/42782/1/9241546263_eng.pdf?ua=1

21 Zemouri C, Wi TE, Kiarie J, Seuc A, Mogasale V, Latif A, et al. The performance of the vaginal discharge syndromic management in treating vaginal and cervical infection: a systematic review and meta-analysis. PloS One. 2016;11(10):e0163365.

22 Simms I, Warburton F, Westrom L. Diagnosis of pelvic inflammatory disease: time for a rethink. Sex Transm Infect. 2003;79(6):491–4.

23 DiCarlo RP, Martin DH. The clinical diagnosis of genital ulcer disease in men. Clin Infect Dis. 1997;25(2):292–8.

24 Turner KM, Adams EJ, Lamontagne DS, Emmett L, Baster K, Edmunds WJ. Modelling the effectiveness of chlamydia screening in England. Sex Transm Infect. 2006;82(6):496–502.

25 Ku L, St Louis M, Farshy C, Aral S, Turner CF, Lindberg LD, et al. Risk behaviors, medical care, and chlamydial infection

among young men in the United States. Am J Public Health. 2002;92(7):1140–3.

26 Zakher B, Cantor AG, Pappas M, Daeges M, Nelson HD. Screening for gonorrhea and Chlamydia: a systematic review for the U.S. Preventive Services Task Force. Ann of Intern Med. 2014;161(12):884–93.

27 Juchau SV, Nackman R, Ruppart D. Comparison of Gram stain with DNA probe for detection of Neisseria gonorrhoeae in urethras of symptomatic males. J of Clin Microbiol. 1995;33(11):3068–9.

28 Nelson HD, Zakher B, Cantor A, Deagas M, Pappas M. U.S. Preventive Services Task Force Evidence Syntheses, formerly Systematic Evidence Reviews. Screening for Gonorrhea and Chlamydia: Systematic Review to Update the US Preventive Services Task Force Recommendations. Rockville (MD): Agency for Healthcare Research and Quality (US); 2014.

29 Iwen PC, Walker RA, Warren KL, Kelly DM, Linder J, Hinrichs SH. Effect of off-site transportation on detection of Neisseria gonorrhoeae in endocervical specimens. Arch of Path Lab Med. 1996;120(11):1019–22.

30 Kingston MA, Bansal D, Carlin EM. "Shelf life" of Trichomonas vaginalis. Int J STD AIDS. 2003;14(1):28–9.

31 Nye MB, Schwebke JR, Body BA. Comparison of APTIMA Trichomonas vaginalis transcription-mediated amplification to wet mount microscopy, culture, and polymerase chain reaction for diagnosis of trichomoniasis in men and women. Am J of Obstet & Gynecol. 2009;200(2):188.e1–7.

32 Lewis DA. Diagnostic tests for chancroid. Sex Transm Infect. 2000;76(2): 137–41.

33 Morse SA, Trees DL, Htun Y, Radebe F, Orle KA, Dangor Y, et al. Comparison of clinical diagnosis and standard laboratory and molecular methods for the diagnosis of genital ulcer disease in Lesotho: association with human immunodeficiency virus infection. J Infect Dis. 1997;175(3):583–9.

34 Bagg J, Mannings A, Munro J, Walker DM. Rapid diagnosis of oral herpes simplex or zoster virus infections by immunofluorescence: comparison with Tzanck cell preparations and viral culture. Brit Dental J. 1989;167(7):235–8.

35 Espy MJ, Uhl JR, Mitchell PS, Thorvilson JN, Svien KA, Wold AD, et al. Diagnosis of herpes simplex virus infections in the clinical laboratory by LightCycler PCR. J Clin Microbiol. 2000;38(2):795–9.

36 Tan TY, Zou H, Ong DC, Ker KJ, Chio MT, Teo RY, et al. Development and clinical validation of a multiplex real-time PCR assay for herpes simplex and varicella zoster virus. Diagnostic molecular pathology: the Am J Surgical Path, part B. 2013;22(4):245–8.

37 LeGoff J, Pere H, Belec L. Diagnosis of genital herpes simplex virus infection in the clinical laboratory. Virology J. 2014;11:83.

38 Binnicker MJ, Espy MJ, Irish CL. Rapid and direct detection of herpes simplex virus in cerebrospinal fluid by use of a commercial real-time PCR assay. J Clin Microbiol. 2014;52(12):4361–2.

39 Larson S, Johnson R. diagnostic tests. In Larsen S, Pope V, Johnson R, Kennedy E, eds A Manual of Tests for Syphilis. Washington, D. C.: American Public Health Association; 1998:1–52.

40 Haas JS, Bolan G, Larsen SA, Clement MJ, Bacchetti P, Moss AR. Sensitivity of treponemal tests for detecting prior treated syphilis during human immunodeficiency virus infection. J Infect Dis. 1990;162(4):862–6.

41 Joyanes P, Borobio MV, Arquez JM, Perea EJ. The association of false-positive rapid plasma reagin results and HIV infection. Sex Transm Dis. 1998;25(10): 569–71.

42 Discordant results from reverse sequence syphilis screening—five laboratories, United States, 2006–2010. MMWR Morb Mortal Wkly Rep. 2011;60(5):133–7.

43 Luger A, Schmidt BL, Steyrer K, Schonwald E. Diagnosis of neurosyphilis by examination of the cerebrospinal fluid. Brit J Venereal Dis. 1981;57(4):232–7.

44 Gayet-Ageron A, Lautenschlager S, Ninet B, Perneger TV, Combescure C. Sensitivity, specificity and likelihood ratios of PCR in the diagnosis of syphilis: a systematic review and meta-analysis. Sex Transm Infect. 2013;89(3):251–6.

45 Jensen JS, Hansen HT, Lind K. Isolation of Mycoplasma genitalium strains from the male urethra. J Clin Microbiol. 1996;34(2):286–91.

46 O'Farrell N. Donovanosis. Sex Trans Infect. 2002;78(6):452–7.

47 Cristillo AD, Bristow CC, Peeling R, Van Der Pol B, de Cortina SH, Dimov IK, et al. Point-of-care sexually transmitted infection diagnostics: proceedings of the STAR Sexually Transmitted Infection-Clinical Trial Group Programmatic Meeting. Sex Transm Dis. 2017;44(4):211–8.

48 Plourde PJ, Tyndall M, Agoki E, Ombette J, Slaney LA, D'Costa LJ, et al. Single-dose cefixime versus single-dose ceftriaxone in the treatment of antimicrobial-resistant Neisseria gonorrhoeae infection. J Infect Dis. 1992;166(4):919–22.

49 Workowski KA, Berman SM. Sexually transmitted diseases treatment guidelines, 2006. MMWR Recommendations and reports. MMWR Morb Mort Wkly Rep. Recommendations and reports. 2006;55(Rr-11):1–94.

50 Aplasca De Los Reyes MR, Pato-Mesola V, Klausner JD, Manalastas R, Wi T, Tuazon CU, et al. A randomized trial of ciprofloxacin versus cefixime for treatment of gonorrhea after rapid emergence of gonococcal ciprofloxacin resistance in the Philippines. Clin Infect Dis. 2001;32(9):1313–8.

51 Workowski KA, Bolan GA. Sexually transmitted diseases treatment guidelines, 2015. MMWR Recomm Rep. 2015;64(RR-03):1–137.

52 Romanowski B, Talbot H, Stadnyk M, Kowalchuk P, Bowie WR. Minocycline compared with doxycycline in the treatment of nongonococcal urethritis and mucopurulent cervicitis. Ann of Internal Med. 1993;119(1):16–22.

53 Lau CY, Qureshi AK. Azithromycin versus doxycycline for genital chlamydial infections: a meta-analysis of randomized clinical trials. Sex Transm Dis. 2002;29(9):497–502.

54 Geisler WM, Uniyal A, Lee JY, Lensing SY, Johnson S, Perry RC, et al. Azithromycin versus Doxycycline for Urogenital Chlamydia trachomatis Infection. N Engl J Med. 2015;373(26):2512–21.

55 Khosropour CM, Manhart LE, Colombara DV, Gillespie CW, Lowens MS, Totten PA, et al. Suboptimal adherence to doxycycline and treatment outcomes among men with non-gonococcal urethritis: a prospective cohort study. Sex Transm Infect. 2014;90(1):3–7.

56 Hooton TM, Rogers ME, Medina TG, Kuwamura LE, Ewers C, Roberts PL, et al. Ciprofloxacin compared with doxycycline for nongonococcal urethritis. Ineffectiveness against Chlamydia trachomatis due to relapsing infection. JAMA. 1990;264(11):1418–21.

57 Fong IW, Linton W, Simbul M, Thorup R, McLaughlin B, Rahm V, et al. Treatment of nongonococcal urethritis with ciprofloxacin. Am J Med. 1987;82(4a):311–6.

58 Mogabgab WJ, Holmes B, Murray M, Beville R, Lutz FB, Tack KJ. Randomized comparison of ofloxacin and doxycycline for chlamydia and ureaplasma urethritis and cervicitis. Chemother. 1990;36(1):70–6.

59 Rastogi S, Kapur S, Salhan S, Mittal A. Chlamydia trachomatis infection in pregnancy: risk factor for an adverse outcome. Brit J of Biomed Sci. 1999;56(2):94–8.

60 Berman SM, Harrison HR, Boyce WT, Haffner WJ, Lewis M, Arthur JB. Low birth weight, prematurity, and postpartum endometritis. Association with prenatal cervical Mycoplasma hominis and

Chlamydia trachomatis infections. JAMA. 1987;257(9):1189–94.

61 Turrentine MA, Newton ER. Amoxicillin or erythromycin for the treatment of antenatal chlamydial infection: a meta-analysis. Obstet Gynecol. 1995;86(6): 1021–5.

62 Kacmar J, Cheh E, Montagno A, Peipert JF. A randomized trial of azithromycin versus amoxicillin for the treatment of Chlamydia trachomatis in pregnancy. Infect Dis Obstet Gynecol. 2001;9(4):197–202.

63 Jacobson GF, Autry AM, Kirby RS, Liverman EM, Motley RU. A randomized controlled trial comparing amoxicillin and azithromycin for the treatment of Chlamydia trachomatis in pregnancy. Am J Obstet Gynecol. 2001;184(7):1352–4; discussion 4–6.

64 Savaris RF, Fuhrich DG, Duarte RV, Franik S, Ross J. Antibiotic therapy for pelvic inflammatory disease. Cochrane Database Syst Rev. 2017;4:Cd010285.

65 Taylor-Robinson D, Jensen JS. Mycoplasma genitalium: from Chrysalis to multicolored butterfly. Clin Microbiol Rev. 2011;24(3):498–514.

66 Lis R, Rowhani-Rahbar A, Manhart LE. Mycoplasma genitalium infection and female reproductive tract disease: a meta-analysis. Clin Infect Dis. 2015;61(3):418–26.

67 Mena LA, Mroczkowski TF, Nsuami M, Martin DH. A randomized comparison of azithromycin and doxycycline for the treatment of Mycoplasma genitalium-positive urethritis in men. Clin Infect Dis. 2009;48(12):1649–54.

68 Schwebke JR, Rompalo A, Taylor S, Sena AC, Martin DH, Lopez LM, et al. Re-evaluating the treatment of nongonococcal urethritis: emphasizing emerging pathogens—a randomized clinical trial. Clin Infect Dis. 2011;52(2):163–70.

69 Li Y, Le WJ, Li S, Cao YP, Su XH. Meta-analysis of the efficacy of moxifloxacin in treating Mycoplasma genitalium infection. Int J STD AIDS. 2017:956462416688562.

70 Pitsouni E, Iavazzo C, Athanasiou S, Falagas ME. Single-dose azithromycin versus erythromycin or amoxicillin for Chlamydia trachomatis infection during pregnancy: a meta-analysis of randomised controlled trials. Internat J Antimicrobial Agents. 2007;30(3):213–21.

71 Ness RB, Soper DE, Holley RL, Peipert J, Randall H, Sweet RL, et al. Effectiveness of inpatient and outpatient treatment strategies for women with pelvic inflammatory disease: results from the Pelvic Inflammatory Disease Evaluation and Clinical Health (PEACH) Randomized Trial. Am J Obstet & Gynecol. 2002;186(5):929–37.

72 Thin RN, Symonds MA, Booker R, Cook S, Langlet F. Double-blind comparison of a single dose and a five-day course of metronidazole in the treatment of trichomoniasis. Brit J Venereal Dis. 1979;55(5):354–6.

73 Hager WD, Brown ST, Kraus SJ, Kleris GS, Perkins GJ, Henderson M. Metronidazole for vaginal trichomoniasis. Seven-day vs. single-dose regimens. JAMA. 1980;244(11):1219–20.

74 Sobel JD, Nyirjesy P, Brown W. Tinidazole therapy for metronidazole-resistant vaginal trichomoniasis. Clin Infect Dis. 2001;33(8):1341–6.

75 duBouchet L, Spence MR, Rein MF, Danzig MR, McCormack WM. Multicenter comparison of clotrimazole vaginal tablets, oral metronidazole, and vaginal suppositories containing sulfanilamide, aminacrine hydrochloride, and allantoin in the treatment of symptomatic trichomoniasis. Sex Transm Dis. 1997;24(3):156–60.

76 Lukehart SA, Hook EW, 3rd, Baker-Zander SA, Collier AC, Critchlow CW, Handsfield HH. Invasion of the central nervous system by Treponema pallidum: implications for diagnosis and treatment. Ann Intern Med. 1988;109(11):855–62.

77 Ghanem KG, Moore RD, Rompalo AM, Erbelding EJ, Zenilman JM, Gebo KA. Lumbar puncture in HIV-infected patients with syphilis and no neurologic symptoms. Clin Infect Dis. 2009;48(6):816–21. doi: 10.1086/597096

78 Clement ME, Okeke NL, Hicks CB. Treatment of syphilis: a systematic review. JAMA. 2014;312(18):1905–17. doi: 10.001/jama.2014.13259

79 Mohr JA, Griffiths W, Jackson R, Saadah H, Bird P, Riddle J. Neurosyphilis and penicillin levels in cerebrospinal fluid. JAMA. 1976;236(19):2208–9.

80 Bai ZG, Wang B, Yang K, Tian JH, Ma B, Liu Y, et al. Azithromycin versus penicillin G benzathine for early syphilis. Cochrane Database Syst Rev. 2012(6):CD007270. doi: 10.1002/14651858.CD007270.pub2

81 Stamm LV. Syphilis: antibiotic treatment and resistance. Epidemiol Infect. 2015;143(8):1567–74. doi: 10.017/S0950268814002830. Epub 2014 Oct 31.

82 Zhou P, Gu Z, Xu J, Wang X, Liao K. A study evaluating ceftriaxone as a treatment agent for primary and secondary syphilis in pregnancy. Sex Transm Dis. 2005;32(8):495–8.

83 Katanami Y, Hashimoto T, Takaya S, Yamamoto K, Kutsuna S, Takeshita N, et al. Amoxicillin and Ceftriaxone as Treatment Alternatives to penicillin for maternal syphilis. Emerg Infect Dis. 2017;23(5):827–9. doi: 10.3201/eid2305.161936

84 Gordon SM, Eaton ME, George R, Larsen S, Lukehart SA, Kuypers J, et al. The response of symptomatic neurosyphilis to high-dose intravenous penicillin G in patients with human immunodeficiency virus infection. N Engl J Med. 1994;331(22):1469–73.

85 Andrade R, Rodriguez-Barradas MC, Yasukawa K, Villarreal E, Ross M, Serpa JA. Single Dose Versus 3 Doses of Intramuscular Benzathine Penicillin for Early Syphilis in HIV: A Randomized Clinical Trial. Clin Infect Dis. 2017;64(6):759–64. doi: 10.1093/cid/ciw862

86 Rolfs RT, Joesoef MR, Hendershot EF, Rompalo AM, Augenbraun MH, Chiu M, et al. A randomized trial of enhanced therapy for early syphilis in patients with and without human immunodeficiency virus infection. The Syphilis and HIV Study Group. N Engl J Med. 1997;337(5):307–14.

87 Sena AC, Zhang XH, Li T, Zheng HP, Yang B, Yang LG, et al. A systematic review of syphilis serological treatment outcomes in HIV-infected and HIV-uninfected persons: rethinking the significance of serological non-responsiveness and the serofast state after therapy. BMC Infect Dis. 2015;15:479. doi:10.1186/s12879-015-1209-0

88 Sena AC, Wolff M, Martin DH, Behets F, Van Damme K, Leone P, et al. Predictors of serological cure and Serofast State after treatment in HIV-negative persons with early syphilis. Clin Infect Dis. 2011;53(11):1092–9. doi: 10.3/cid/cir671. Epub 2011 Oct 12.

89 Marra CM, Maxwell CL, Tantalo LC, Sahi SK, Lukehart SA. Normalization of serum rapid plasma reagin titer predicts normalization of cerebrospinal fluid and clinical abnormalities after treatment of neurosyphilis. Clin Infect Dis. 2008;47(7):893–9. doi: 10.1086/591534

90 Butler T. The Jarisch-Herxheimer reaction after antibiotic treatment of spirochetal infections: a review of recent cases and our understanding of pathogenesis. Am J Trop Med Hyg. 2017;96(1):46–52. doi: 10.4269/ajtmh.16-0434 Epub 2016 Oct 24.

91 Gupta R, Warren T, Wald A. Genital herpes. Lancet. 2008;370(9605): 2127–37.

92 Johnston C, Corey L. Current concepts for genital herpes simplex virus infection: diagnostics and pathogenesis of genital tract shedding. Clin Microbiol Rev. 2016;29(1):149–61. doi: 10.1128/CMR.00043-15

93 Patel R, Tyring S, Strand A, Price MJ, Grant DM. Impact of suppressive antiviral therapy on the health related quality of life of patients with recurrent genital herpes infection. Sex Transm Infect. 1999;75(6):398–402.

94 Heslop R, Roberts H, Flower D, Jordan V. Interventions for men and women with their first episode of genital herpes. Cochrane Database Syst Rev. 2016(8):CD010684. doi: 10.1002/14651858.CD010684.pub2

95 Le Cleach L, Trinquart L, Do G, Maruani A, Lebrun-Vignes B, Ravaud P, et al. Oral antiviral therapy for prevention of genital herpes outbreaks in immunocompetent and nonpregnant patients. Cochrane Database Syst Rev. 2014(8):CD009036. doi: 10.1002/14651858.CD009036.pub2

96 Chi CC, Wang SH, Delamere FM, Wojnarowska F, Peters MC, Kanjirath PP. Interventions for prevention of herpes simplex labialis (cold sores on the lips). Cochrane Database Syst Rev. 2015(8):CD010095. doi: 10.1002/14651858.CD010095.pub2

97 Bacon TH, Levin MJ, Leary JJ, Sarisky RT, Sutton D. Herpes simplex virus resistance to acyclovir and penciclovir after two decades of antiviral therapy. Clin Microbiol Rev. 2003;16(1):114–28.

98 Corey L, Wald A, Patel R, Sacks SL, Tyring SK, Warren T, et al. Once-daily valacyclovir to reduce the risk of transmission of genital herpes. N Engl J Med. 2004;350(1):11–20.

99 Pasternak B, Hviid A. Use of acyclovir, valacyclovir, and famciclovir in the first trimester of pregnancy and the risk of birth defects. JAMA. 2010;304(8):859–66.

100 Brown ZA, Selke S, Zeh J, Kopelman J, Maslow A, Ashley RL, et al. The acquisition of herpes simplex virus during pregnancy. N Engl J Med. 1997;337(8):509–15.

101 Prober CG, Sullender WM, Yasukawa LL, Au DS, Yeager AS, Arvin AM. Low risk of herpes simplex virus infections in neonates exposed to the virus at the time of vaginal delivery to mothers with recurrent genital herpes simplex virus infections. N Engl J Med. 1987;316(5):240–4.

102 Sheffield JS, Hollier LM, Hill JB, Stuart GS, Wendel GD. Acyclovir prophylaxis to prevent herpes simplex virus recurrence at delivery: a systematic review. Obstet Gynecol. 2003;102(6):1396–403.

103 Freeman EE, Weiss HA, Glynn JR, Cross PL, Whitworth JA, Hayes RJ. Herpes simplex virus 2 infection increases HIV acquisition in men and women: systematic review and meta-analysis of longitudinal studies. AIDS. 2006;20(1):73–83.

104 Gray RH, Wawer MJ, Brookmeyer R, Sewankambo NK, Serwadda D, Wabwire-Mangen F, et al. Probability of HIV-1 transmission per coital act in monogamous, heterosexual, HIV-1-discordant couples in Rakai, Uganda. Lancet. 2001;357(9263):1149–53.

105 Celum C, Wald A, Hughes J, Sanchez J, Reid S, Delany-Moretlwe S, et al. Effect of aciclovir on HIV-1 acquisition in herpes simplex virus 2 seropositive women and men who have sex with men: a randomised, double-blind, placebo-controlled trial. Lancet. 2008;371(9630): 2109–19.

106 Watson-Jones D, Weiss HA, Rusizoka M, Changalucha J, Baisley K, Mugeye K, et al. Effect of herpes simplex suppression on incidence of HIV among women in Tanzania.[see comment]. N Engl J Med. 2008;358(15):1560–71.

107 Celum C, Wald A, Lingappa JR, Magaret AS, Wang RS, Mugo N, et al. Acyclovir and transmission of HIV-1 from persons infected with HIV-1 and HSV-2. N Engl J Med. 2010;362(5):427–39.

108 Barnabas RV, Webb EL, Weiss HA, Wasserheit JN. The role of coinfections in HIV epidemic trajectory and positive prevention: a systematic review and meta-analysis. AIDS. 2011;25(13):1559–73. doi: 10.097/QAD.0b013e3283491e3e

109 Tan DH, Murphy K, Shah P, Walmsley SL. Herpes simplex virus type 2 and HIV disease progression: a systematic review of observational studies. BMC Infect Dis. 2013;13(1):502.

110 Ballard RC, da L'Exposto F, Dangor Y, Fehler HG, Miller SD, Koornhof HJ. A comparative study of spectinomycin and erythromycin in the treatment of chancroid. J Antimicrob Chemother. 1990;26(3):429–34.

111 Ison CA, Dillon JA, Tapsall JW. The epidemiology of global antibiotic

resistance among Neisseria gonorrhoeae and Haemophilus ducreyi. Lancet. 1998;351 Suppl 3:8–11.

112 Ernst AA, Marvez-Valls E, Martin DH. Incision and drainage versus aspiration of fluctuant buboes in the emergency department during an epidemic of chancroid. Sex Transm Dis. 1995;22(4):217–20.

113 Leeyaphan C, Ong JJ, Chow EP, Kong FY, Hocking JS, Bissessor M, et al. Systematic review and meta-analysis of doxycycline efficacy for rectal lymphogranuloma venereum in men who have sex with men. Emerg Infect Dis. 2016;22(10):1778–84. doi: 10.3201/eid2210.160986. Epub 2016 Oct 15.

114 Leeyaphan C, Ong JJ, Chow EP, Dimovski K, Kong FY, Hocking JS, et al. Treatment outcomes for rectal lymphogranuloma venereum in men who have sex with men using doxycycline, azithromycin, or both: a review of clinical cases. Sex Transm Dis. 2017;44(4):245–8. doi: 10.1097/OLQ.0000000000000578

115 Mechai F, de Barbeyrac B, Aoun O, Merens A, Imbert P, Rapp C. Doxycycline failure in lymphogranuloma venereum. Sex Transm Infect. 2010;86(4):278–9. doi: 10.1136/sti.2009.042093

116 O'Farrell N, Moi H. 2016 European guideline on donovanosis. Int J STD AIDS. 2016;27(8):605–7. doi: 10.1177/0956462416633626. Epub 2016 Feb 15.

117 Handsfield HH. Clinical presentation and natural course of anogenital warts. Am J Med. 1997;102(5A):16–20.

118 Werner RN, Westfechtel L, Dressler C, Nast A. Self-administered interventions for anogenital warts in immunocompetent patients: a systematic review and meta-analysis. Sex Transm Infect. 2017;93(3):155–61. doi: 10.1136/sextrans-2016-052768. Epub 2016 Nov 1.

119 Thurgar E, Barton S, Karner C, Edwards SJ. Clinical effectiveness and cost-effectiveness of interventions for the treatment of anogenital warts: systematic review and economic evaluation. Health Technol Assess. 2016;2016 Mar;20(24):v–vi.

120 Lyng J, Christensen J. A double-blind study of the value of treatment with a single dose tinidazole of partners to females with trichomoniasis. Acta Obstet Gynecol Scand. 1981;60(2):199–201.

121 Shain RN, Perdue ST, Piper JM, Holden AE, Champion JD, Newton ER, et al. Behaviors changed by intervention are associated with reduced STD recurrence: the importance of context in measurement. Sex Transm Dis. 2002;29(9):520–9.

122 Hook EW, 3rd, Stephens J, Ennis DM. Azithromycin compared with penicillin G benzathine for treatment of incubating syphilis. Ann Intern Med. 1999;131(6):434–7.

123 Ferreira A, Young T, Mathews C, Zunza M, Low N. Strategies for partner notification for sexually transmitted infections, including HIV. Cochrane Database Syst Rev. 2013(10):Cd002843.

124 Ahmed S, Lutalo T, Wawer M, Serwadda D, Sewankambo NK, Nalugoda F, et al. HIV incidence and sexually transmitted disease prevalence associated with condom use: a population study in Rakai, Uganda. AIDS. 2001;15(16):2171–9.

125 Holmes KK, Levine R, Weaver M. Effectiveness of condoms in preventing sexually transmitted infections. Bull World Health Organ. 2004;82(6):454–61.

126 Roddy RE, Zekeng L, Ryan KA, Tamoufe U, Tweedy KG. Effect of nonoxynol-9 gel on urogenital gonorrhea and chlamydial infection: a randomized controlled trial. JAMA. 2002;287(9):1117–22.

127 Roddy RE, Zekeng L, Ryan KA, Tamoufe U, Weir SS, Wong EL. A controlled trial of nonoxynol 9 film to reduce male-to-female transmission of sexually transmitted diseases. N Engl J Med. 1998;339(8):504–10.

128 Kreiss J, Ngugi E, Holmes K, Ndinya-Achola J, Waiyaki P, Roberts PL, et al. Efficacy of nonoxynol 9 contraceptive sponge use in preventing heterosexual

acquisition of HIV in Nairobi prostitutes. JAMA. 1992;268(4):477–82.

129   Joura EA, Kjaer SK, Wheeler CM, Sigurdsson K, Iversen OE, Hernandez-Avila M, et al. HPV antibody levels and clinical efficacy following administration of a prophylactic quadrivalent HPV vaccine. Vaccine. 2008;26(52):6844–51.

130   Koutsky LA, Ault KA, Wheeler CM, Brown DR, Barr E, Alvarez FB, et al. A controlled trial of a human papillomavirus type 16 vaccine. N Engl J Med. 2002;347(21):1645–51.

131   Villa LL, Ault KA, Giuliano AR, Costa RL, Petta CA, Andrade RP, et al. Immunologic responses following administration of a vaccine targeting human papillomavirus Types 6, 11, 16, and 18. Vaccine. 2006;24(27–28):5571–83.

132   Villa LL, Costa RL, Petta CA, Andrade RP, Ault KA, Giuliano AR, et al. Prophylactic quadrivalent human papillomavirus (types 6, 11, 16, and 18) L1 virus-like particle vaccine in young women: a randomised double-blind placebo-controlled multicentre phase II efficacy trial. Lancet Oncol. 2005;6(5):271–8.

133   Harper DM, Franco EL, Wheeler C, Ferris DG, Jenkins D, Schuind A, et al. Efficacy of a bivalent L1 virus-like particle vaccine in prevention of infection with human papillomavirus types 16 and 18 in young women: a randomised controlled trial. Lancet. 2004;364(9447):1757–65.

134   Quadrivalent vaccine against human papillomavirus to prevent high-grade cervical lesions. N Engl J Med. 2007;356(19):1915–27.

135   Paavonen J, Jenkins D, Bosch FX, Naud P, Salmeron J, Wheeler CM, et al. Efficacy of a prophylactic adjuvanted bivalent L1 virus-like-particle vaccine against infection with human papillomavirus types 16 and 18 in young women: an interim analysis of a phase III double-blind, randomised controlled trial. Lancet. 2007;369(9580):2161–70.

136   Joura EA, Leodolter S, Hernandez-Avila M, Wheeler CM, Perez G, Koutsky LA, et al. Efficacy of a quadrivalent prophylactic human papillomavirus (types 6, 11, 16, and 18) L1 virus-like-particle vaccine against high-grade vulval and vaginal lesions: a combined analysis of three randomised clinical trials. Lancet. 2007;369(9574):1693–702.

137   Garland SM, Hernandez-Avila M, Wheeler CM, Perez G, Harper DM, Leodolter S, et al. Quadrivalent vaccine against human papillomavirus to prevent anogenital diseases. N Engl J Medicine. 2007;356(19):1928–43.

138   Hildesheim A, Herrero R, Wacholder S, Rodriguez AC, Solomon D, Bratti MC, et al. Effect of human papillomavirus 16/18 L1 viruslike particle vaccine among young women with preexisting infection: a randomized trial. JAMA. 2007;298(7):743–53.

139   Giuliano AR, Palefsky JM, Goldstone S, Moreira ED, Jr., Penny ME, Aranda C, et al. Efficacy of quadrivalent HPV vaccine against HPV Infection and disease in males. N Engl J Med. 2011;364(5):401–11.

140   Palefsky JM, Giuliano AR, Goldstone S, Moreira ED, Jr., Aranda C, Jessen H, et al. HPV vaccine against anal HPV infection and anal intraepithelial neoplasia. N Engl J Med. 2011;365(17):1576–85.

141   O'Connor E, Lin JS, Burda BU, Henderson JT, Walsh ES, Whitlock EP. U.S. Preventive Services Task Force Evidence Syntheses, formerly Systematic Evidence Reviews. Behavioral Sexual Risk Reduction Counseling in Primary Care to Prevent Sexually Transmitted Infections: An Updated Systematic Evidence Review for the US Preventive Services Task Force. Rockville (MD): Agency for Healthcare Research and Quality (US); 2014.

Chapter 12

Human Immunodeficiency Virus (HIV)

Ali Amini, Monique Andersson, Ravindra Gupta, and Brian Angus

12.1 Primary HIV Infection

> ### Case Presentation 1
>
> A 52-year-old homosexual man is feeling unwell with fever, malaise, a diffuse maculo-papular rash, and lymphadenopathy. He holidays regularly in Thailand and has had unprotected receptive anal sexual inter-course with a regular Thai partner as well as contact with five commercial sex workers in Bangkok. You suspect he has primary HIV infection, and ask how best to make the diagnosis and whether he should be treated with antiretroviral drugs immediately.

12.1.1 Diagnostic Confirmation

Primary HIV infection (PHI) is important both for the individual and at a population level given the high early risk of transmission and implications for contact tracing.

Routine universal laboratory screening is now recommended given appreciation of the limited diagnostic utility of clinical features [1]. A meta-analysis (16 studies; 24,745 patients) evaluating the accuracy of clinical assessment in identifying 1,253 persons with early HIV (defined as infection within 6 months), found only a modest association with the presence of genital ulcers (Likelihood Ratio [LR] 5.4, 95% Confidence Interval [CI] 2.5–12), weight loss (LR 4.7, 95% CI 2.1–7.2), vomiting (LR 4.6, 95% CI 2.5–8.0), and swollen lymph nodes (LR 4.6, 95% CI 1.3–8.0) [2]. In a prospective Swiss cohort ($n = 290$; 93% men), atypical manifestations of PHI were found in 30% and included GI or neurological complaints. PHI was only suspected in 38% initially [3].

Laboratory testing algorithms recommend screening with a fourth-generation assay for p24 antigen and HIV-1/HIV-2 IgG/M antibodies, followed by a confirmatory immunoassay able to differentiate HIV-1 and HIV-2 [4,5]. The HIV-1 western blot and HIV-1 indirect immunofluorescence assay (IFA) are no longer recommended for confirmation of reactive initial immunoassay results, given false negative results during seroconversion, with the majority of HIV-2 infections misclassified by western blot. Fourth-generation assays add a significant diagnostic yield in acute infection, identifying 134 of 168 patients with acute infection (negative third-generation rapid test, positive individual HIV-RNA testing) from a multi-site prospective American cohort of 86,836 individuals [6]. In acute infection, fourth-generation tests were 79.8% sensitive (95% CI 72.9–85.6) and 99.9% specific (95% CI 99.9–99.9), while pooled RNA-testing was 97.6% sensitive (95% CI 94.0–99.4) and 100% specific (95% CI 100–100). Missed acute infections only

Evidence-Based Infectious Diseases, Third Edition. Edited by Dominik Mertz, Fiona Smaill, and Nick Daneman.
© 2018 John Wiley & Sons Ltd. Published 2018 by John Wiley & Sons Ltd.

detectable by RNA ($n = 34$) were presumably in the early window period prior to peak viremia and p24 development, with lower median viral load (6,019 copies/mL) than those detectable with fourth-generation assays (750,000 copies/mL, p <0.001). Reassuringly, fourth-generation assays diagnosed all cases of established HIV infection (detectable by rapid tests) correctly, in addition to identifying all 19 false positives. Compared with rapid HIV testing alone, HIV Ag/Ab combination testing increased the relative HIV diagnostic yield (both established, $n = 1,158$, and acute HIV infections) by 10.4% (95% CI 8.8–12.2) and pooled HIV RNA testing increased the relative HIV diagnostic yield by 12.4% (95% CI 10.7–14.3).

Nucleic acid testing (NAT) for HIV-1 RNA can be used in suspected seroconversion in the window period, especially with non-confirmatory serology, if there is a high index of suspicion or population prevalence.

Rapid point-of-care tests are available, but are generally not recommended in high prevalence settings where laboratory facilities exist, given concerns regarding missed acute infection. The latest meta-analysis (18 studies, 110,122 testing episodes) found that rapid tests had a pooled sensitivity of 94.5% (95% CI 87.4–97.7) and specificity of 93.7% (95% CI 88.7–96.5), compared to fourth-generation laboratory immunoassays and NAT, respectively [7]. Venous blood is preferable to finger-stick or oral fluid. A sub-analysis of oral fluid samples in five studies, all in high income countries, found a pooled sensitivity of 82.1% (95% CI 78.0–85.6), agreeing with results of a previous meta-analysis (24 studies) where only 60% of studies used a perfect accepted reference standard [8]; sensitivity was about 2% lower with oral (98.0%, 95% CI 95.9–99.1) than blood-based specimens (99.7%, 95% CI 97.3–100.0), with similar specificity (oral 99.7%, 95% CI 99.5–99.9; blood 99.9%, 95% CI 99.8–100.0). Finally, although new fourth-generation rapid tests are now available, these are not recommended in cases where acute infection is suspected. A systematic review (four studies, 17,831 persons) of the latest fourth-generation rapid tests in acute infection found zero sensitivity of the p24 antigen component [9]; 26 cases of acute HIV were missed, and specificity was similar across all studies (98.3–99.9%).

12.1.2 Asymptomatic HIV

International guidelines now strongly recommend immediate initiation of antiretroviral therapy (ART) among newly diagnosed adults, irrespective of CD4 count, given evidence of reduced HIV and non-HIV related illness [10,11]. The American NA-ACCORD analysis [12] found a significant reduction in mortality in patients initiated at CD4 cell counts both above 350 and 500 cells/mm^3. The European ART-CC analysis, however, found no clear reduction in mortality or AIDS in patients initiated early at CD4 above 350 cells/mm^3 [13].

Three trials have randomized patients with CD4 counts above 350 cells/mm^3 to start or defer treatment. The HIV Prevention Trials Network (HPTN) 052 trial [14] enrolled discordant couples ($n = 1,763$) from nine low- and middle-income countries with CD4 counts between 350 and 550 cells/mm^3, randomized equally to immediate or delayed therapy after development of symptoms or a decline in CD4 (below 250 cells/mm^3), with median CD4 count at initiation 442 cells/mm^3 and 230 cells/mm^3, respectively. The study reported significant benefit in terms of transmission (hazard ratio [HR] 0.04, 95% CI 0.01–0.27) and clinical endpoints, predominantly extra-pulmonary TB (HR 0.59, 95% CI 0.40–0.88) in the early therapy group, although the lower CD4 count in the deferred arm could obviously overestimate the benefits of therapy compared to starting at less than 350 cells/mm^3. A strong public health benefit was confirmed in the 2016 study update with sustained reduction in transmission [15].

Critical evidence was from the seminal Strategic Timing of Antiretroviral Treatment (START) Trial [16]. ART-naïve asymptomatic adults ($n = 4,685$; 27% women; 55%

MSM) with CD4 cell counts above 500 cells/ mm^3 (median CD4 cell count 651 cells/mm^3) in 35 countries were randomized to immediate ($n = 2,326$) or deferred ART ($n = 2,359$) until the development of AIDS or CD4 below 350 cells/mm^3 (median 408 cells/mm^3 at initiation). After a median three years follow-up, there was a 57% reduction in the combined primary end point (death, serious AIDS, or non-AIDS related event) in the immediate-initiation group (HR 0.43, 95% CI 0.30–0.620), mainly attributable to rates of AIDS events, notably TB and malignancy (lymphoma or Kaposi's). This was irrespective of age, sex, region (high compared to low- and middle-income countries), viral load, or CD4, with most events occurring when CD4 was above 500 cells/mm^3 in both groups. There were no differences in high-risk grade 4 events or unscheduled hospital admissions. Of note, the majority were initiated on tenofovir-containing regimens. Importantly, the absolute risk of deferring treatment was small (4.1%; 1.38 events per 100 person-years) compared to early therapy (1.8%; 0.60 events per 100 person years) over three years follow-up. Nevertheless, ART initiation at CD4 counts of >500 cells/mm^3 was clearly beneficial, such that individuals committing to therapy should start irrespective of CD4 count.

12.1.3   Early Treatment in PHI

There is no RCT evidence comparing long term impacts of immediate to deferred therapy in PHI. Guidelines are influenced by evidence from chronic infection, with experts recommending expedited treatment, particularly in symptomatic patients within 12 weeks of transmission, in order to reduce onward transmission and symptoms, preserve immune function and prevent rapid progression [10,11]. There is accumulating evidence for more rapid and enhanced recovery in surrogate markers of progression and immune reconstitution, such as CD4 counts [17,18] and CD4/CD8 ratio [19,20], reflecting decreased immune activation and

inflammation for those initiating treatment close to HIV acquisition.

Studies have also highlighted the superiority of early treatment in reducing the HIV reservoir size, defined by HIV DNA levels and resting CD4+ T cells able to generate replication-competent virus [21], and treatment during acute infection could prevent development of escape mutants in latently infected cytotoxic T lymphocytes (CTL) [22].

12.1.4   Drug Resistance, Baseline Genotyping, and Clinical Impact

12.1.4.1   Epidemiology

Resistance is common after treatment failure using non-nucleoside reverse transcriptase inhibitors (NNRTI). A retrospective global cohort of 1,926 patients (36 countries; 1998–2015) failing WHO recommended first-line tenofovir-containing NNRTI-based regimens had tenofovir resistance mutations in 20% (Europe) to 57% (sub-Saharan Africa) [23]. Most patients (65%) with tenofovir resistance had resistance to other drugs in the regimen.

The prevalence of pre-treatment/transmitted drug resistance (TDR) among drug-naïve patients therefore unsurprisingly differs between regions. Data from the START study demonstrated significant prevalence of pre-treatment resistance in Australia (17.5%), France (16.7%), United States (12.6%), and Spain (12.6%) [24]. A meta-analysis (2001–2011; 162 studies; 42 countries) examining the prevalence among over 20,000 treatment-naïve patients in resource-limited settings found the largest annual increase of resistance in East Africa (29%) and Southern Africa (15%) after ART rollout [25].

12.1.4.2   Baseline Genotyping

Baseline genotypic resistance testing (sequencing of reverse transcriptase and protease protein encoding pol gene) is considered cost-effective [26] and recommended in all patients with HIV at diagnosis, regardless of whether ART is planned, to exclude transmitted drug resistance [10,27]. Without drug selection pressure some mutations may become undetectable over time, although there is evidence that most persist. A U.K. cohort (331 patients, mostly MSM) found that 24% of mutations persisted 18 months after initial testing, with mutations K70R (7/14 patients), M184V (16/34), T215Y (13/25), and Y181C (10/20) most likely to disappear; multivariate analysis confirmed that non-subtype B virus mutations reverted to wild type more frequently [28].

There is currently limited evidence to recommend testing for integrase strand-transfer inhibitor (INSTI) resistance, with experts recommending testing patients with other TDR mutants, a history of possible transmission from a partner with INSTI resistance, or a high background population resistance above 3% [10]. Tropism testing is suggested if use of a CCR5 antagonist is contemplated [27].

12.1.4.3 Clinical Impact

Analysis of 10,056 European ART-naïve patients undergoing baseline testing (1998–2008) found that virological failure was three times higher among those with resistance to at least one drug compared to those with a fully active regimen at one year [29].

Transmission rates of resistant virus are possibly underestimated. Minority viral populations below 25%, not detected by standard sequencing technologies, are associated with increased virological failure, and can persist without selection pressure. In a pooled analysis of seven studies of 240 treatment and baseline-resistance naïve patients (detected by standard commercial assays), NNRTI minority variants at baseline were found more commonly in patients subsequently developing virological failure and NNRTI resistance [30].

12.1.5 Prognostic Features for Progression of Disease

Early initiation of ART impacts disease progression as shown by the START study [18]. Should a patient decide not to start treatment, progression varies depending on viral characteristics, host genetics, and environmental factors. Baseline viral load has limited predictive value for the rate progression [31], although early studies suggested that high viral load was associated with an increased risk of death and a more rapid fall in CD4 count [32]. An analysis of outcomes for people starting HAART showed only a small effect of viral load influencing outcome [33]. During 61,798 person-years of follow-up, there were 1,303 AIDS events and 1,005 deaths. The risk of disease progression at one to five years after beginning treatment was calculated according to five key baseline variables: CD4 count, viral load, age, transmission category, and CDC stage. Overall, a CD4 count <200 cells/mm^3, viral load >5 log (100,000 copies/mL), age >50, being an injecting drug user, and being in CDC stage 3 predicted a poorer outcome. (There is a useful online risk calculator at http://www.art-cohort-collaboration.org.)

12.1.6 Summary

Fourth-generation laboratory based immunoassays are sensitive and specific for detection of both acute and established HIV, with some incremental yield using NAT in primary HIV infection. Rapid tests, including newer fourth-generation versions, are suboptimal and should be supplemented in the diagnosis of PHI. Guidelines now suggest universal treatment irrespective of CD4 count. The increase in transmitted drug resistance means that baseline genotyping is recommended to guide therapy.

Case Presentation 1 (continued)

The patient tests positive for HIV antibody on multiple immunoassays. His CD4 count is 560 cells/mm^3 with a HIV viral load of 100,000 copies/mL by PCR which is Clade E and found to be wild type. He is HBV, HCV, and VDRL negative. He commences treatment and has a calculated risk of AIDS after starting HAART of 7.4% (95% CI 6.3–8.6) and of death of 3.2% (95% CI 2.5–3.9) at the end of year 3 of treatment.

12.2 Tuberculosis

Case Presentation 2

A 38-year-old female asylum seeker from Ethiopia is admitted directly from an airport health screening clinic. She has an abnormal chest radiograph with a cough, hemoptysis, and weight loss. On examination she has a fever of 38.2 °C. She looks pale and has widespread lymphadenopathy and hepatosplenomegaly. Her blood count shows a hemoglobin of 8.4 g/dL, white cell count of 4.3×10^9/L, platelets of 166×10^9/L. Her chest radiograph shows left apical infiltration. She tests seropositive for HIV-1 infection, hepatitis B surface, and core antibody positive, but she is HBV-antigen negative. She is hepatitis C seronegative and VDRL negative. CD4 count is 310 cells/mm^3, viral load 70,000 copies/mL. You suspect she has *Mycobacterium tuberculosis* infection complicating HIV infection. You question how best to confirm the diagnosis of tuberculosis (TB) and what your treatment options are.

Of the global caseload, 13% or around 1.1 million people are estimated to have tuberculosis–HIV co-infection, with 80% of these in Africa. HIV-associated tuberculosis deaths accounted for about 25% of the total (34). Worryingly 480,000 new cases of multidrug-resistant (MDR) tuberculosis are estimated worldwide, resulting in about 210,000 deaths. MDR tuberculosis was reported in about 3.5% of new cases and 20.5% of re-treated cases [35].

12.2.1 Diagnosis

The gold standard for diagnosis is now an automated liquid culture (limit of detection of ∼10 organisms per mL) of sputum. Samples can be also be directly tested with the Gene Xpert MTB/RIF and Hain MTBDRplus assays, which include *rpoB* gene sequencing for rifampicin resistance. The sensitivity of Xpert is around 89% in smear-positive and 67% in smear-negative pulmonary tuberculosis,

with high specificity. However, if MDR tuberculosis prevalence is less than 10%, the positive predictive value for *rpoB* gene sequencing is likely to be less than 85%, and so confirmatory testing with culture is advised [36].

Sputum samples are just as likely to be AFB positive in HIV-positive as HIV-negative patients [37]. Induced sputum may increase the yield [38]. Concentration methods of liquefied sputum in a large cohort of consecutive patients with suspected pulmonary TB showed that the overall sensitivity increased from 54.2% using conventional direct microscopy to 63.1% after concentration ($p = 0.015$) [39]. In HIV-positive patients, sensitivity increased from 38.5%–50.0% ($p = 0.0034$).

12.2.2 Treatment

The efficacy of a six-month short-course quadruple drug regimen of chemotherapy for pulmonary TB in the presence of HIV infection was confirmed in a study performed in Kinshasa, Zaire [40]. After six months, the rates of treatment failure between HIV-positive and HIV-negative participants were similar at 3.8% and 2.7%, respectively. At 24 months, the HIV-positive patients who received six months' extended treatment of rifampicin and isoniazid twice weekly had a relapse rate of 1.9%, as compared with 9% among the HIV-positive patients who received placebo for the second six months ($p = 0.01$). Extended treatment, however, did not improve survival.

A prospective cohort study comparing a daily regimen of ethambutol, isoniazid, rifampicin, and pyrazinamide for two months, followed by ethambutol and isoniazid three times weekly for six months (2EHRZ/6E3H3); or the same initial intensive phase as the first regimen, followed by four months or six months of daily rifampicin and isoniazid (2EHRZ/4HR) and (2EHRZ/6HR) showed that the 2EHRZ/6E3H3 regimen was safe and effective but had a significant risk of relapse [41]. The relapse rate was 18.2 per 100 person-years observation (PYO) for the intermittent ethambutol arm compared to 9.7/100 PYO ($p = 0.0063$) and 4.8/100 PYO ($p = 0.0001$)

in patients treated with 2 EHRZ/4HR or 2EHRZ/6HR, respectively.

Treatment of MDR tuberculosis regimen is difficult with increased number of drugs (at least 4) and prolonged duration (up to 24 months) based on phenotypic drug resistance patterns [42]. There is little controlled trial data.

12.2.3 Antituberculosis Prophylaxis

Without prophylaxis, people who are HIV-positive and tuberculin skin test-positive have a 50% or more lifetime risk of developing active TB compared with a 10% lifetime risk in people who are HIV-positive but tuberculin skin test-negative [43]. Two systematic reviews have found that anti-TB prophylaxis reduces the rate of developing active TB and death in the short term in people who are HIV-positive and tuberculin skin test-positive. A Cochrane review identified 11 well-conducted RCTs in 8,130 HIV-positive adults from Haiti, Kenya, United States, Zambia, Spain, and Uganda [44]. All evaluated isoniazid (6–12 months) either compared with placebo or combination therapy (3 months). Mean follow-up was two to three years, and the main outcomes, stratified by tuberculin skin test positivity, were TB (either microbiologic or clinical) and death. Among tuberculin skin test-positive adults, anti-TB prophylaxis significantly reduced the incidence of TB (Relative Risk [RR] compared with placebo 0.38, 95% CI 0.25–0.57) and was associated with a trend toward reducing the risk of death (RR compared with placebo 0.80, 95% CI 0.63–1.02). Among tuberculin skin test-negative adults, there was no significant difference in risk of TB (RR compared with placebo 0.83, 95% CI 0.58–1.18) or death. There was a significant increase in adverse drug reactions requiring cessation of treatment on treatment compared with placebo (RR 2.49, 95% CI 1.64–3.77).

A meta-analysis concluded that RZ is equivalent to INH in terms of efficacy and mortality in the treatment of latent tuberculosis infection. However, this regimen increases the risk of severe adverse effects compared with INH in non-HIV-infected persons [45].

There is insufficient evidence about the long-term effects of prophylaxis on rates of TB and death, and recent studies have found no evidence of benefit in people who are HIV-positive but tuberculin skin test-negative [46].

12.2.4 Summary

TB remains one of the most common causes of illness in the world, both in HIV-infected and uninfected individuals. The diagnostic and therapeutic approach should be the same. Anti-TB chemoprophylaxis may be useful in HIV-positive people who are also tuberculin skin test-positive. However, in areas with constantly high rates of TB exposure, the impact of this is not clear.

Case Presentation 2 (continued)

Her sputum is positive for acid-fast bacilli and she is commenced on rifampicin, isoniazid, pyrazinamide, and ethambutol orally for six months. Sputum culture is positive for *Mycobacterium tuberculosis* which is sensitive to rifampicin, pyrazinamide, and ethambutol but resistant to isoniazid and streptomycin.

The main concern in this patient is to treat her TB infection effectively. She is at some risk of hepatotoxicity (see later). Since this patient's CD4 count is adequate, it may be reasonable not to commence any other potentially hepatotoxic drugs or drugs that potentially may interact with her anti-TB therapy immediately; starting ART can probably be safely deferred. Careful consideration needs to be given to the risk of the patient having multidrug-resistant tuberculosis (MDR-TB). Findings from a meta-analysis of 29 papers found that MDRTB cases were more likely to be foreign born (OR 2.46, 95%

CI 1.86–3.24), younger than 65 years (OR 2.53, 95% CI 1.74–4.83), male (OR 1.38, 95% CI 1.16–1.65), and HIV positive (OR 3.52, 95% CI 2.48–5.01) [47].

12.3 *Pneumocystis Jiroveci (carinii)* Pneumonia

Case Presentation 3

A 42-year-old Zimbabwean nurse presents to the Accident and Emergency Department. He is short of breath on exertion and has a fever of 39 °C, pulse 110 per minute, and a blood pressure of 110/76 mmHg. Pulse oximetry shows an oxygen saturation of 83% on room air. You suspect *Pneumocystis jiroveci* pneumonia (PCP) and wonder how best to investigate and manage him.

PCP remains the most common AIDS-related opportunistic infection (OI), usually occurring among those not receiving primary care (48).

12.3.1 Diagnosis

Kovacs et al. [49] described the differences between the clinical characteristics of PCP in 49 HIV-infected and in 39 HIV-negative persons. At presentation, patients with AIDS had a longer median duration of symptoms (28 vs. 5 days) and higher median room air arterial oxygen tension (69 vs. 52 mmHg, 9.2–6.9 kPa). In HIV-positive patients presenting with respiratory symptoms, the sensitivity of induced sputum for the diagnosis of *P. carinii* was 13% and of BAL 77%. In the sub-group of patients with an adequate induced sputum sample, the sensitivity of induced sputum was 28% [50]. The sensitivity of different stains for detection of *P. carinii* in induced sputum ranges from 92–97% and for bronchoalveolar lavage (BAL) from 81–90% (51). PCR seems to be more sensitive than any of these methods [52,53] although still not in routine clinical use.

Serum beta-D-glucan has a sensitivity of 92% but a specificity of only 86% for detecting PCP, yet may be helpful if positive while awaiting for a bronchoscopy specimen [54].

Typical radiographic features of PCP are bilateral, symmetrical ground-glass opacities, but a wide variety of radiographic findings are observed. In 34 patients, high-resolution computed tomography of the lung showed ground-glass opacities sparing the lung periphery (41% of episodes) or displaying a mosaic pattern (29%), or being nearly homogeneous (24%), ground-glass opacities associated with air-space consolidation (21%), associated with cystic formation (21%), associated with linear-reticular opacities (18%), patchily and irregularly distributed (15%), associated with solitary or multiple nodules (9%), and associated with parenchymal cavity lesions (6%) [55].

12.3.2 Treatment

In the pre-AIDS era, co-trimoxazole (trimethoprim-sulfamethoxazole, TMP-SMX) was shown to be as effective as pentamidine in children with PCP and with fewer side effects [56]. In a study of PCP in HIV, 31 (86%) patients treated with co-trimoxazole and 20 (61%) with pentamidine survived and were without respiratory support at completion of treatment (95% CI for the difference in response, 5 to 45; $p = 0.03$) [57]. Co-trimoxazole caused a rash (44%) and anemia (39%) more frequently ($p = 0.03$), whereas pentamidine caused nephrotoxicity (64%), hypotension (27%), or hypoglycemia (21%) more frequently ($p = 0.01$).

There is evidence from RCTs that corticosteroids are a useful adjunct to therapy in severe PCP. Six studies were included in a meta-analysis [58]. Risk ratios for overall mortality for adjunctive corticosteroids were 0.54 (95% CI 0.38–0.79) at one month and 0.67 (95% CI 0.49–0.93) at three to four months of follow-up. Numbers needed to treat, to prevent one death, are nine patients in a setting without highly active antiretroviral therapy (HAART) available and

22 patients with HAART available. Only the three largest trials provided data on the need for mechanical ventilation with a risk ratio of 0.37 (95% CI 0.20–0.70) in favor of adjunctive corticosteroids.

12.3.3 Alternative Treatments

The combination of clindamycin plus primaquine appears to be the most effective alternative treatment for patients with PCP who are unresponsive to first line therapy [59]. In a meta-analysis of 27 published clinical drug trials, case series, and case reports, 497 patients with microbiologically confirmed PCP (456 with HIV), whose initial antipneumocystis treatment had failed and who required alternative drug therapy, were reviewed. Efficacies of salvage regimens were as follows: clindamycin-primaquine 42–44 (88–92%) of 48 patients, atovaquone 4/5 (80%), eflornithine hydrochloride 40/70 (57%), co-trimoxazole 27/51 (53%), pentamidine 64/164 (39%), and trimetrexate 47/159 (30%).

12.3.4 Summary

PCP remains the most common AIDS-related OI and co-trimoxazole, and if severe, steroids are recommended for its treatment.

Case Presentation 3 (continued)

PCP is suspected on CXR and confirmed on silver staining of BAL fluid, and he recovers well with intravenous co-trimoxazole therapy and steroids. He is continued on oral co-trimoxazole as secondary prophylaxis.

12.4 Antiretroviral Regimen Selection and Adherence

Case Presentation 4

A 28-year-old homeless, intravenous drug user is admitted with widespread psoriasis to the dermatology ward. He is found to have diffuse generalized lymphadenopathy and oral candidiasis. He is tested for HIV and found to be seropositive. His CD4 count is 120 cells/mm^3 and the viral load is >500,000 copies/mL. He is hepatitis C antibody-positive, but HCV RNA-negative. He is hepatitis B surface antigen-negative and HBs antibody and HBc antibody positive. He wants to know what treatment you would recommend for HIV, and you consider what might be useful in helping him to adhere to the treatment plan.

12.4.1 Which Drugs to Start?

The question of which definitive drugs to start in the treatment of naive patients is still unanswered [10] and unlikely to be addressed in a large enough trial due to the huge number of combinations now available. Furthermore virological efficacy is pre-established for most drugs, and trials now are powered on toxicity and reduced adherence. The following were ranked as critical outcomes in the BHIVA grading process: viral suppression at week 48/96, proportion with virological failure, proportion developing resistance, proportion discontinuing for adverse events, proportion with grade 3/4 adverse events. Current guidelines recommend that all patients with HIV commence ART irrespective of CD4 count. Current first-line ART combination strategies are the result of historic developments in antiviral therapy. The 2015 BHIVA guidelines [10] recommend a preferred nucleoside reverse transcriptase inhibitor (NRTI) backbone of tenofovir DF and emtricitabine with an alternative of abacavir and lamivudine. The third agent choice is from the other classes: either the boosted protease inhibitors atazanavir/ritonavir or darunavir/ritonavir (DRV/r), or the NNRTIs efavirenz or rilpivirine, or integrase inhibitors raltegravir or dolutegravir or elvitegravir/cobicistat.

Antiretroviral therapy can slow the progression of liver disease in HCV co-infection, and for most HCV/HIV co-infected patients, even those with cirrhosis, the benefits of ART outweigh the risks of liver toxicity.

12.4.2 Number of Drugs in First-Line Regimen

There is evidence that three drugs are better than two, and two are better than monotherapy [60]. There were 20,404 patients included in the 54 RCTs with 66 comparison groups included in the analysis. For both the clinical outcomes and surrogate markers, combinations with up to, and including, three drugs (HAART) were progressively and significantly more effective. The odds ratio for disease progression or death for triple therapy compared with double therapy was 0.6 (95% CI 0.5–0.8). There was heterogeneity in effect sizes probably related to the different drugs used and differences in trial design.

A Cochrane review has shown that in HIV-infected adults who have responded to an initial three- or four-drug regimen, a two-drug maintenance regimen is associated with a higher risk of virologic failure compared with three or four drugs (OR 5.55, 95% CI 3.14–9.80) [61].

Other induction-maintenance regimens have been studied. The Forte trial compared induction with four drugs and maintenance with three drugs (2 NRTIs, 1 NNRTI, and 1 protease inhibitor (PI) for 24 to 32 weeks, until viral load <50 copies/mL, followed by two NRTIs and one NNRTI, compared with a standard three drug regimen consisting of dual NRTI and a single NNRTI) [62]. More patients in the three-drug arm had virologic failure at 24 weeks, and after 48 weeks more patients in the induction/maintenance arm had viral loads below 50 copies/mL.

In the ESS40013 study, patients were treated with AZT, 3TC, abacavir, and efavirenz for 48 weeks, then randomized to continue with the four-drug regimen or to drop efavirenz [63]. There were no significant differences in the proportions of patients with viral loads below 50 copies/mL and time to treatment failure between the two arms of

the study 48 weeks after withdrawal of efavirenz from the maintenance arm, but the three drug regimen was better tolerated.

12.4.3 Choice of NRTI Backbone

The choice of NRTI backbone depends on this patient's HLA type and evidence of renal disease. Pharmacogenomic screening for HLA-B*5701 is recommended, especially in white populations. In a double-blind, prospective randomized study of 1,956 patients who had not previously received abacavir, the risk of an abacavir hypersensitivity reaction was reduced in patients who had prospective HLA-B*5701 screening (immunologically confirmed hypersensitivity reaction 0% vs. 2.7% in the control group, $p < 0.001$) [64]. As well, there was a significantly lower incidence of clinically diagnosed hypersensitivity reaction in the prospectively screened group (3.4%) than in the control group (7.8%) ($p < 0.001$).

There are contradictorily reported associations between abacavir and increased cardiovascular disease (CVD) [65–67], while tenofovir DF is associated with renal disease [68], which is reduced in the new formulation of tenofovir AF.

A number of studies have been conducted to compare tenofovir DF/emtricitabine with abacavir/lamivudine as the NRTI backbone [69,70]. None have shown differences in clinical endpoints, although 48-week virologic suppression rates favored tenofovir for higher baseline viral loads [70]. Bone mineral density outcomes were better for abacavir/lamivudine over tenofovir DF/emtricitabine [71]. In HBV co-infection, tenofovir DF and emtricitabine are active against HBV, and so are recommended in combination.

12.4.4 Choice of the Third Agent

The choice of the third agent for this patient is influenced by his social circumstances (homelessness and intravenous drug use) and his hepatitis C co-infection. A history of psychiatric illness would preclude the use of efavirenz as it is associated with increased neuropsychiatric toxicity in such patients.

However, in low resource settings, efavirenz remains the main first choice. ACTG 5142 recruited 757 antiretroviral-naive people with a viral load >2,000 copies/mL and any CD4 count (median 182 cells/mm^3) [72]. The open-label design randomized study participants to standard doses of efavirenz or lopinavir/ritonavir with lamivudine and a second NRTI, or to 533/133 mg of lopinavir/ritonavir twice daily plus standard-dose efavirenz. The time to virologic failure proved significantly faster in people who started lopinavir/ritonavir as the third agent rather than efavirenz ($p = 0.006$).

The results of the five-year FIRST trial CPCRA 058 that compared a PI plus NRTI versus NNRTI plus NRTI versus a three-class strategy supported the results of ACTG 5142 in finding a better virologic response to first line NNRTIs than PIs (HR 1.42, 95% CI 1.23–1.64) [73]. However, the study found no difference between NNRTI and PI regimens in a composite endpoint including CD4 drop, progression to AIDS, and death (NNRTI versus PI hazard ratios (HRs) for the composite endpoint were 1.02 [95% CI 0.79–1.31], 1.07 [0.80–1.41], 0.95 [0.66–1.37], and 0.66 [0.56–0.78], respectively).

In the recent BHIVA guidelines [10], efavirenz is demoted to an alternative to other newer drugs due mainly to its increased toxicity. In a comparison of the NNRTI rilpivirine with efavirenz (74–76), there was no significant difference in overall virological success at weeks 48 or 96. There were, however, differences in drug resistance and viral failure favouring efavirenz especially if viral load was above 100,000 copies/mL, but rilpivirine was associated with fewer discontinuations for adverse events.

Efavirenz was however found to be inferior to the integrase inhibitor dolutegravir (DTG) in the SINGLE study [77]. In 833 subjects, there was superior virological control in the DTG/abacavir/lamivudine group than in the efavirenz/tenofovir/emtricitabine group at week 48 (88% vs. 81% < 50 copies/ml,

$p = 0.003$). Those taking DTG-ABC-3TC also had a significantly shorter median time to viral suppression (28 vs. 84 days, $p < 0.001$), as well as greater increases in CD4+ T-cell count (267 vs. 208 cells/mm^3, $p < 0.001$). Only 2% discontinued therapy in the DTG-ABC-3TC group compared to 10% in the EFV-TDF-FTC group mainly due to rash and neuropsychiatric events (abnormal dreams, anxiety, dizziness, and somnolence). However, insomnia was more common in the DTG group.

In fact, most studies now confirm dolutegravir to be superior to the comparator agent. For example, compared to boosted darunavir in the FLAMINGO study [78], the proportion of participants with undetectable HIV RNA was 80% in the DTG arm versus 68% in the DRV/r arm at week 96. This was especially true in people with a high baseline viral load (82% vs. 52%). The main drug-related adverse events were diarrhoea, nausea, and headache, which were significantly more common in the DRV/r (24%) group than DTG (10%). Dolutegravir was also non-inferior to the twice-a-day integrase inhibitor raltegravir in the SPRING-2 study [79]. At week 96, 81% in the dolutegravir group and 76% in the raltegravir group had an undetectable viral load (adjusted difference 4.5%, 95% CI 1.1%–10.0%).

12.4.5 Drug-drug Interactions Associated with HAART

Aside from virologic and immunologic efficacy, there are other considerations when selecting combinations for individual patients. Importantly, drug-drug interactions between rifampicin as part of antituberculosis therapy and the boosted protease inhibitors are a key consideration in selecting regimens for TB/HIV co-infected patients. Dose adjustment is also required with integrase inhibitors.

There are complex interactions between antiretroviral drugs and with other drugs. It is always worth checking and new interactions are still being described. The website http://www.hiv-druginteractions.org is a useful resource for ARVs, and for hepatitis C directly acting antiviral drugs (DAA), use http://hcvguidelines.org/. Dolutegravir does not interact with methadone [80].

12.4.6 Therapeutic Drug Monitoring

There are no randomized controlled data to support therapeutic drug monitoring routinely, but in a pharmacologic sub-study of VIRADAPT, the impact of plasma protease inhibitor trough levels on changes in HIV RNA were assessed in 81 patients treated with genotype guided therapy [81]. Multivariate analysis showed PI plasma concentrations to be an independent predictor of evolution of HIV-RNA drug resistance ($p = 0.017$).

12.4.7 Compliance/Adherence

Compliance has been shown to be an important factor in the long-term outcome of treatment. It may be that the easiest drug combination to comply with will be the most effective irrespective of drug potency or resistance profile. Adherence to any long-term drug regimen is difficult; however, it is of particular importance in the treatment of HIV because of the propensity of the virus to mutate and escape drug control. Good adherence can predict for viral suppression and the development of viral resistance is associated with low blood drug levels that are usually because of poor adherence [82,83]. After controlling for potential confounding variables, patients who were less than 95% adherent to medications were 3.5 times more likely to have treatment failure (HIV-1 RNA >50 copies/mL) than subjects with adherence rates of 95–100%. The strongest predictor of adherence was adverse clinical events (e.g., dermatologic, gastrointestinal symptoms): patients with adverse events were 12.8 times less likely to have 95–100% adherence [84].

To assess the effect of HAART adherence on survival in HIV-infected patients, a cohort study was performed on 1,219 patients who began ART during the period 1990–1999.

In multivariate analysis, adherence was associated with a significant difference with respect to mortality (non-adherence: RH 3.87, 95% CI 1.77–8.46) [85]. A systematic review of 76 studies showed that once or twice a day was better than more frequent dosing (compliance with one dose: 79% ± 14%; two doses: 69% ± 15%; three doses: 65% ± 16%; four doses: 51% ± 20% ($p < 0.001$ among dose schedules, no significant difference between one and two doses) [86].

The principal factors associated with non-adherence for HAART appear to be mainly patient-related, including homelessness and substance and alcohol abuse, reflecting the types of individuals affected by HIV [87]. Other factors may also contribute, such as inconvenient dosing frequency, dietary restrictions, pill burden, side effects [88], patient healthcare provider relationships, and the system of care [89].

Text messaging interventions improved adherence overall (odds ratio [OR] 1.48, 95% credible interval [CrI] 1.00–2.16), including in Low and Middle Income Countries (LMIC) (1.49, 1.04–2.09) [90]. Multiple interventions were better than single interventions. Cognitive behavioral therapy (CBT) (1.46, 1.05–2.12) and supportive interventions (1.28, 1.01–1.71) were superior overall in a global network, but no technique was shown to improve viral response in LMIC. Overall, it was found that the beneficial effects of interventions waned over time.

A systematic review on the effectiveness of patient support and education to improve adherence to HAART identified 19 RCTs involving 2,159 participants [91]. Study interventions included cognitive behavioral therapy, motivational interviewing, medication management strategies, and interventions indirectly targeting adherence, such as programs to reduce risky sexual behaviors. There is evidence that interventions targeting practical medication management skills and those delivered over at least 12 weeks were associated with improved adherence. Interventions administered to individuals were more effective than group interventions. There was no evidence that interventions targeting women or patients with a history of alcoholic abuse were effective. Overall, effective adherence interventions have not been shown to be associated with improved virologic or immunologic outcomes.

12.4.8 Toxicity

Toxicity is also a determinant of a successful regimen both in terms of tolerability and adherence. Liver enzyme elevation (LEE) defined as transaminases greater than five times baseline or >100 IU/L is commonly observed after combination HAART is begun. Hepatitis B surface antigen (HBsAg) positivity, the use of NRTI, age greater than 40 years, an absolute CD4 count of <310 cells/mm^3, and coexisting hepatitis C infection have all been shown to be significantly associated with hepatotoxicity [92,93].

In a retrospective study of 394 patients, 7% were HBsAg-positive and 14% were anti-HCV-positive [94]. Patients with chronic hepatitis had a higher risk for LEE compared with patients without co-infection: 37% versus 12%, respectively. After adjustment for higher baseline transaminases, the presence of HBsAg or anti-HCV remained associated with an increased risk of LEE (RR 2.78, 95% CI 1.50–5.16 and RR 2.46, 95% CI 1.43–4.24, respectively). In patients with LEE, transaminases declined whether HAART was continued or modified.

In the Swiss cohort, a prospective analysis revealed 1,157 patients (37.2%) were co-infected with HCV, 1,015 of whom (87.7%) had a history of intravenous drug use [94]. In multivariate Cox's regression, the probability of progression to a new AIDS-defining clinical event or to death was independently associated with HCV seropositivity (HR 1.7, 95% CI 1.26–2.30), and with active intravenous drug use (HR 1.38, 95% CI 1.02–1.88). Virologic response to HAART and the probability of treatment change were not associated with HCV serostatus. In contrast, HCV seropositivity was associated with a smaller CD4 cell recovery (HR for a CD4 cell count

increase of at least 50 cells/mm^3 0.79, 95% CI 0.72–0.87). Newer agents are better tolerated but long term data is lacking [95].

There is a significantly elevated risk of severe liver disease in persons who are co-infected with HIV and HCV. A meta-analysis to quantify the effect of HIV co-infection on progressive liver disease in persons with HCV revealed eight studies that included outcomes of histologic cirrhosis or decompensated liver disease [96]. These studies yielded a combined adjusted RR of 2.92 (95% CI 1.70–5.01). Studies that examined decompensated liver disease had a combined RR of 6.14 (95% CI 2.86–13.20), whereas studies that examined histologic cirrhosis had a pooled RR of 2.07 (95% CI 1.40–3.07). Current guidelines suggest that there should be no special considerations between treating HCV mono or co-infected patients. Use of Directly Acting Antivirals for HCV should be guided by HCV genotype, hepatic fibrosis stage, and previous treatment [97].

12.4.9 Summary

There is no randomized trial evidence as to which drug regimen is most efficacious clinically. There is convincing evidence that three drugs are better than two or one. Dual nucleosides are the standard backbone in HAART. There seems to be little to choose between NNRTIs and boosted PIs when considering the third agent; however, integrase inhibitors seem to have better tolerability. In this case, dolutegravir may be preferred due to the simplicity of one tablet once a day in a co-formulation with abacavir-lamivudine if the patient is HLA-B*5701 negative. Dolutegravir is well tolerated and has few interactions including with recreational drugs.

Adherence to HAART is critically important, and to facilitate this, drug regimens are becoming simpler, many with once-a-day drugs and no food or fluid restrictions. Once-a-day medications can be given as directly observed therapy combined, for example, with methadone [98] although there are important interactions with methadone and HAART [99]. There is still no consensus on how best to measure adherence. The studies to try to improve adherence through social means and education have been disappointing. Hepatotoxicity remains a challenge especially in the many patients who have coexisting liver disease who may be taking other hepatotoxic drugs. There is a high incidence of substance abuse and psychiatric illness among HIV-positive patients, which complicates the ability to take treatment [100].

Case Presentation 4 (continued)

After discussion and social support, he is commenced on a once-a-day combination of abacavir/lamivudine and dolutegravir. His drug use is also stabilized on methadone with appropriate counselling. He is at risk of opportunistic infections and so he is also started on co-trimoxazole initially. He develops a widespread maculopapular rash with nausea and vomiting. A diagnosis of co-trimoxazole hypersensitivity is made. What are the options for patients who cannot tolerate TMX/SMX?

12.5 Opportunistic Infection Prophylaxis

Although the risk of opportunistic infection has fallen in recent years, it increases dramatically once a patient's CD4 count is less than 200 cells/mm^3 [48]. In the United Kingdom, around 39% of patients presented with a CD4 < 350 cells/mm^3 in 2015 [101].

12.5.1 Prophylaxis for PCP

There have been two systematic reviews analyzing the data on therapy for PCP prophylaxis: Ioannidis et al. searching in 1995 and covering 35 RCTs [102], and Bucher et al. from 1997 [103] covering 22 trials. Both of these were before the widespread introduction of HAART. Since then, the incidence of OIs in HIV patients has fallen so much that

further studies are unlikely. The main focus has been on stopping prophylaxis after immune restoration.

The first systematic review [102] found that prophylaxis with co-trimoxazole or aerosolized pentamidine reduced the incidence of PCP more than placebo (RR 0.32, 95% CI 0.23–0.46) and that co-trimoxazole was more effective at preventing PCP than aerosolized pentamidine (RR 0.58, 95% CI 0.45–0.75). The second [103] found that co-trimoxazole was significantly more effective in preventing PCP than dapsone/pyrimethamine (RR 0.49, 95% CI 0.26–0.92). While this also showed that co-trimoxazole compared with dapsone (with or without pyrimethamine) was more effective, the result did not reach statistical significance (RR 0.61, 95% CI 0.34–1.10).

There is no significant difference in the rate of PCP infection between lower dose (160/800 mg 3 times weekly or 80/400 mg daily) and higher dose (160/800 mg daily) co-trimoxazole, although severe adverse effects (predominantly rash, fever, and hematologic effects leading to discontinuation within 1 year) occurred in more people taking higher doses of co-trimoxazole than lower doses (25% vs. 15%) [102].

One RCT of 545 people in sub-Saharan Africa with symptomatic disease (second or third clinical stage disease in the WHO staging system) regardless of CD4 cell count, comparing co-trimoxazole with placebo, found no significant difference in incidence of PCP or toxoplasmosis. Patients taking co-trimoxazole were less likely to suffer a serious event (death or hospital admission, irrespective of the cause) than those on placebo regardless of their initial CD4 cell count (84 vs. 124, HR 0.57, 95% CI 0.43–0.75, $p < 0.001$). This implies that in Africa the greater effect of co-trimoxazole is on preventing bacterial infections, not PCP [104].

The gradual initiation of co-trimoxazole may improve tolerance of the regimen (17% vs. 33% at 12 weeks) [105]. Dapsone, aerosolized pentamidine, and atovaquone are effective in persons intolerant of co-trimoxazole [106,107].

12.5.2 Concomitant Coverage for Toxoplasmosis

Co-trimoxazole was more effective at preventing toxoplasmosis than aerosolized pentamidine (RR 0.78, 95% CI 0.55–1.11), but there was no significant difference between co-trimoxazole and dapsone/pyrimethamine (RR 1.17, 95% CI 0.68–2.04) [103]. Aerosolized pentamidine is not recommended for toxoplasmosis prophylaxis. Toxoplasmosis risk is probably clinically meaningful only with CD4 < 100 cells/mm^3 and positive toxoplasma serology [108].

12.5.3 Summary

Co-trimoxazole is the recommended prophylactic agent for PCP, with an efficacy of around 80%. Patients who experience adverse events (grade 3 or less) may tolerate gradual reintroduction of co-trimoxazole or administering drug at a reduced dose.

Case Presentation 4 (continued)

The patient is commenced on dapsone along with abacavir, lamivudine, and dolutegravir. His viral load falls to undetectable, and CD4 count climbs to 320 cells/mm^3 within six months. He has some problems with recurrent oral cold sores. You wonder how to manage his herpes infection and when his PCP prophylaxis can be safely stopped.

12.6 Treatment of Herpes Simplex

In the case of severe or frequent recurrences of orolabial herpes, episodic or suppressive therapy may be considered. Topical antiviral agents should be avoided. For severe mucocutaneous disease it is suggested that acyclovir be administered intravenously. Famciclovir and valacyclovir are effective for the suppression of herpes simplex virus (HSV) [109] and valacyclovir has been shown to be equivalent to acyclovir [110].

12.7 Stopping Opportunistic Infection prophylaxis

12.7.1 Stopping *Pneumocystis* Prophylaxis

In the meta-analysis of 14 randomized and nonrandomized studies with 3,584 subjects who had discontinued prophylaxis when their CD4 count was sustained >200 cells/mm^3 for three months, eight cases of PCP occurred during 3,449 person-years (0.23 cases per 100 person-years; 95% CI 0.10–0.46) [111]. Neither of the two RCTs identified in the review found any cases of PCP after discontinuation [112,113]. A total of 146 patients were enrolled in a randomized study of stopping secondary prophylaxis (77 in the treatment discontinuation arm) [114]. After >2 years, one definitive and one presumptive case of PCP were observed, both of which occurred in patients who discontinued therapy.

Nineteen patients with suppressed viral loads but CD4 counts below 200 cells/mm^3 were followed after prophylaxis was discontinued. Eleven had been taking daily TMP-SMX, seven were receiving monthly aerosolized pentamidine, and one patient never received any prophylaxis [115]. The median CD4 count at the time of discontinuation and at the most recent determination was 120 (range 34–184) and 138 (range 6–201) cells/mm^3, respectively. At the time of reporting, patients had been off PCP prophylaxis for a median of 9.0 (range 3–39) months (261 patient-months). No patient developed PCP. This is significantly different from the risk of developing PCP with a CD4 count of <200 cells/mm^3 in untreated HIV infection (rate difference 9.2%, 95% CI 5.7–12.8%, $p < 0.05$).

There is also no change in incidence of other bacterial infections after stopping prophylaxis [116].

12.7.2 Toxoplasmosis Prophylaxis

The efficacy of a thrice-weekly regimen was similar to that of a daily regimen in the prevention of relapses of toxoplasma encephalitis in a RCT in 124 Spanish patients.

Administration of antiretroviral therapy was the only factor associated with a lower incidence of relapse [117].

Two RCT's guide when to stop prophylaxis. The first, which was included in the systematic review, found no cases of toxoplasma encephalitis at six months in people discontinuing prophylaxis (see PCP above) [113]. The second RCT (381 people with a satisfactory response to HAART) compared discontinuation with continuation of toxoplasma prophylaxis [118]. After a median of 10 months it found no episodes of toxoplasma encephalitis in either group. Maintenance therapy can be discontinued after six months of successful suppression of HIV viral replication and elevation of CD4 count to >200 cells/ul.

12.8 Other Opportunistic Infections

Case Presentation 4 (continued)

He returns after six months with CD4 now 400 cells/mm^3 and viral load undetectable. However, after the death of a close friend, it soon becomes apparent that he has developed a chaotic lifestyle, abusing substances, and has problems with taking regular medication. He decides not to attend the clinic for a while and is lost to follow-up. After three years he returns with a CD4 count of 50 cells/mm^3 and an increasing viral load. The patient decides not to continue with therapy and is adamant that he no longer wants any in the future. He is admitted with increasing confusion, fever, and neck stiffness. Fundoscopy reveals CMV retinitis but no papilledema. His CD4 count is 10 cells/mm^3. You consider the possible conditions he is at risk of and how best to manage him.

Table 12.1 lists the usual pathogens related to CD4 count.

Cryptococcal meningitis should be excluded by lumbar puncture. CSF examination (Gram stain or India Ink) may reveal yeast forms and cryptococcal antigen (CrAg) may be detected. The opening pressure is elevated in 60–80% of patients with cryptococcal meningitis [119].

Case Presentation 4 (continued)

The opening pressure is 33 mm of CSF, and CSF is positive for *Cryptococcus* with a white cell count of 115, mainly lymphocytes; a CSF protein of 0.98 g/L (normal <0.45 g/L), and a glucose of 0.6 mmol/L. A diagnosis of cryptococcal meningitis is made.

12.8.1 Treatment of Cryptococcal Meningitis

In a double-blind multi-center study, patients with a first episode of AIDS-associated cryptococcal meningitis were randomly assigned to treatment with higher dose amphotericin B (0.7 mg/kg per day) with or without flucytosine (100 mg/kg per day) for two weeks (step 1), followed by eight weeks of treatment with itraconazole (400 mg per day) or fluconazole (400 mg per day) (step 2) [120]. At two weeks, the CSF cultures were negative in 60% of the 202 patients receiving amphotericin B plus flucytosine and in 51% of the 179 receiving amphotericin B alone ($p = 0.06$). The clinical outcome did not differ significantly between the two groups. Overall mortality was 5.5% in the first two weeks and 3.9% in the next eight weeks, with no significant difference between the groups. In a multivariate analysis, the addition of flucytosine during the initial two weeks and treatment with fluconazole for the next eight weeks were independently associated with CSF sterilization.

There is one direct comparison between amphotericin B deoxycholate (0.7 mg/kg per day) and liposomal amphotericin (AmBisome) (4 mg/kg per day) in 27 patients showing that AmBisome therapy resulted in earlier negative CSF cultures [121]. The liposomal amphotericin was less nephrotoxic and this has been confirmed in other studies in HIV-positive patients [122].

In a randomized trial comparing amphotericin B and fluconazole, treatment was successful in 25 of the 63 amphotericin B recipients (40%; 95% CI 26–53) and in 44 of the 131 fluconazole recipients (34%, 95% CI 25–42, $p = 0.40$) [123]. There was no significant

Table 12.1 Pathogens related to CD4 counts.

CD4 count	Infection	Non-infectious complications
>500	Acute HIV syndrome	Progressive generalized lymphadenopathy
	Candida vaginitis	Polymyositis
		Aseptic meningitis
		Guillain–Barré syndrome
200–500	Pneumococcal and other bacterial pneumonia	Carcinoma in situ
	Pulmonary tuberculosis	Cervical cancer
	Kaposi sarcoma	Lymphocytic interstitial pneumonitis
	Herpes zoster	Mononeuritis multiplex
	Thrush	Anemia
	Cryptosporidiosis, self-limiting	Idiopathic thrombocytopenia purpura
	Oral hairy leukoplakia	
<200	*Pnemocystis carinii* pneumonia	Wasting
	Candida esophagitis	B-cell lymphoma
	Disseminated/chronic herpes simplex	Cardiomyopathy
	Toxoplasmosis	Peripheral neuropathy
	Cryptococcosis	HIV-associated dementia
	Disseminated histoplasmosis	CNS lymphoma
	Disseminated coccidiomycosis	HIV-associated nephropathy
	Chronic cryptosporidiosis	
	Progressive multifocal leukoencephalopathy (PMLE)	
	Microsporidiosis	
	Miliary/extrapulmonary tuberculosis	
<50	CMV disease	
	Disseminated *Mycobacteruim avium* complex	

Reproduced by permission of Bartlett, JG, Gallant JE. Medical Management of HIV Infection. Johns Hopkins University 2007.

difference between the groups in overall mortality owing to cryptococcosis (amphotericin vs. fluconazole, 9 of 63 [4%] vs. 24 of 131 [8%], $p = 0.48$); however, mortality during the first two weeks of therapy was higher in the fluconazole group (15% vs. 8%, $p = 0.25$). Multivariate analyses identified abnormal mental status (lethargy, somnolence, or obtundation) as the most important predictive factor of death during therapy ($p < 0.0001$). In Africa, 30 patients were randomized to receive combination therapy with fluconazole (200 mg once a day for 2 months) and flucytosine (150 mg/kg per day)

for the first two weeks, and 28 to receive fluconazole alone. Patients in both groups who survived for two months continued fluconazole as maintenance therapy at a dose of 200 mg three times per week for four months. The combination therapy prevented death within two weeks and significantly increased the survival rate among patients (32%) at six months over that among patients receiving monotherapy (12%) ($p = 0.022$) [124].

Oral itraconazole (200 mg twice a day) for six weeks was less effective than amphotericin B (0.3 mg/kg per day) plus flucytosine

(150 mg/kg daily) in 28 patients [125]. Maintenance therapy with fluconazole has been shown to be superior to amphotericin B with less toxicity and lower rates of relapse [126].

The standard guidelines for treatment of cryptococcal meningitis have recommended two weeks of amphotericin B at a dose of 0.7 mg/kg per day (with flucytosine) followed by fluconazole at a dose of 400 mg per day for another eight weeks. However liposomal amphotericin B (4 mg/kg/day) is the preferred preparation because of the reduced risk of nephrotoxicity.

The importance of controlling the raised intracranial pressure associated with cryptococcal meningitis by repeated lumbar puncture or CSF drainage was established in a retrospective analysis of 221 patients in the van der Horst study [120]. After receiving antifungal therapy, those patients whose CSF pressure was reduced by >10 mm or did not change had more frequent clinical response at two weeks than did those whose pressure increased >10 mm ($p = 0.001$). Patients with pretreatment opening pressure of <250 mmHg had increased short-term survival compared with those with higher pressure [119]. This was confirmed in a small prospective study of 10 patients with raised ICP treated with CSF drainage [127]. Recurrent lumbar punctures or ventriculoperitoneal shunting should be considered in those with persistent raised ICP.

A double bind placebo controlled study on the effect of dexamethasone or placebo in patients with HIV presenting with cryptococcal meningitis showed increased mortality in the dexamethasone group, and steroid treatment is generally not recommended for this infection [128].

12.8.2 Prophylaxis Against Fungal Infection

Five studies were identified in a Cochrane review of interventions for the primary prevention of cryptococcal disease [129]. The authors concluded that prophylaxis with either itraconazole or fluconazole was effective

(RR 0.21, 95% CI 0.09–0.46 compared with placebo; $n = 1,316$); however, neither had a clear effect on overall mortality. One RCT found that there were more relapses of successfully treated cryptococcal meningitis with itraconazole compared with fluconazole (13/57, 23% vs. 2/51, 4%; ARR 19%, 95% CI 6.2–31.7; RR 0.17, 95% CI 0.04–0.71; NNT 5, 95% CI 3–16) [130].

A Cochrane review included nine studies of interventions for the prevention of oropharyngeal candidiasis [131]. Fluconazole was effective in preventing clinical episodes compared with placebo (RR 0.61, 95% CI 0.5–0.74) and compared with no treatment (RR 0.16, 95% CI 0.08–0.34). In a RCT comparing dosing regimen, there was no difference in the rate of invasive fungal infections between fluconazole 200 mg daily with 400 mg once weekly over a follow-up of 74 weeks (8% vs. 6%; ARR 2.2%, 95% CI 1.7% –6.1) [132]. However, the incidence of oral candidiasis was twice as common in people taking the weekly dose.

There is one open-label uncontrolled study (44 people), which found that itraconazole may be effective in preventing the relapse of histoplasmosis [133].

12.8.3 Mycobacterium Avium Complex Infection

12.8.3.1 Mycobacterium Avium Complex Treatment

HIV-positive patients ($n = 246$) with disseminated *Mycobacterium avium* complex (MAC) received either clarithromycin 500 mg twice a day, azithromycin 250 mg every day, azithromycin 600 mg every day, or each combined with ethambutol, for 24 weeks. The azithromycin 250 mg arm of the study was dropped after an interim analysis showed a lower rate of clearance of bacteremia. At 24 weeks of therapy, the likelihood of patients developing two consecutive negative cultures (46% vs. 56%, $p = 0.24$) or one negative culture (59% vs. 61%, $p = 0.80$) was similar for azithromycin 600 mg ($n = 68$) and clarithromycin ($n = 57$), respectively. The likelihood of relapse was 39% versus 27%

($p = 0.21$) on azithromycin compared with clarithromycin, respectively. Of the six patients who experienced relapse, none of those randomized to receive azithromycin developed isolates resistant to macrolides, compared with two of three patients randomized to receive clarithromycin. Mortality was similar in patients comprising each arm of the study (69% vs. 63%, HR 1.1, 95% CI 0.7–1.7) [134]. Although clarithromycin is associated with more rapid clearance of MAC from the blood [135], azithromycin is better tolerated and has fewer drug interactions [136]. HIV patients with disseminated MAC disease ($n = 85$) were randomized to receive a three-drug regimen of clarithromycin, rifabutin or clofazimine, and ethambutol. Two dosages of clarithromycin, 500 or 1,000 mg twice daily, were compared [137]. After a mean follow-up of 4.5 months, 10 (22%) of 45 patients receiving clarithromycin at 500 mg twice daily had died (70 deaths per 100 person-years) compared with 17 (43%) of 40 patients receiving clarithromycin at 1,000 mg twice daily (158 deaths per 100 person-years) (RR 2.43, 95% CI 1.11–5.34, $p = 0.02$). After 10.4 months, 20 (49%) of 41 patients receiving rifabutin had died (81 deaths per 100 person-years) compared with 23 (52%) of 44 patients receiving clofazimine (94 deaths per 100 person-years) (RR 1.20, 95% CI 0.65–2.19, $p = 0.56$). Bacteriologic outcomes were similar among treatment groups. In treating MAC disease in HIV patients, the recommended maximum dose of clarithromycin is 500 mg twice daily.

12.8.3.2 Prophylaxis

Prospective cohort studies have found that the risk of disseminated MAC disease increases substantially with a lower CD4 count, but was clinically important only for CD4 < 50 cells/mm^3 [108].

A RCT study comparing clarithromycin with placebo enrolled 194 patients: 111 patients were started on clarithromycin and 83 placebo. MAC infection developed in 19 of 333 patients (6%) receiving clarithromycin and 53 of 334 (16%) in the placebo group

(adjusted hazard ratio 0.31, 95% CI 0.18–.53, $p < 0.001$). During the follow up period of 10 months, 32% of patients in the clarithromycin group died and 41% in the placebo group died (hazard ratio, 0.75, $p = 0.026$) [138].

Azithromycin once weekly reduced the incidence of MAC more than placebo (11% vs. 25%, $p = 0.004$). Gastrointestinal side effects were more likely with azithromycin than with placebo, but they were rarely severe enough to cause discontinuation of treatment (8% vs. 2% in the two arms, $p = 0.14$) [139].

A Cochrane review of interventions for the prevention of Mycobacterium avium in patients with HIV included eight studies and concluded azithromycin or clarithromycin are the prophylactic agents of choice (140).

12.8.3.3 Stopping MAC Prophylaxis

In 643 HIV-1-infected patients, with a previous CD4 cell count <50 cells/mm^3 and a sustained increase to >100 cells/mm^3 during HAART, given azithromycin 1200 mg once weekly ($n = 321$), or matching placebo ($n = 322$), there were two cases of MAC infection among the 321 patients assigned to placebo (incidence rate, 0.5 events per 100 person-years; 95% CI 0.06–1.83 events per 100 person-years) compared with no cases among the 322 patients assigned to azithromycin (95% CI 0–0.92 events per 100 person years), resulting in a treatment difference of 0.5 events per 100 person-years (95% CI 0.20–1.21 events per 100 person-years) for placebo versus azithromycin [141]. Both cases were atypical in that MAC was localized to the vertebral spine. Patients receiving azithromycin were more likely than those receiving placebo to discontinue treatment with the study drug permanently because of adverse events (8% vs. 2%. HR 0.24, 95% CI 0.10–0.57).

A second RCT compared azithromycin with placebo in 520 people without previous MAC disease with CD4 > 100 cells/mm^3 in response to HAART. There were no episodes of confirmed MAC disease in either group over a median follow-up of 12 months [142]. Patients responding to ARVs can discontinue with CD4 count rises above 100 cells/mm^3. A cut-off of above 50 cells/mm^3 is supported by some data [138].

12.8.3.4 Summary

Clarithromycin or azithromycin are recommended to reduce the incidence of MAC. Data supports stopping prophylaxis in patients responding to ART with CD4 counts above 100 cells/mm.^{3}

12.9 Cytomegalovirus (CMV) Infection

12.9.1 Treatment of Cytomegalovirus

Ganciclovir and foscarnet have been the mainstays of treatment of CMV disease [143]. With the availability of oral valganciclovir, this drug was compared with intravenous ganciclovir as induction therapy for newly diagnosed CMV retinitis in 160 patients with AIDS. After four weeks, all patients received valganciclovir as maintenance therapy. Of the patients who could be evaluated, 7 of 70 assigned to intravenous ganciclovir (10.0%) and 7 of 71 assigned to oral valganciclovir (9.9%) had progression of CMV retinitis during the first four weeks (difference in proportions, 0.1 percentage point, 95% CI –9.7–10.0); 47 of 61 patients (77.0%) assigned to intravenous ganciclovir and 46 of 64 (71.9%) assigned to valganciclovir had a satisfactory response to induction therapy (difference in proportions, 5.2 percentage points, 95% CI 20.4–10.1). The median times to progression of retinitis were 125 days in the group assigned to intravenous ganciclovir and 160 days in the group assigned to oral valganciclovir. The frequency and severity of adverse events were similar in the two treatment groups [144]. A double-blind placebo-controlled trial of 62 patients with biopsy proven CMV colitis showed a significant reduction in CMV-positive colonic and urine cultures were seen with ganciclovir ($p = 0.034$ and $p < 0.001$, respectively, compared with placebo. New extra-colonic CMV disease developed in 23%

of 30 placebo patients and 9% of ganciclovir patients ($p = 0.026$) [145]. Ganciclovir and foscarnet are equivalent in efficacy, but renal side effects are an important limitation of foscarnet [146].

12.9.2 Prophylaxis for Cytomegalovirus

No prophylaxis is needed for gastrointestinal CMV, unless there is evidence of relapse [146]. Maintenance therapy for CMV retinitis can be stopped where there is response to ART with CD4 > 100 cells/mm^3 and undetectable viral load.

Case Presentation 4 (continued)

The patient improves with amphotericin and is discharged home on oral fluconazole; however, he presents again three months later with increasing confusion. CT scan shows no focal lesions and CSF obtained by lumbar puncture shows neither evidence of cryptococcal infection nor any white cells. You review the causes of confusion in late HIV disease.

12.10 AIDS Dementia Complex

There is little currently data to support any specific ART combination in the management of patients with AIDS dementia complex.

12.11 Progressive Multifocal Leukoencephalopathy (PMLE)

PMLE affects between 4–8% of patients with advanced HIV disease, and survival after the diagnosis of leukoencephalopathy averages only about three months. With effective administration of ART, the prognosis for these patients has substantially improved. Diagnosis is based on MRI findings. More advanced neuroimaging techniques may provide greater diagnostic accuracy [147]. PCR of CSF yielded sensitivity and specificity values of up to 100% and 90%, respectively [148], in the pre-ART era, but post-ART, the sensitivity has fallen to around 50% [149]. This probably reflects reduced viral replication and increased viral clearance. PMLE may present in patients on ART, in the setting of initiating ART, or as part of an immune reconstitution syndrome.

Case Presentation 4 (continued)

CSF samples are sent for JC virus PCR and this is positive. MRI scans show typical changes of PMLE. Lymph node biopsy does not show any evidence of lymphoma nor of Mycobacterium avium-intracellulare. He deteriorates further and dies in a hospice two months later.

There is no specific therapy for PMLE or JC virus infection. The mainstay of therapy is to reverse immunosuppression. ART halts the progression of disease in around 50% of patients. Most often neurological deficits persists, but some patients experience improvement [150,151].

Acknowledgements

The authors are indebted to the work contained in Clinical Evidence in HIV (http://clinicalevidence.bmj.com/ceweb/conditions/hiv/0902/0902_contribdetails.jsp) by Professor Margaret Johnson, Professor David Wilkinson, and Professor Andrew Phillips, published by BMJ Publishing Group Ltd, as a basis for this work.

References

1 Moyer VA, U. S. Preventive Services Task Force. Screening for HIV: U.S. Preventive Services Task Force Recommendation Statement. Ann Intern Med. 2013 Jul 02;159(1):51–60. PubMed PMID: 23698354.

2 Wood E, Kerr T, Rowell G, Montaner JS, Phillips P, Korthuis PT, et al. Does this adult patient have early HIV infection?: The Rational Clinical Examination systematic review. JAMA. 2014 Jul 16;312(3):278–85. PubMed PMID: 25027143.

3 Braun DL, Kouyos RD, Balmer B, Grube C, Weber R, Gunthard HF. Frequency and spectrum of unexpected clinical manifestations of primary HIV-1 infection. Clin Infect Dis. 2015 Sep 15;61(6):1013–21. PubMed PMID: 25991469.

4 Gokengin D, Geretti AM, Begovac J, Palfreeman A, Stevanovic M, Tarasenko O, et al. 2014 European guideline on HIV testing. Int J STD AIDS. 2014 Sep;25(10):695–704. PubMed PMID: 24759563.

5 Centers for Disease Control and Prevention and Association of Public Health Laboratories. Laboratory testing for the diagnosis of HIV infection: updated recommendations. Available at http://stackscdcgov/view/cdc/23447. 2014 Published June 27, 2014.

6 Peters PJ, Westheimer E, Cohen S, Hightow-Weidman LB, Moss N, Tsoi B, et al. Screening yield of HIV antigen/antibody combination and pooled HIV RNA testing for acute HIV infection in a high-prevalence population. JAMA. 2016 Feb 16;315(7):682–90. PubMed PMID: 26881371.

7 Tan WS, Chow EP, Fairley CK, Chen MY, Bradshaw CS, Read TR. Sensitivity of HIV rapid tests compared with fourth-generation enzyme immunoassays or HIV RNA tests. AIDS. 2016 Jul 31;30(12):1951–60. PubMed PMID: 27124900.

8 Pai NP, Balram B, Shivkumar S, Martinez-Cajas JL, Claessens C, Lambert G, et al. Head-to-head comparison of accuracy of a rapid point-of-care HIV test with oral versus whole-blood specimens: a systematic review and meta-analysis. Lancet Infect Dis. 2012 May;12(5):373–80. PubMed PMID: WOS:000303422700017.

9 Lewis JM, Macpherson P, Adams ER, Ochodo E, Sands A, Taegtmeyer M. Field accuracy of fourth-generation rapid diagnostic tests for acute HIV-1: a systematic review. AIDS. 2015 Nov 28;29(18):2465–71. PubMed PMID: 26558545. Pubmed Central PMCID: PMC4645957.

10 Churchill D, Waters L, Ahmed N, Angus B, Boffito M, Bower M, et al. British HIV Association guidelines for the treatment of HIV-1-positive adults with antiretroviral therapy 2015. HIV Med. 2016 Aug;17 Suppl 4:s2–s104. PubMed PMID: 27568911.

11 Gunthard HF, Saag MS, Benson CA, del Rio C, Eron JJ, Gallant JE, et al. Antiretroviral drugs for treatment and prevention of HIV infection in adults: 2016 Recommendations of the International Antiviral Society-USA Panel. JAMA. 2016 Jul 12;316(2):191–210. PubMed PMID: 27404187. Pubmed Central PMCID: PMC5012643.

12 Kitahata MM, Gange SJ, Abraham AG, Merriman B, Saag MS, Justice AC, et al. Effect of early versus deferred antiretroviral therapy for HIV on survival. N Engl J Med. 2009 Apr 30;360(18):1815–26. PubMed PMID: 19339714. Pubmed Central PMCID: PMC2854555.

13 When To Start Consortium, Sterne JA, May M, Costagliola D, de Wolf F, Phillips AN, et al. Timing of initiation of antiretroviral therapy in AIDS-free HIV-1-infected patients: a collaborative analysis of 18 HIV cohort studies. Lancet. 2009 Apr 18;373(9672):1352–63. PubMed PMID: 19361855. Pubmed Central PMCID: PMC2670965.

14 Cohen MS, Chen YQ, McCauley M, Gamble T, Hosseinipour MC, Kumarasamy N, et al. Prevention of HIV-1 infection with early antiretroviral therapy. N Engl J Med. 2011 Aug 11;365(6):493–505. PubMed PMID: 21767103. Pubmed Central PMCID: PMC3200068.

15 Cohen MS, Chen YQ, McCauley M, Gamble T, Hosseinipour MC, Kumarasamy N, et al. Antiretroviral therapy for the prevention of HIV-1 transmission. N Engl J Med. 2016 Sep 01;375(9):830–9. PubMed PMID: 27424812. Pubmed Central PMCID: PMC5049503.

16 Insight Start Study Group, Lundgren JD, Babiker AG, Gordin F, Emery S, Grund B, et al. Initiation of antiretroviral therapy in early asymptomatic HIV infection. N Engl J Med. 2015 Aug 27;373(9):795–807. PubMed PMID: 26192873. Pubmed Central PMCID: PMC4569751.

17 Tyrer F, Walker AS, Gillett J, Porter K, UK Register HIV Seroconverters. The relationship between HIV seroconversion illness, HIV test interval and time to AIDS in a seroconverter cohort. Epidemiol Infect. 2003 Dec;131(3):1117–23. PubMed PMID: WOS:000188995600013.

18 Spartac Trial Investigators, Fidler S, Porter K, Ewings F, Frater J, Ramjee G, et al. Short-course antiretroviral therapy in primary HIV infection. N Engl J Med. 2013 Jan 17;368(3):207–17. PubMed PMID: 23323897. Pubmed Central PMCID: PMC4131004.

19 Rosenberg ES, Altfeld M, Poon SH, Phillips MN, Wilkes BM, Eldridge RL, et al. Immune control of HIV-1 after early treatment of acute infection. Nature. 2000 Sep 28;407(6803):523–6. PubMed PMID: 11029005.

20 Thornhill J, Inshaw J, Kaleebu P, Cooper D, Ramjee G, Schechter M, et al. Brief report: enhanced normalization of CD4/CD8 ratio with earlier antiretroviral therapy at primary HIV infection. J Acquir Immune Defic Syndr. 2016 Sep 01;73(1):69–73. PubMed PMID: 27070122. Pubmed Central PMCID: PMC4981213.

21 Ananworanich J, Dube K, Chomont N. How does the timing of antiretroviral therapy initiation in acute infection affect HIV reservoirs? Curr Opin HIV AIDS. 2015 Jan;10(1):18–28. PubMed PMID: 25415421. Pubmed Central PMCID: PMC4271317.

22 Deng K, Pertea M, Rongvaux A, Wang L, Durand CM, Ghiaur G, et al. Broad CTL response is required to clear latent HIV-1

due to dominance of escape mutations. Nature. 2015 Jan 15;517(7534):381–5. PubMed PMID: 25561180. Pubmed Central PMCID: PMC4406054.

23 TenoRes Study Group. Global epidemiology of drug resistance after failure of WHO recommended first-line regimens for adult HIV-1 infection: a multicentre retrospective cohort study. Lancet Infect Dis. 2016 May;16(5):565–75. PubMed PMID: 26831472. Pubmed Central PMCID: 4835583.

24 Baxter JD, Dunn D, White E, Sharma S, Geretti AM, Kozal MJ, et al. Global HIV-1 transmitted drug resistance in the INSIGHT Strategic Timing of AntiRetroviral Treatment (START) trial. HIV Med. 2015 Apr;16 Suppl 1(S1):77–87. PubMed PMID: 25711326. Pubmed Central PMCID: PMC4341921.

25 Gupta RK, Jordan MR, Sultan BJ, Hill A, Davis DH, Gregson J, et al. Global trends in antiretroviral resistance in treatment-naive individuals with HIV after rollout of antiretroviral treatment in resource-limited settings: a global collaborative study and meta-regression analysis. Lancet. 2012 Oct 06;380(9849):1250–8. PubMed PMID: 22828485. Pubmed Central PMCID: PMC3790969.

26 Sax PE, Islam R, Walensky RP, Losina E, Weinstein MC, Goldie SJ, et al. Should resistance testing be performed for treatment-naive HIV-infected patients? A cost-effectiveness analysis. Clin Infect Dis. 2005 Nov 01;41(9):1316–23. PubMed PMID: 16206108.

27 Hirsch MS, Gunthard HF, Schapiro JM, Brun-Vezinet F, Clotet B, Hammer SM, et al. Antiretroviral drug resistance testing in adult HIV-1 infection: 2008 recommendations of an International AIDS Society-USA panel. Clin Infect Dis. 2008 Jul 15;47(2):266–85. PubMed PMID: 18549313.

28 Castro H, Pillay D, Cane P, Asboe D, Cambiano V, Phillips A, et al. Persistence of HIV-1 transmitted drug resistance mutations. J Infect Dis. 2013 Nov 01;208(9):1459–63. PubMed PMID: 23904291. Pubmed Central PMCID: PMC3789571.

29 Wittkop L, Gunthard HF, de Wolf F, Dunn D, Cozzi-Lepri A, de Luca A, et al. Effect of transmitted drug resistance on virological and immunological response to initial combination antiretroviral therapy for HIV (EuroCoord-CHAIN joint project): a European multicohort study. Lancet Infect Dis. 2011 May;11(5):363–71. PubMed PMID: 21354861.

30 Li JZ, Paredes R, Ribaudo HJ, Kozal MJ, Svarovskaia ES, Johnson JA, et al. Impact of minority nonnucleoside reverse transcriptase inhibitor resistance mutations on resistance genotype after virologic failure. J Infect Dis. 2013 Mar 15;207(6):893–7. PubMed PMID: 23264671. Pubmed Central PMCID: PMC3571444.

31 Rodriguez B, Sethi AK, Cheruvu VK, Mackay W, Bosch RJ, Kitahata M, et al. Predictive value of plasma HIV RNA level on rate of CD4 T-cell decline in untreated HIV infection. JAMA. 2006 Sep 27;296(12):1498–506. PubMed PMID: 17003398.

32 Mellors JW, Munoz A, Giorgi JV, Margolick JB, Tassoni CJ, Gupta P, et al. Plasma viral load and CD4(+) lymphocytes as prognostic markers of HIV-1 infection. Ann Intern Med. 1997 Jun 15;126(12):946–54. PubMed PMID: WOS:A1997XE54900006.

33 May M, Sterne JA, Sabin C, Costagliola D, Justice AC, Thiebaut R, et al. Prognosis of HIV-1-infected patients up to 5 years after initiation of HAART: collaborative analysis of prospective studies. AIDS. 2007 May 31;21(9):1185–97. PubMed PMID: 17502729. Pubmed Central PMCID: 3460385.

34 World Health Organization. Global Tuberculosis Report, 2016. World Health Organization, Geneva: WHO, 2016.

35 Dheda K, Barry CE, 3rd, Maartens G. Tuberculosis. Lancet. 2016 Mar 19;387(10024):1211–26. PubMed PMID: 26377143.

36 van Zyl-Smit RN, Binder A, Meldau R, Mishra H, Semple PL, Theron G, et al. Comparison of quantitative techniques including Xpert MTB/RIF to evaluate mycobacterial burden. PLoS One. 2011;6(12):e28815. PubMed PMID: 22216117. Pubmed Central PMCID: 3245241.

37 Long R, Scalcini M, Manfreda J, Jean-Baptiste M, Hershfield E. The impact of HIV on the usefulness of sputum smears for the diagnosis of tuberculosis. Am J Public Health. 1991 Oct;81(10):1326–8. PubMed PMID: 1928536. Pubmed Central PMCID: PMC1405318.

38 Parry CM, Kamoto O, Harries AD, Wirima JJ, Nyirenda CM, Nyangulu DS, et al. The use of sputum induction for establishing a diagnosis in patients with suspected pulmonary tuberculosis in Malawi. Tuber Lung Dis. 1995 Feb;76(1):72–6. PubMed PMID: 7718851.

39 Bruchfeld J, Aderaye G, Palme IB, Bjorvatn B, Kallenius G, Lindquist L. Sputum concentration improves diagnosis of tuberculosis in a setting with a high prevalence of HIV. Trans R Soc Trop Med Hyg. 2000 Nov-Dec;94(6):677–80. PubMed PMID: 11198655.

40 Perriens JH, St Louis ME, Mukadi YB, Brown C, Prignot J, Pouthier F, et al. Pulmonary tuberculosis in HIV-infected patients in Zaire. A controlled trial of treatment for either 6 or 12 months. N Engl J Med. 1995 Mar 23;332(12):779–84. PubMed PMID: 7862181.

41 Okwera A, Johnson JL, Luzze H, Nsubuga P, Kayanja H, Cohn DL, et al. Comparison of intermittent ethambutol with rifampicin-based regimens in HIV-infected adults with PTB, Kampala. Int J Tuberc Lung Dis. 2006 Jan;10(1):39–44. PubMed PMID: 16466035. Pubmed Central PMCID: PMC2869085.

42 World Health Organization. WHO treatment guidelines for drug-resistant tuberculosis—2016 update. World Health Organization, Geneva 2016.

43 Selwyn PA, Hartel D, Lewis VA, Schoenbaum EE, Vermund SH, Klein RS, et al. A prospective study of the risk of tuberculosis among intravenous drug users with human immunodeficiency virus infection. N Engl J Med. 1989 Mar 02;320(9):545–50. PubMed PMID: 2915665.

44 Woldehanna S, Volmink J. Treatment of latent tuberculosis infection in HIV infected persons. Cochrane Database Syst Rev. 2004;10.1002/14651858.CD000171.pub2(1):CD000171. PubMed PMID: 14973947.

45 Gao XF, Wang L, Liu GJ, Wen J, Sun X, Xie Y, et al. Rifampicin plus pyrazinamide versus isoniazid for treating latent tuberculosis infection: a meta-analysis. Int J Tuberc Lung Dis. 2006 Oct;10(10):1080–90. PubMed PMID: 17044199.

46 Mohammed A, Myer L, Ehrlich R, Wood R, Cilliers F, Maartens G. Randomised controlled trial of isoniazid preventive therapy in South African adults with advanced HIV disease. Int J Tuberc Lung Dis. 2007 Oct;11(10):1114–20. PubMed PMID: 17945069.

47 Faustini A, Hall AJ, Perucci CA. Risk factors for multidrug resistant tuberculosis in Europe: a systematic review. Thorax. 2006 Feb;61(2):158–63. PubMed PMID: 16254056. Pubmed Central PMCID: PMC2104570.

48 Kaplan JE, Hanson D, Dworkin MS, Frederick T, Bertolli J, Lindegren ML, et al. Epidemiology of human immunodeficiency virus-associated opportunistic infections in the United States in the era of highly active antiretroviral therapy. Clin Infect Dis. 2000 Apr;30 Suppl 1(Suppl 1):S5–14. PubMed PMID: 10770911.

49 Kovacs JA, Hiemenz JW, Macher AM, Stover D, Murray HW, Shelhamer J, et al. Pneumocystis carinii pneumonia: a comparison between patients with the acquired immunodeficiency syndrome and patients with other immunodeficiencies. Ann Intern Med. 1984 May;100(5):663–71. PubMed PMID: 6231873.

50 Miller RF, Kocjan G, Buckland J, Holton J, Malin A, Semple SJ. Sputum induction for

the diagnosis of pulmonary disease in HIV positive patients. J Infect. 1991 Jul;23(1):5–15. PubMed PMID: 1885913.

51 Cregan P, Yamamoto A, Lum A, VanDerHeide T, MacDonald M, Pulliam L. Comparison of four methods for rapid detection of Pneumocystis carinii in respiratory specimens. J Clin Microbiol. 1990 Nov;28(11):2432–6. PubMed PMID: 1701444. Pubmed Central PMCID: PMC268201.

52 Ribes JA, Limper AH, Espy MJ, Smith TF. PCR detection of Pneumocystis carinii in bronchoalveolar lavage specimens: analysis of sensitivity and specificity. J Clin Microbiol. 1997 Apr;35(4):830–5. PubMed PMID: 9157136. Pubmed Central PMCID: PMC229684.

53 Huggett JF, Taylor MS, Kocjan G, Evans HE, Morris-Jones S, Gant V, et al. Development and evaluation of a real-time PCR assay for detection of Pneumocystis jirovecii DNA in bronchoalveolar lavage fluid of HIV-infected patients. Thorax. 2008 Feb;63(2):154–9. PubMed PMID: 17693588.

54 Tasaka S, Hasegawa N, Kobayashi S, Yamada W, Nishimura T, Takeuchi T, et al. Serum indicators for the diagnosis of pneumocystis pneumonia. Chest. 2007 Apr;131(4):1173–80. PubMed PMID: 17426225.

55 Fujii T, Nakamura T, Iwamoto A. Pneumocystis pneumonia in patients with HIV infection: clinical manifestations, laboratory findings, and radiological features. J Infect Chemother. 2007 Feb;13(1):1–7. PubMed PMID: 17334722.

56 Hughes WT, Feldman S, Chaudhary SC, Ossi MJ, Cox F, Sanyal SK. Comparison of pentamidine isethionate and trimethoprim-sulfamethoxazole in the treatment of Pneumocystis carinii pneumonia. J Pediatr. 1978 Feb;92(2):285–91. PubMed PMID: 304478.

57 Sattler FR, Cowan R, Nielsen DM, Ruskin J. Trimethoprim-sulfamethoxazole compared with pentamidine for treatment of Pneumocystis carinii pneumonia in the acquired immunodeficiency syndrome. A prospective, noncrossover study. Ann Intern Med. 1988 Aug 15;109(4):280–7. PubMed PMID: 3260759.

58 Briel M, Boscacci R, Furrer H, Bucher HC. Adjunctive corticosteroids for Pneumocystis jiroveci pneumonia in patients with HIV infection: a meta-analysis of randomised controlled trials. BMC Infect Dis. 2005 Nov 07;5:101. PubMed PMID: 16271157. Pubmed Central PMCID: PMC1309617.

59 Smego RJ, Nagar S, Maloba B, Popara M. A meta-analysis of salvage therapy for Pneumocystis carinii pneumonia. Arch Intern Med. 2001 Jun 25;161(12):1529–33. PubMed PMID: 11427101.

60 Jordan R, Gold L, Cummins C, Hyde C. Systematic review and meta-analysis of evidence for increasing numbers of drugs in antiretroviral combination therapy. BMJ. 2002 Mar 30;324(7340):757. PubMed PMID: 11923157. Pubmed Central PMCID: PMC100314.

61 Rutherford GW, Sangani PR, Kennedy GE. Three- or four- versus two-drug antiretroviral maintenance regimens for HIV infection. Cochrane Database Syst Rev. 2003;10.1002/14651858. CD002037(4):CD002037. PubMed PMID: 14583945.

62 Asboe D, Williams IG, Goodall RL, Darbyshire JH, Hooker MH, Babiker AG, et al. A virological benefit from an induction/maintenance strategy: the Forte trial. Antivir Ther. 2007;12(1):47–54. PubMed PMID: 17503747.

63 Markowitz M, Hill-Zabala C, Lang J, DeJesus E, Liao Q, Lanier ER, et al. Induction with abacavir/lamivudine/zidovudine plus efavirenz for 48 weeks followed by 48-week maintenance with abacavir/lamivudine/zidovudine alone in antiretroviral-naive HIV-1-infected patients. J Acquir Immune Defic Syndr. 2005 Jul 01;39(3):257–64. PubMed PMID: 15980684.

64 Mallal S, Phillips E, Carosi G, Molina JM, Workman C, Tomazic J, et al. HLA-B*5701

screening for hypersensitivity to abacavir. N Engl J Med. 2008 Feb 07;358(6):568–79. PubMed PMID: 18256392.

65 Obel N, Farkas DK, Kronborg G, Larsen CS, Pedersen G, Riis A, et al. Abacavir and risk of myocardial infarction in HIV-infected patients on highly active antiretroviral therapy: a population-based nationwide cohort study. HIV Med. 2010 Feb;11(2):130–6. PubMed PMID: 19682101.

66 Worm SW, Sabin C, Weber R, Reiss P, El-Sadr W, Dabis F, et al. Risk of myocardial infarction in patients with HIV infection exposed to specific individual antiretroviral drugs from the 3 major drug classes: the data collection on adverse events of anti-HIV drugs (D:A:D) study. J Infect Dis. 2010 Feb 01;201(3):318–30. PubMed PMID: 20039804.

67 Bedimo RJ, Westfall AO, Drechsler H, Vidiella G, Tebas P. Abacavir use and risk of acute myocardial infarction and cerebrovascular events in the highly active antiretroviral therapy era. Clin Infect Dis. 2011 Jul 01;53(1):84–91. PubMed PMID: 21653308.

68 Yombi JC, Pozniak A, Boffito M, Jones R, Khoo S, Levy J, et al. Antiretrovirals and the kidney in current clinical practice: renal pharmacokinetics, alterations of renal function and renal toxicity. AIDS. 2014 Mar 13;28(5):621–32. PubMed PMID: 24983540.

69 Smith KY, Patel P, Fine D, Bellos N, Sloan L, Lackey P, et al. Randomized, double-blind, placebo-matched, multicenter trial of abacavir/lamivudine or tenofovir/emtricitabine with lopinavir/ritonavir for initial HIV treatment. AIDS. 2009 Jul 31;23(12):1547–56. PubMed PMID: 19542866.

70 Sax PE, Tierney C, Collier AC, Daar ES, Mollan K, Budhathoki C, et al. Abacavir/lamivudine versus tenofovir DF/emtricitabine as part of combination regimens for initial treatment of HIV: final results. J Infect Dis. 2011 Oct 15;204(8):1191–201. PubMed PMID: 21917892. Pubmed Central PMCID: 3173503.

71 McComsey GA, Kitch D, Daar ES, Tierney C, Jahed NC, Tebas P, et al. Bone mineral density and fractures in antiretroviral-naive persons randomized to receive abacavir-lamivudine or tenofovir disoproxil fumarate-emtricitabine along with efavirenz or atazanavir-ritonavir: Aids Clinical Trials Group A5224s, a substudy of ACTG A5202. J Infect Dis. 2011 Jun 15;203(12):1791–801. PubMed PMID: 21606537. Pubmed Central PMCID: 3100514.

72 Riddler SA, Haubrich R, DiRienzo AG, Peeples L, Powderly WG, Klingman KL, et al. Class-sparing regimens for initial treatment of HIV-1 infection. N Engl J Med. 2008 May 15;358(20):2095–106. PubMed PMID: 18480202. Pubmed Central PMCID: PMC3885902.

73 MacArthur RD, Novak RM, Peng G, Chen L, Xiang Y, Hullsiek KH, et al. A comparison of three highly active antiretroviral treatment strategies consisting of non-nucleoside reverse transcriptase inhibitors, protease inhibitors, or both in the presence of nucleoside reverse transcriptase inhibitors as initial therapy (CPCRA 058 FIRST Study): a long-term randomised trial. Lancet. 2006 Dec 16;368(9553):2125–35. PubMed PMID: 17174704.

74 Porter DP, Kulkarni R, Fralich T, Miller MD, White KL. 96-week resistance analyses of the STaR study: rilpivirine/emtricitabine/tenofovir DF versus efavirenz/emtricitabine/tenofovir DF in antiretroviral-naive, HIV-1-infected subjects. HIV Clin Trials. 2015 Jan-Feb;16(1):30–8. PubMed PMID: 25777187.

75 Molina JM, Clumeck N, Orkin C, Rimsky LT, Vanveggel S, Stevens M, et al. Week 96 analysis of rilpivirine or efavirenz in HIV-1-infected patients with baseline viral load </= 100 000 copies/mL in the pooled ECHO and THRIVE phase 3, randomized, double-blind trials. HIV Med. 2014 Jan;15(1):57–62. PubMed PMID: 23980523.

76 Nelson MR, Elion RA, Cohen CJ, Mills A, Hodder SL, Segal-Maurer S, et al. Rilpivirine versus efavirenz in HIV-1-infected subjects receiving emtricitabine/tenofovir DF: pooled 96-week data from ECHO and THRIVE Studies. HIV Clin Trials. 2013 May-Jun;14(3):81–91. PubMed PMID: 23835510.

77 Walmsley SL, Antela A, Clumeck N, Duiculescu D, Eberhard A, Gutierrez F, et al. Dolutegravir plus abacavir-lamivudine for the treatment of HIV-1 infection. N Engl J Med. 2013 Nov 07;369(19):1807–18. PubMed PMID: 24195548.

78 Molina JM, Clotet B, van Lunzen J, Lazzarin A, Cavassini M, Henry K, et al. Once-daily dolutegravir is superior to once-daily darunavir/ritonavir in treatment-naive HIV-1-positive individuals: 96 week results from FLAMINGO. J Int AIDS Soc. 2014;17(4 Suppl 3):19490. PubMed PMID: 25393999. Pubmed Central PMCID: 4224885.

79 Raffi F, Jaeger H, Quiros-Roldan E, Albrecht H, Belonosova E, Gatell JM, et al. Once-daily dolutegravir versus twice-daily raltegravir in antiretroviral-naive adults with HIV-1 infection (SPRING-2 study): 96 week results from a randomised, double-blind, non-inferiority trial. Lancet Infect Dis. 2013 Nov;13(11):927–35. PubMed PMID: 24074642.

80 Song I, Mark S, Chen S, Savina P, Wajima T, Peppercorn A, et al. Dolutegravir does not affect methadone pharmacokinetics in opioid-dependent, HIV-seronegative subjects. Drug and Alcohol Dependence. 2013 Dec 01;133(2):781–4. PubMed PMID: 24018316.

81 Durant J, Clevenbergh P, Garraffo R, Halfon P, Icard S, Del Giudice P, et al. Importance of protease inhibitor plasma levels in HIV-infected patients treated with genotypic-guided therapy: pharmacological data from the Viradapt Study. AIDS. 2000 Jul 07;14(10):1333–9. PubMed PMID: 10930147.

82 Paterson DL, Swindells S, Mohr J, Brester M, Vergis EN, Squier C, et al. Adherence to protease inhibitor therapy and outcomes in patients with HIV infection. Ann Intern Med. 2000 Jul 04;133(1):21–30. PubMed PMID: 10877736.

83 Nieuwkerk PT, Sprangers MA, Burger DM, Hoetelmans RM, Hugen PW, Danner SA, et al. Limited patient adherence to highly active antiretroviral therapy for HIV-1 infection in an observational cohort study. Arch Intern Med. 2001 Sep 10;161(16):1962–8. PubMed PMID: 11525698.

84 Ickovics JR, Cameron A, Zackin R, Bassett R, Chesney M, Johnson VA, et al. Consequences and determinants of adherence to antiretroviral medication: results from Adult AIDS Clinical Trials Group protocol 370. Antivir Ther. 2002 Sep;7(3):185–93. PubMed PMID: 12487386.

85 Garcia de Olalla P, Knobel H, Carmona A, Guelar A, Lopez-Colomes JL, Cayla JA. Impact of adherence and highly active antiretroviral therapy on survival in HIV-infected patients. J Acquir Immune Defic Syndr. 2002 May 01;30(1):105–10. PubMed PMID: 12048370.

86 Claxton AJ, Cramer J, Pierce C. A systematic review of the associations between dose regimens and medication compliance. Clin Ther. 2001 Aug;23(8):1296–310. PubMed PMID: 11558866.

87 Bamberger JD, Unick J, Klein P, Fraser M, Chesney M, Katz MH. Helping the urban poor stay with antiretroviral HIV drug therapy. Am J Public Health. 2000 May;90(5):699–701. PubMed PMID: 10800416. Pubmed Central PMCID: PMC1446238.

88 Nieuwkerk P, Gisolf E, Sprangers M, Danner S, Prometheus Study Group. Adherence over 48 weeks in an antiretroviral clinical trial: variable within patients, affected by toxicities and independently predictive of virological

response. Antivir Ther. 2001 Jun;6(2):97–103. PubMed PMID: 11491422.

89 Chesney MA. Factors affecting adherence to antiretroviral therapy. Clin Infect Dis. 2000 Jun;30 Suppl 2:S171–6. PubMed PMID: 10860902.

90 Kanters S, Park JJ, Chan K, Socias ME, Ford N, Forrest JI, et al. Interventions to improve adherence to antiretroviral therapy: a systematic review and network meta-analysis. Lancet HIV. 2017 Jan;4(1):e31–e40. PubMed PMID: 27863996.

91 Rueda S, Park-Wyllie LY, Bayoumi AM, Tynan AM, Antoniou TA, Rourke SB, et al. Patient support and education for promoting adherence to highly active antiretroviral therapy for HIV/AIDS. Cochrane Database Syst Rev. 2006 Jul 19; 3, (3):CD001442. PubMed PMID: 16855968.

92 Hernandez LV, Gilson I, Jacobson J, Affi A, Puetz TR, Dindzans VJ. Antiretroviral hepatotoxicity in human immunodeficiency virus-infected patients. Aliment Pharmacol Ther. 2001 Oct;15(10):1627–32. PubMed PMID: 11564003.

93 Gisolf EH, Dreezen C, Danner SA, Weel JL, Weverling GJ, Prometheus Study G. Risk factors for hepatotoxicity in HIV-1-infected patients receiving ritonavir and saquinavir with or without stavudine. Prometheus Study Group. Clin Infect Dis. 2000 Nov;31(5):1234–9. PubMed PMID: 11073757.

94 den Brinker M, Wit FW, Wertheim-van Dillen PM, Jurriaans S, Weel J, van Leeuwen R, et al. Hepatitis B and C virus co-infection and the risk for hepatotoxicity of highly active antiretroviral therapy in HIV-1 infection. AIDS. 2000 Dec 22;14(18):2895–902. PubMed PMID: 11153671.

95 Surgers L, Lacombe K. Hepatoxicity of new antiretrovirals: a systematic review. Clin Res Hepatol Gastroenterol. 2013 Apr;37(2):126–33. PubMed PMID: 23522569.

96 Graham CS, Baden LR, Yu E, Mrus JM, Carnie J, Heeren T, et al. Influence of human immunodeficiency virus infection on the course of hepatitis C virus infection: a meta-analysis. Clin Infect Dis. 2001 Aug 15;33(4):562–9. PubMed PMID: 11462196.

97 Rockstroh JK, Hardy WD. Current treatment options for hepatitis C patients co-infected with HIV. Expert Rev Gastroenterol Hepatol. 2016 Jun;10(6):689–95. PubMed PMID: 26799571.

98 Clarke S, Keenan E, Ryan M, Barry M, Mulcahy F. Directly observed antiretroviral therapy for injection drug users with HIV infection. AIDS Read. 2002 Jul;12(7):305–7, 12–6. PubMed PMID: 12161852.

99 Clarke SM, Mulcahy FM. Antiretroviral therapy for drug users. Int J STD AIDS. 2000 Oct;11(10):627–31. PubMed PMID: 11057932.

100 Chander G, Himelhoch S, Moore RD. Substance abuse and psychiatric disorders in HIV-positive patients: epidemiology and impact on antiretroviral therapy. Drugs. 2006;66(6):769–89. PubMed PMID: 16706551.

101 Cuong C, Kirwan P, Brown A, Gill N, Delpech V. HIV official statistics overview: HIV diagnoses, late diagnoses and numbers accessing treatment and care London: Public Health England Publications 2016.

102 Ioannidis JP, Cappelleri JC, Skolnik PR, Lau J, Sacks HS. A meta-analysis of the relative efficacy and toxicity of Pneumocystis carinii prophylactic regimens. Arch Intern Med. 1996 Jan 22;156(2):177–88. PubMed PMID: 8546551.

103 Bucher HC, Griffith L, Guyatt GH, Opravil M. Meta-analysis of prophylactic treatments against Pneumocystis carinii pneumonia and toxoplasma encephalitis in HIV-infected patients. J Acquir Immune Defic Syndr Hum Retrovirol.

1997 Jun 01;15(2):104–14. PubMed PMID: 9241108.

104 Anglaret X, Chene G, Attia A, Toure S, Lafont S, Combe P, et al. Early chemoprophylaxis with trimethoprim-sulphamethoxazole for HIV-1-infected adults in Abidjan, Cote d'Ivoire: a randomised trial. Cotrimo-CI Study Group. Lancet. 1999 May 01;353(9163): 1463–8. PubMed PMID: 10232311.

105 Para MF, Finkelstein D, Becker S, Dohn M, Walawander A, Black JR. Reduced toxicity with gradual initiation of trimethoprim-sulfamethoxazole as primary prophylaxis for Pneumocystis carinii pneumonia: AIDS Clinical Trials Group 268. J Acquir Immune Defic Syndr. 2000 Aug 01;24(4):337–43. PubMed PMID: 11015150.

106 Chan C, Montaner J, Lefebvre EA, Morey G, Dohn M, McIvor RA, et al. Atovaquone suspension compared with aerosolized pentamidine for prevention of Pneumocystis carinii pneumonia in human immunodeficiency virus-infected subjects intolerant of trimethoprim or sulfonamides. J Infect Dis. 1999 Aug;180(2):369–76. PubMed PMID: 10395851.

107 El-Sadr WM, Murphy RL, Yurik TM, Luskin-Hawk R, Cheung TW, Balfour HH, Jr., et al. Atovaquone compared with dapsone for the prevention of Pneumocystis carinii pneumonia in patients with HIV infection who cannot tolerate trimethoprim, sulfonamides, or both. Community Program for Clinical Research on AIDS and the AIDS Clinical Trials Group. N Engl J Med. 1998 Dec 24;339(26):1889–95. PubMed PMID: 9862944.

108 Gallant JE, Moore RD, Chaisson RE. Prophylaxis for opportunistic infections in patients with HIV infection. Ann Intern Med. 1994 Jun 01;120(11):932–44. PubMed PMID: 8172439.

109 Schacker T, Hu HL, Koelle DM, Zeh J, Saltzman R, Boon R, et al. Famciclovir for the suppression of symptomatic and asymptomatic herpes simplex virus reactivation in HIV-infected persons. A double-blind, placebo-controlled trial. Ann Intern Med. 1998 Jan 01;128(1):21–8. PubMed PMID: 9424977.

110 Conant MA, Schacker TW, Murphy RL, Gold J, Crutchfield LT, Crooks RJ, et al. Valaciclovir versus aciclovir for herpes simplex virus infection in HIV-infected individuals: two randomized trials. Int J STD AIDS. 2002 Jan;13(1):12–21. PubMed PMID: 11802924.

111 Trikalinos TA, Ioannidis JP. Discontinuation of Pneumocystis carinii prophylaxis in patients infected with human immunodeficiency virus: a meta-analysis and decision analysis. Clin Infect Dis. 2001 Dec 01;33(11):1901–9. PubMed PMID: 11692302.

112 Lopez Bernaldo de Quiros JC, Miro JM, Pena JM, Podzamczer D, Alberdi JC, Martinez E, et al. A randomized trial of the discontinuation of primary and secondary prophylaxis against Pneumocystis carinii pneumonia after highly active antiretroviral therapy in patients with HIV infection. Grupo de Estudio del SIDA 04/98. N Engl J Med. 2001 Jan 18;344(3):159–67. PubMed PMID: 11172138.

113 Mussini C, Pezzotti P, Govoni A, Borghi V, Antinori A, d'Arminio Monforte A, et al. Discontinuation of primary prophylaxis for Pneumocystis carinii pneumonia and toxoplasmic encephalitis in human immunodeficiency virus type I-infected patients: the changes in opportunistic prophylaxis study. J Infect Dis. 2000 May;181(5):1635–42. PubMed PMID: 10823763.

114 Mussini C, Pezzotti P, Antinori A, Borghi V, Monforte A, Govoni A, et al. Discontinuation of secondary prophylaxis for Pneumocystis carinii pneumonia in human immunodeficiency virus-infected patients: a randomized trial by the CIOP Study Group. Clin Infect Dis. 2003 Mar 01;36(5):645–51. PubMed PMID: 12594647.

115 D'Egidio GE, Kravcik S, Cooper CL, Cameron DW, Fergusson DA, Angel JB. Pneumocystis jiroveci pneumonia prophylaxis is not required with a CD4+ T-cell count < 200 cells/microl when viral replication is suppressed. AIDS. 2007 Aug 20;21(13):1711–5. PubMed PMID: 17690568.

116 Eigenmann C, Flepp M, Bernasconi E, Schiffer V, Telenti A, Bucher H, et al. Low incidence of community-acquired pneumonia among human immunodeficiency virus-infected patients after interruption of Pneumocystis carinii pneumonia prophylaxis. Clin Infect Dis. 2003 Apr 01;36(7):917–21. PubMed PMID: 12652393.

117 Podzamczer D, Miro JM, Ferrer E, Gatell JM, Ramon JM, Ribera E, et al. Thrice-weekly sulfadiazine-pyrimethamine for maintenance therapy of toxoplasmic encephalitis in HIV-infected patients. Spanish Toxoplasmosis Study Group. Eur J Clin Microbiol Infect Dis. 2000 Feb;19(2):89–95. PubMed PMID: 10746493.

118 Miro JM, Lopez JC, Podzamczer D, Pena JM, Alberdi JC, Martinez E, et al. Discontinuation of primary and secondary Toxoplasma gondii prophylaxis is safe in HIV-infected patients after immunological restoration with highly active antiretroviral therapy: results of an open, randomized, multicenter clinical trial. Clin Infect Dis. 2006 Jul 01;43(1): 79–89. PubMed PMID: 16758422.

119 Graybill JR, Sobel J, Saag M, van Der Horst C, Powderly W, Cloud G, et al. Diagnosis and management of increased intracranial pressure in patients with AIDS and cryptococcal meningitis. The NIAID Mycoses Study Group and AIDS Cooperative Treatment Groups. Clin Infect Dis. 2000 Jan;30(1):47–54. PubMed PMID: 10619732.

120 van der Horst CM, Saag MS, Cloud GA, Hamill RJ, Graybill JR, Sobel JD, et al. Treatment of cryptococcal meningitis associated with the acquired immunodeficiency syndrome. National Institute of Allergy and Infectious Diseases Mycoses Study Group and AIDS Clinical Trials Group. N Engl J Med. 1997 Jul 03;337(1):15–21. PubMed PMID: 9203426.

121 Leenders AC, Reiss P, Portegies P, Clezy K, Hop WC, Hoy J, et al. Liposomal amphotericin B (AmBisome) compared with amphotericin B both followed by oral fluconazole in the treatment of AIDS-associated cryptococcal meningitis. AIDS. 1997 Oct;11(12):1463–71. PubMed PMID: 9342068.

122 Coker RJ, Viviani M, Gazzard BG, Du Pont B, Pohle HD, Murphy SM, et al. Treatment of cryptococcosis with liposomal amphotericin B (AmBisome) in 23 patients with AIDS. AIDS. 1993 Jun;7(6):829–35. PubMed PMID: 8363759.

123 Saag MS, Powderly WG, Cloud GA, Robinson P, Grieco MH, Sharkey PK, et al. Comparison of amphotericin B with fluconazole in the treatment of acute AIDS-associated cryptococcal meningitis. The NIAID Mycoses Study Group and the AIDS Clinical Trials Group. N Engl J Med. 1992 Jan 09;326(2):83––9. PubMed PMID: 1727236.

124 Mayanja-Kizza H, Oishi K, Mitarai S, Yamashita H, Nalongo K, Watanabe K, et al. Combination therapy with fluconazole and flucytosine for cryptococcal meningitis in Ugandan patients with AIDS. Clin Infect Dis. 1998 Jun;26(6):1362–6. PubMed PMID: 9636863.

125 de Gans J, Portegies P, Tiessens G, Eeftinck Schattenkerk JK, van Boxtel CJ, van Ketel RJ, et al. Itraconazole compared with amphotericin B plus flucytosine in AIDS patients with cryptococcal meningitis. AIDS. 1992 Feb;6(2):185–90. PubMed PMID: 1313682.

126 Powderly WG, Saag MS, Cloud GA, Robinson P, Meyer RD, Jacobson JM, et al. A controlled trial of fluconazole or amphotericin B to prevent relapse of

cryptococcal meningitis in patients with the acquired immunodeficiency syndrome. The NIAID AIDS Clinical Trials Group and Mycoses Study Group. N Engl J Med. 1992 Mar 19;326(12):793–8. PubMed PMID: 1538722.

127 Fessler RD, Sobel J, Guyot L, Crane L, Vazquez J, Szuba MJ, et al. Management of elevated intracranial pressure in patients with Cryptococcal meningitis. J Acquir Immune Defic Syndr Hum Retrovirol. 1998 Feb 01;17(2):137–42. PubMed PMID: 9473014.

128 Beardsley J, Wolbers M, Kibengo FM, Ggayi AB, Kamali A, Cuc NT, et al. Adjunctive Dexamethasone in HIV-Associated Cryptococcal Meningitis. N Engl J Med. 2016 Feb 11;374(6):542–54. PubMed PMID: 26863355. Pubmed Central PMCID: PMC4778268.

129 Chang LW, Phipps WT, Kennedy GE, Rutherford GW. Antifungal interventions for the primary prevention of cryptococcal disease in adults with HIV. Cochrane Database Syst Rev. 2005 Jul 20;3(3):CD004773. PubMed PMID: 16034947.

130 Saag MS, Cloud GA, Graybill JR, Sobel JD, Tuazon CU, Johnson PC, et al. A comparison of itraconazole versus fluconazole as maintenance therapy for AIDS-associated cryptococcal meningitis. National Institute of Allergy and Infectious Diseases Mycoses Study Group. Clin Infect Dis. 1999 Feb;28(2):291–6. PubMed PMID: 10064246.

131 Pienaar ED, Young T, Holmes H. Interventions for the prevention and management of oropharyngeal candidiasis associated with HIV infection in adults and children. Cochrane Database Syst Rev. 2006 Jul 19;10.1002/14651858. CD003940.pub2(3):CD003940. PubMed PMID: 16856025.

132 Havlir DV, Dube MP, McCutchan JA, Forthal DN, Kemper CA, Dunne MW, et al. Prophylaxis with weekly versus daily fluconazole for fungal infections in patients with AIDS. Clin Infect Dis. 1998 Dec;27(6):1369–5. PubMed PMID: 9868644.

133 Wheat J, Hafner R, Wulfsohn M, Spencer P, Squires K, Powderly W, et al. Prevention of relapse of histoplasmosis with itraconazole in patients with the acquired immunodeficiency syndrome. Ann Intern Med. 1993 Apr 15;118(8):610–6. PubMed PMID: 8383934.

134 Dunne M, Fessel J, Kumar P, Dickenson G, Keiser P, Boulos M, et al. A randomized, double-blind trial comparing azithromycin and clarithromycin in the treatment of disseminated Mycobacterium avium infection in patients with human immunodeficiency virus. Clin Infect Dis. 2000 Nov;31(5):1245–52. PubMed PMID: 11073759.

135 Ward TT, Rimland D, Kauffman C, Huycke M, Evans TG, Heifets L. Randomized, open-label trial of azithromycin plus ethambutol vs. clarithromycin plus ethambutol as therapy for Mycobacterium avium complex bacteremia in patients with human immunodeficiency virus infection. Veterans Affairs HIV Research Consortium. Clin Infect Dis. 1998 Nov;27(5):1278–85. PubMed PMID: 9827282.

136 Koletar SL, Berry AJ, Cynamon MH, Jacobson J, Currier JS, MacGregor RR, et al. Azithromycin as treatment for disseminated Mycobacterium avium complex in AIDS patients. Antimicrobial agents and chemotherapy. 1999 Dec;43(12):2869–72. PubMed PMID: 10582873. Pubmed Central PMCID: 89578.

137 Cohn DL, Fisher EJ, Peng GT, Hodges JS, Chesnut J, Child CC, et al. A prospective randomized trial of four three-drug regimens in the treatment of disseminated Mycobacterium avium complex disease in AIDS patients: excess mortality associated with high-dose clarithromycin. Terry Beirn Community Programs for Clinical Research on AIDS. Clin Infect Dis. 1999

Jul;29(1):125–33. PubMed PMID: 10433575.

138 Pierce M, Crampton S, Henry D, Heifets L, LaMarca A, Montecalvo M, et al. A randomized trial of clarithromycin as prophylaxis against disseminated Mycobacterium avium complex infection in patients with advanced acquired immunodeficiency syndrome. N Engl J Med. 1996 Aug 08;335(6):384–91. PubMed PMID: 8663871.

139 Oldfield ECr, Fessel WJ, Dunne MW, Dickinson G, Wallace MR, Byrne W, et al. Once weekly azithromycin therapy for prevention of Mycobacterium avium complex infection in patients with AIDS: a randomized, double-blind, placebo-controlled multicenter trial. Clin Infect Dis. 1998 Mar;26(3):611–9. PubMed PMID: 9524832.

140 Uthman MM, Uthman OA, Yahaya I. Interventions for the prevention of mycobacterium avium complex in adults and children with HIV. Cochrane Database Syst Rev. 2013 Apr 30;10.1002/14651858.CD007191. pub2(4):CD007191. PubMed PMID: 23633339.

141 Currier JS, Williams PL, Koletar SL, Cohn SE, Murphy RL, Heald AE, et al. Discontinuation of Mycobacterium avium complex prophylaxis in patients with antiretroviral therapy-induced increases in CD4+ cell count. A randomized, double-blind, placebo-controlled trial. AIDS Clinical Trials Group 362 Study Team. Ann Intern Med. 2000 Oct 03;133(7):493–503. PubMed PMID: 11015162.

142 El-Sadr WM, Burman WJ, Grant LB, Matts JP, Hafner R, Crane L, et al. Discontinuation of prophylaxis against Mycobacterium avium complex disease in HIV-infected patients who have a response to antiretroviral therapy. Terry Beirn Community Programs for Clinical Research on AIDS. N Engl J Med. 2000 Apr 13;342(15):1085–92. PubMed PMID: 10766581.

143 Moyle G, Harman C, Mitchell S, Mathalone B, Gazzard BG. Foscarnet and Ganciclovir in the treatment of CMV retinitis in AIDS patients: a randomised comparison. J Infect. 1992 Jul;25(1):21–7. PubMed PMID: 1326012.

144 Martin DF, Sierra-Madero J, Walmsley S, Wolitz RA, Macey K, Georgiou P, et al. A controlled trial of valganciclovir as induction therapy for cytomegalovirus retinitis. N Engl J Med. 2002 Apr 11;346(15):1119–26. PubMed PMID: 11948271.

145 Dieterich DT, Kotler DP, Busch DF, Crumpacker C, Du Mond C, Dearmand B, et al. Ganciclovir treatment of cytomegalovirus colitis in AIDS: a randomized, double-blind, placebo-controlled multicenter study. J Infect Dis. 1993 Feb;167(2):278–82. PubMed PMID: 8380610.

146 Blanshard C, Benhamou Y, Dohin E, Lernestedt JO, Gazzard BG, Katlama C. Treatment of AIDS-associated gastrointestinal cytomegalovirus infection with foscarnet and ganciclovir: a randomized comparison. J Infect Dis. 1995 Sep;172(3):622–8. PubMed PMID: 7658052.

147 da Pozzo S, Manara R, Tonello S, Carollo C. Conventional and diffusion-weighted MRI in progressive multifocal leukoencephalopathy: new elements for identification and follow-up. Radiol Med. 2006 Oct;111(7):971–7. PubMed PMID: 17021685.

148 Garcia de Viedma D, Alonso R, Miralles P, Berenguer J, Rodriguez-Creixems M, Bouza E. Dual qualitative-quantitative nested PCR for detection of JC virus in cerebrospinal fluid: high potential for evaluation and monitoring of progressive multifocal leukoencephalopathy in AIDS patients receiving highly active antiretroviral therapy. J Clin Microbiol. 1999 Mar;37(3):724–8. PubMed PMID: 9986840. Pubmed Central PMCID: PMC84536.

149 Marzocchetti A, Di Giambenedetto S, Cingolani A, Ammassari A, Cauda R, De

Luca A. Reduced rate of diagnostic positive detection of JC virus DNA in cerebrospinal fluid in cases of suspected progressive multifocal leukoencephalopathy in the era of potent antiretroviral therapy. J Clin Microbiol. 2005 Aug;43(8):4175–7. PubMed PMID: 16081969. Pubmed Central PMCID: PMC1233964.

150 Antinori A, Cingolani A, Lorenzini P, Giancola ML, Uccella I, Bossolasco S, et al. Clinical epidemiology and survival of progressive multifocal leukoencephalopathy in the era of highly active antiretroviral therapy: data from the Italian Registry Investigative Neuro AIDS (IRINA). J Neurovirol. 2003;9 Suppl 1:47–53. PubMed PMID: 12709872.

151 Berenguer J, Miralles P, Arrizabalaga J, Ribera E, Dronda F, Baraia-Etxaburu J, et al. Clinical course and prognostic factors of progressive multifocal leukoencephalopathy in patients treated with highly active antiretroviral therapy. Clin Infect Dis. 2003 Apr 15;36(8):1047–52. PubMed PMID: 12684918.

Chapter 13

Hepatitis

Lise Bondy and Michael S. Silverman

13.1 Hepatitis A

> **Case Presentation 1**
>
> A 23-year-old man who works in an organic juice bar presents with malaise, vomiting, dark urine, and anorexia. He traveled to Mexico one month ago and did not seek any pre-travel advice. On examination, he has mild jaundice and right upper quadrant tenderness. His ALT is 1200 U/L, AST 900 U/L, and total bilirubin is 79 umol/L. His hepatitis A IgM is positive. You wonder about his risk of complications from this infection, and what can be done to protect customers at the juice bar.

Hepatitis A is a RNA virus classified as a picornavirus. It is spread through the fecal-oral route. It has been associated with outbreaks of food-borne illness. Groups at increased risk include international travelers, men who have sex with men (MSM), and people who inject drugs (PWID). The incubation period is 15–50 days. Duration of symptoms is typically less than two months [1]. Patients shed virus for two to three weeks prior to onset of illness, and one week after symptom onset. In children younger than 6, less than 30% are symptomatic, and in those with clinical illness, the symptoms are generally mild [1].

In resource limited settings, most people are infected by the age of 10.

In older children or adults, acute hepatitis with jaundice, right upper quadrant pain, and vomiting are common. Transaminases may be above 1,000. Fulminant liver failure may occur, but is rare (approximately 1%) and occurs most commonly among those with chronic liver disease [2]. Acute infection is diagnosed using hepatitis A IgM. Treatment is supportive. Infection can be prevented by two doses of hepatitis A vaccine 6–12 months apart. The vaccine can also be used for post-exposure prophylaxis within two weeks of exposure. After exposure, immune globulin may be offered to patients over forty, immunocompromised patients, children under 12 months of age, and those with chronic liver disease. Rarely, a prolonged cholestatic hepatitis or a relapsing course can occur in the six months after infection.

> **Case Presentation 1 (continued)**
>
> Public health is notified and the patient is excluded from work for one week after the onset of his symptoms. A public information campaign ensues, and contact tracing is performed. A free vaccination clinic is offered. The patient makes an uneventful recovery, although reports several months of fatigue. No secondary cases of hepatitis A are reported.

Evidence-Based Infectious Diseases, Third Edition. Edited by Dominik Mertz, Fiona Smaill, and Nick Daneman.
© 2018 John Wiley & Sons Ltd. Published 2018 by John Wiley & Sons Ltd.

Table 13.1 Comparison of hepatitis viruses.

	Hep A	Hep B	Hep C	Hep D	Hep E
Mode of transmission	Fecal-oral	Perinatal, sexual, parenteral, blood product	Predominantly parenteral	Parenteral	Fecal-oral
Virus type	RNA	DNA	RNA	RNA	RNA
Prevention	Vaccine, sanitation programs	Vaccine, screening of blood supply, needle and syringe programs	Screening of blood supply, needle and syringe programs, possibly treatment as prevention	Vaccine, screening of blood supply, needle and syringe programs	Sanitation programs, avoidance of consumption of undercooked pork
Treatment	Supportive	Nucleos(t)ide analogs, Interferon alpha	Direct acting antivirals (DAAs)	Interferon alpha may be used	Ribavirin may be effective

13.2 Hepatitis B

Case Presentation 2

A 47-year-old woman who emigrated from China eight years ago presents to your office. She recently found a new family physician, who sent a hepatitis B surface antigen (HBsAg), which has returned as positive. She denies any personal or family history of viral hepatitis or liver disease. She believes that she had screening bloodwork upon immigration to Canada. She is asymptomatic. Her ALT is 34 U/L, hepatitis B virus (HBV) DNA is 2.34E + 3 IU/mL, and she is hepatitis B e antigen (HBeAg) negative and anti-HBe-positive. She has a boyfriend, and they are sexually active. You wonder if she requires treatment for hepatitis B, if she requires ultrasound screening for hepatocellular carcinoma, and what recommendations should be made regarding condom use with her boyfriend.

Hepatitis B is an enormously successful virus. Approximately one-third of the world's population has been exposed to this virus [3]. It represents a major infectious cause of mortality worldwide and is an oncogenic virus. It is transmitted perinatally, percutaneously,

Table 13.2 Chronic Hepatitis B[+].

Stage	Immune tolerant	Immune active	Inactive
ALT*	normal	elevated	normal
e Antigen	+	+ or −	−
DNA (IU/ml)	>200,000	>2,000 may be >200,000	<2,000
Fibrosis**	None	Present	+/−
Treatment	None (controversial)	Yes	None

[+]Surface Antigen Positive OR Surface Antigen negative but core Antibody AND Hepatitis B DNA positive (i.e., occult HBV—very rare).
*Normal ALT is ≤30 for males and ≤19 for females.
**All patients with cirrhosis and detectable HBV DNA should be treated.

and sexually. Infections in healthy adults often clear spontaneously. Infections in neonates and young children are asymptomatic and more likely to become chronic. The incubation period is 45–150 days [1]. Acute infection is characterized by elevated transaminases and positive Hep B core IgM. Hepatitis B is difficult to eradicate due to the persistence of covalently closed circular DNA (cccDNA) in the nucleus. The virus evades immune control by producing a large amount of surface antigen that acts as a decoy and prevents the virus from being cleared.

Patients with positive HBeAg tend to have higher levels of HBV DNA. Younger patients who are in the immune tolerant phase of infection generally are HBeAg positive/anti-HBe negative, have high levels of HBV DNA, normal ALT, and normal liver histology.

In young adulthood, people generally enter the immune active stage. This is characterized by a rise in the liver enzymes and fluctuating levels of HBV DNA. They may convert from eAg positive/eAb-negative to eAg-negative/eAb-positive. This immune active stage can persistent over several years, and the inflammation caused by the immune system's attempt to clear HBV from the hepatocytes can lead to progressive liver damage and cirrhosis.

People of Asian descent are more likely to have pre-core mutants that are e antigen negative and may be associated with more progressive disease. Among Chinese patients with chronic hepatitis B (generally perinatally acquired), 40–50% of men and 15% of women died of a liver related death from liver failure or hepatocellular carcinoma [4].

Extra-hepatic complications of hepatitis B include polyarteritis nodosa and glomerular disease.

Among Hepatitis B infected patients, it is recommended that Asian men over 40 and Asian women over 50 are screened for hepatocellular carcinoma every 6–12 months with an ultrasound [5,6]. African people are recommended, in some guidelines, to start screening in their twenties. All patients with cirrhosis, no matter their age, need lifelong ultrasound screening for hepatocellular carcinoma.

Chronic hepatitis B is defined as a positive hepatitis B surface antigen that persists for six months or longer. Chronic inactive hepatitis B is characterized by low levels of hepatitis B DNA (<2,000 IU/ml) and persistently normal liver enzymes. These patients generally do not require treatment and should be followed longitudinally. It is important to note that hepatitis B infection in these

patients is inactive due to immune control, and any treatment that causes immune suppression can cause potentially life-threatening reactivation.

All pregnant women should be screened for hepatitis B infection due to the risk of perinatal transmission. Neonates born to pregnant women should commence the hepatitis B vaccine series within 12 hours of delivery [7]. Many countries administer hepatitis B immune globulin as well, and this is an expensive intervention. Women should be encouraged to breastfeed. Pregnant women with a viral load greater than 10^6 IU/ml should be offered tenofovir in the second trimester to reduce the risk of transmission [8].

Hepatitis B immunization should be offered to all neonates or children of school age, and adults in at risk groups (household contacts or sexual partners of individuals with hepatitis B, PWIDs, MSM, HIV, dialysis patients, chronic liver disease, etc.). Generally, a series of three doses at zero, one, and six months is used. A double dose vaccine series is typically recommended for patients on hemodialysis. Patients with HIV do not respond as well to single strength vaccine and may also be offered double dose vaccine. A hepatitis B surface antibody level above 10 IU/L is considered to be seroprotective [7].

Screening for hepatitis B should be done for all patients from endemic areas, nonvaccinated patients whose parents are from HBV-endemic countries, household contacts/sexual partners of those with HBV, patients on hemodialysis, HIV-positive patients, all pregnant women, patients needing immunosuppressive therapy, health care workers, people who use drugs, people with elevated transaminases of unknown etiology, people with multiple sexual partners, and MSM [6].

Hepatitis B reactivation with immune suppression may occur. All patients about to receive immunosuppressive therapy should receive screening with HBsAg, HBcAb, and HBsAb. Patients who are HBsAg positive should receive preventive therapy against reactivation with a nucleos(t)ide analogue during the duration of immunosuppression and for six months after. Patients with isolated HBcAb positivity should be offered antiviral therapy if they are to receive B-cell targeted biologic therapy such as rituximab and/or bone marrow transplantation. Generally, therapy is continued for 12 months after the last dose of rituximab. Patients at risk of hepatitis B reactivation should be screened q3 monthly with ALT +/− HBV DNA.

Not all patients with hepatitis B require treatment. Generally, all patients with cirrhosis and a detectable viral load should receive therapy. Patients with immune active disease, especially those with evidence of progressive fibrosis on liver biopsy or non-invasive measures of fibrosis such as Fibroscan, should be treated. Patients with chronic inactive hepatitis B who are going to receive immunosuppression such as chemotherapy also require treatment.

Available treatments include interferon and nucleoside/tide analogues. Response to interferon is generally determined by genotype, with patients with Genotypes A and B responding better than those with Genotypes C and D. Generally, interferon is administered for 12 months and has numerous side effects, including triggering autoimmune syndromes, cytopenias, depression, and fatigue. It should not be used in patients with decompensated cirrhosis. The goal of interferon therapy is sustained loss of hepatitis B surface antigen, which is a functional cure.

Nucleos(t)ide analogs suppress replication of hepatitis B by inhibiting the reverse transcriptase enzyme. The goal of treatment is suppression of hepatitis B DNA and normalization of liver enzymes. Therapy is generally continued long-term and loss of HBsAg is rare with these agents. Lamivudine has a low barrier to resistance and up to 80% of patients develop resistance to this agent after five years of therapy. Adefovir is rarely used due to a high rate of adverse drug reactions. Entecavir has a higher barrier to resistance and resistance is rare in treatment naïve patients. It is well tolerated. Tenofovir Disoproxil Fumarate (TDF) has the highest barrier to resistance, and is often used when patients develop resistance to lamivudine. TDF is also well tolerated. The main concern with this medication is renal and bone toxicity. The dose should be adjusted in those with CrCl less than 60. Tenofovir Alafenamide (TAF) is another pro drug of tenofovir with lower extracellular concentrations, and has recently been approved for monotherapy for hepatitis B and may have less renal and bone toxicity. The NAs are relatively expensive; however, generic forms of lamivudine are now available and a generic form of TDF may be released soon.

Case Presentation 2 (continued)

The patient's Fibroscan shows no evidence of fibrosis. You monitor her liver enzymes every three months and her ALT remains less than 40. Her HBV DNA is persistently low. Hepatitis D serology is negative. You decide not to treat with antiviral medications and to follow the patient in your out-patient clinic. Hepatitis A vaccine series is administered and she is advised to minimize alcohol and maintain a healthy body mass index. Her boyfriend is recommended to see his family physician and receive a hepatitis B vaccine series if he is non-immune. Ultrasound screening every six months for hepatocellular carcinoma is begun at age 50.

13.3 Hepatitis C

Case Presentation 3

A 44-year-old man presents for out-patient assessment for hepatitis C. He was referred by his methadone provider. His hepatitis C antibody was noted to be positive on enrolling in the methadone program. His HIV serology is negative, and his hepatitis B surface antigen is negative, core antibody is positive, and surface antibody is negative. His ALT has been mildly elevated for several years, ranging from 45–57. He previously injected opioids, but has stopped five years ago and has been stable on methadone maintenance therapy. He has ADHD and depression, and has a remote history of a suicide attempt. He consumes 14–18 alcoholic beverages per week and smokes marijuana daily. He has never been treated previously for hepatitis C, as he was concerned about the adverse effects of interferon therapy. He has heard about new therapies for hepatitis C and wonders if he is eligible for treatment. His physical examination is normal and his abdominal ultrasound shows mildly increased echogenicity but no features of portal hypertension. His CBC, creatinine, albumin, bilirubin and INR are normal, and his ALT is 55; AST, 42 ALP, 97. You wonder if he would benefit from therapy for his hepatitis C, and how to stage his liver disease. You have read reports of hepatitis B reactivation on therapy for hepatitis C in patients who have markers of previous hepatitis B infection.

Hepatitis C is a single stranded RNA virus in the flavivirus family which infects hepatocytes. Hepatitis C is one of the leading causes of infectious disease related morbidity and mortality globally. It is the leading indication for liver transplantation in developed countries. It is estimated by the WHO to infect 130–150 million people worldwide and cause 700,000 deaths per year. Mortality from hepatitis C has exceeded that of HIV in developed countries [9,10,11,12]. In fact, in Ontario, Canada, hepatitis C was found to be responsible for more years of life lost than any other infectious pathogen [13].

Hepatitis C is transmitted through blood-to-blood contact. Individuals at higher risk for this infection include people who inject drugs (currently or in the past), men who have sex with men, people living with HIV/AIDS, immigrants and refugees, people who received blood products prior to 1992, people on hemodialysis, children born to hepatitis C positive women, and First Nations people. The so-called "Baby Boomer" generation of individuals born between 1945 and 1965 has a higher prevalence of hepatitis C infection than the general population and many organizations suggest screening for hepatitis C in this group.

Patients can have hepatitis C and yet have normal liver enzyme levels (ALT). Screening for hepatitis C infection is therefore done through an antibody test (serology) [9]. The hepatitis C antibody can usually be detected 4–10 weeks after infection, but in some patients the antibody response can be delayed. The antibody can be detected in >97% of persons by six months after exposure. If the antibody is positive, testing with the polymerase chain reaction (PCR) for hepatitis C RNA should be done to confirm active infection. About 20–30% of individuals will clear the virus spontaneously. The antibody generally stays positive for life and does not confer protective immunity. Individuals can become re-infected with hepatitis C if they are re-exposed.

There are six genotypes of hepatitis C virus, which are spread geographically across the globe [11]. There are numerous quasi-species of hepatitis C. Different genotypes may share only 70% of their nucleotide sequence. Genotype 1 is the most common genotype worldwide, followed by Genotype 3. Genotype 1 contains two subtypes—1a and 1b. Genotype 4 is predominantly found in individuals from North Africa and the Middle East. Genotypes 5 and 6 are rare. Chronic mixed infections with more than one genotype may occur. Superinfection with a second genotype that appears to replace the earlier one can also occur. Genotype 3 infection may be associated with a more rapid progression of liver disease.

Acute hepatitis C may result in symptoms such as jaundice, dark urine, and pale stool in 20% of patients although the majority are asymptomatic. Fulminant liver failure from acute hepatitis C is exceedingly rare. Most patients with chronic hepatitis C infection are also asymptomatic. Extra-hepatic manifestations of chronic hepatitis C may occur. These include cryoglobulinemic vasculitis, which may result in glomerulonephritis or peripheral neuropathy. Even in the absence of cryoglobulinemia, hepatitis C can cause several other forms of glomerulonephritis, including membranoproliferative glomerulonephritis (MPGN) and membranous nephropathy. Other dermatologic complications of hepatitis C include cutaneous necrotising vasculitis, porphyria cutanea tarda, and lichen planus. Circulating cryoglobulins, if measured correctly, can be detected in a large proportion of patients with hepatitis C (up to 50% in some studies) and about 10% of patients with hepatitis C have symptomatic cryoglobulinemia [14,15]. Associations between hepatitis C and an increased risk of type 2 diabetes and some non-Hodgkins lymphomas have been reported.

Between 1–5% of patients infected with hepatitis C will die of liver cancer or liver failure [12]. The majority of people chronically infected with hepatitis C will die with the infection, rather than from the infection.

Remarkable advances have been made in the treatment of hepatitis C with new Direct Acting Antivirals (DAAs) [16,17,18,19]. These drugs target different steps in the life cycle of the hepatitis C virus. Prior to 2011, the only therapy available for hepatitis C was interferon and ribavirin. Interferon stimulates the patient's own immune system to eradicate the virus. Ribavirin has an unknown mechanism of action. When prescribed in combination for 24–48 weeks, interferon and ribavirin eradicated the virus in 20–80% of individuals. Side effects of interferon are myriad, including flu-like illness, neuropsychiatric symptoms, cytopenias, thyroid dysfunction, fatigue, and exacerbation of many autoimmune syndromes. Ribavirin commonly induces rash, hemolytic anemia, and is absolutely contraindicated in pregnancy and for men whose partners are or who may become pregnant due to animal data suggesting the risk of serious birth defects, and fetal loss. Although interferon is now almost never used in the treatment of hepatitis C,

ribavirin still has a role in several patient subgroups.

Overall, the currently available DAAs are safe, well tolerated, and effective. There have been a multitude of well designed, industry-sponsored, randomized controlled trials investigating their efficacy. The main concern with these medications is their cost and accessibility. Patients who are treatment experienced or have cirrhosis may be more difficult to treat.

Patients with HIV co-infection have a faster progression of liver fibrosis due to hepatitis C. They have a lower response rate to therapy with interferon and ribavirin compared to patients with hepatitis C monoinfection. With the new DAAs, this patient group now has similar or higher rates of cure compared with hepatitis C monoinfected patients. The main issues in treating this group are drug-drug interactions with antiretroviral therapy.

The goal of hepatitis C therapy is to achieve a Sustained Virologic Reponse (SVR). This means that at 12 weeks after completion of therapy the viral RNA is not detected in blood. SVR12 correlates well with long-term disease-free progression. The risk of viral relapse after SVR12 is far less than 1%, and therefore, patients that have achieved SVR12 are considered cured of their infection. Some groups suggest checking an additional HCV viral load at 48 weeks post-treatment [12]. Individuals should be counseled that they are not immune from re-infection. If they have ongoing risk factors for hepatitis C acquisition, these should be addressed and the patients should be followed longitudinally. The frequency of monitoring and the ideal screening test (i.e., ALT vs. HCV PCR) are not yet known.

Patients with advanced fibrosis or cirrhosis require long-term follow up after SVR. The risk of hepatic decompensation after SVR is very low if patients do not have another concomitant liver disease such as alcoholic or non-alcoholic fatty liver disease. However, the risk of hepatocellular carcinoma (HCC) in patients with cirrhosis remains elevated after SVR and the current recommendation for patients with advanced fibrosis or cirrhosis (F3-4) is for lifelong surveillance with ultrasound for HCC every six months. Research is underway to determine in which patients and at what time surveillance for HCC can cease post-SVR. Continued endoscopic screening for varices may also be considered [20]. Patients with hepatitis C should be counseled to abstain from alcohol or minimize their alcohol intake. They should be counseled to maintain or attain a healthy BMI. They should be offered hepatitis A and B vaccination.

Therapeutic options for hepatitis C are chosen based on genotype, treatment experience, and the presence of cirrhosis. Prior to therapy, an assessment of fibrosis should be performed as this will impact the duration and choice of therapy in most cases. Normal liver enzymes and a normal ultrasound do not rule out significant fibrosis. Due to the cost of the medications, in most healthcare settings, reimbursement for treatment is based on the presence of moderate to advanced fibrosis, unless there are extra-hepatic manifestations. Fibrosis is graded on the Metavir scale, from F0 (no fibrosis) to F4 (cirrhosis). The traditional gold standard of fibrosis assessment is the liver biopsy. Currently, non-invasive measures of liver fibrosis are in widespread use. The most common method is ultrasound transient elastography (Fibroscan), which measures liver stiffness and gives a result in kilopascals. Other methods used at some centers include the Fibrotest (a serum panel with biomarkers for fibrosis), APRI (AST to Platelet Radio Index), and MR elastography (MRE). Findings on abdominal ultrasound and clinical features of hepatic decompensation are also helpful in staging the severity of liver disease.

The current classes of DAAs include protease inhibitors, nucleos(t)ide and non-nucleoside polymerase inhibitors, and NS5A inhibitors (replication and assembly inhibitors). These medications are always used in combination (regimens include a DAA combined with at least one or more other DAA's or ribavirin or both).

Treatment guidelines and new therapies for hepatitis C are in a stage of rapid change, and we encourage you to consult an online resource such as hcvguidelines.org for the most up to date treatment recommendations. At the time of writing, there are two pan-genotypic options commercially available for hepatitis C. One is sofosbuvir/velpatasvir. This single pill (once daily) regimen is prescribed for 12 weeks for all genotypes. Patients with decompensated cirrhosis should receive 12 weeks plus weight-based ribavirin. The other is Sofosbuvir/daclatasvir. This once daily regimen is currently considerably more expensive and is dosed for 12–24 weeks with or without ribavirin. Other pangenotypic combinations currently under investigation include sofosbuvir/velpatasvir/voxilaprevir and glecaprevir/pibrentasvir.

The following recommendations apply only to patients who are treatment naïve (TN) or treatment experienced (TE) with interferon and ribavirin. Expert consultation should be sought for patients who fail DAA therapy.

There are additional considerations among patients with renal failure. Sofosbuvir-based regimens are not approved in patients with CrCl <30. G/E is approved in renal failure, including dialysis. The PrOD regimen is also well studied in renal failure. Ribavirin can cause severe hemolysis in renal failure and the hemoglobin must be monitored closely. Patients may require transfusion or erythropoietin.

Protease-inhibitor based regimens are not safe for patients with Child-Pugh B or C cirrhosis. Patients with Child-Pugh A cirrhosis, especially those with a history of decompensated liver disease, must be monitored closely on therapy for signs of decompensation (such as rising bilirubin, INR, ascites, or peripheral edema). Consultation with a center with transplantation expertise is recommended.

All patients should be screened for HIV and hepatitis B prior to treatment. There have been reports of reactivation of hepatitis B infection with treatment using interferon free DAA regimens in hepatitis C co-infected patients. Cases have occurred even in patients who are HBsAg negative and core antibody positive. Patients with hepatitis B co-infection should be closely monitored for

Table 13.3 Treatment recommendations.

Genotype 1 infection:
Sofosbuvir/ledipasvir (SOF/LED)
1a or b, non-cirrhotic, treatment naive:
SOF/LED for 8 weeks if VL <6 million, 12 weeks if >6 million OR HIV co-infected
1a or 1b, non-cirrhotic, treatment experienced:
SOF/LED × 12 weeks
1a or 1b, cirrhotic, treatment naïve:
SOF/LED × 12 weeks
1a or 1b, cirrhotic, treatment experienced:
SOF/LED × 24 weeks OR SOF/LED/ribavirin × 12 weeks
Based on the results of the ION trials [21]

Paritaprevir/ritonavir/ombitasvir/dasabuvir (PrOD):
G1a – non-cirrhotic – 12 weeks + ribavirin
G1a – cirrhotic – 24 weeks + ribavirin
G1b – non-cirrhotic or cirrhotic – 12 weeks
Note: Contraindicated in decompensated cirrhosis (Child Pugh B or C).
Based on the results of the TURQUOISE/SAPPHIRE/MALACHITE/PEARL trials [22]

Sofosbuvir/velpatasvir (SOF/VEL) (for TN or TE, cirrhosis or non-cirrhotic):
12 weeks
Based on the results of the ASTRAL trials [23]

Grazoprevir/elbasvir (GZR/EBR):
Genotype 1a – Canadian Recommendations- treatment naive 12 weeks; treatment experienced 16 weeks plus weight based ribavirin
Genotype 1a U.S. Recommendations if treatment naive or treatment experienced perform testing for NS5A resistance associated polymorphisms. If no NS5A resistance associated polymorphisms treat for 12 weeks. If NS5A resistance associated polymorphisms found treat for 16 weeks and add weight based ribavirin.
Genotype 1b – treatment naïve or experienced, cirrhotic or non-cirrhotic – 12 weeks
Note: Contraindicated in decompensated cirrhosis (Child Pugh B or C).
Based on the results of the C-EDGE/C-WORTHY trials [24]

Genotype 2 infection:
12 weeks SOF/VEL (cirrhotic or non-cirrhotic)
12 weeks SOF/DAC (non cirrhotic)
16–24 weeks SOF/DAC (cirrhotic)
Less effective alternative:
12 weeks of SOF/Rib (16 weeks if cirrhotic)

Genotype 3 infection:
SOF/VEL × 12 weeks (cirrhotic or non-cirrhotic) *consider adding ribavirin if TE + cirrhotic
SOF/DAC × 12 weeks (non-cirrhotic)
SOF/DAC (+/– ribavirin) × 24 weeks (cirrhotic)
Less effective alternative:
SOF/RIB × 24 weeks

Genotype 4 infection:
SOF/LED × 12 weeks (+ribavirin if treatment experienced and cirrhotic)
SOF/VEL × 12 weeks
PrO + ribavirin × 12 weeks
GZR/EBR × 12 weeks (16 weeks + RBV if treatment experienced)

Genotype 5 + 6 infection:
SOF/VEL × 12 weeks
SOF/LDV × 12 weeks

Decompensated cirrhosis (Child Pugh B or C): Should be managed by a practitioner with experience with management of this condition, and ideally in a hepatic transplant center
SOF/LED + ribavirin × 12 weeks (for Genotypes 1 and 4)
SOF/VEL + ribavirin × 12 weeks (for Genotypes 1–4)
SOF/DAC + ribavirn × 12 weeks (for Genotypes 1–4) (Using a low initial dose of RBV [600 mg] and increase as tolerated)

evidence of reactivation. Consider initiation of treatment for hepatitis B prior to initiating DAA therapy for hepatitis C in co-infected patients. More research is required to determine the factors that predict reactivation. Use of the ritonavir-containing regimen PrOD in a patient with HIV not on ARVs (or a fully suppressive regimen) could lead to development of HIV drug resistance.

Despite the recent dramatic improvement in treatments for hepatitis C, prevention remains a priority. Approaches to hepatitis C prevention include: screening of blood supply and blood donors, appropriate disposal of sharps and infection control practices in health care settings, addiction treatment including Opiate Substitution Therapy, needle and syringe programs, and safe sex practices, especially in HIV-infected MSM. There is currently no available vaccine. Research in this area is ongoing.

Case Presentation 1 (continued)

You obtain an HCV PCR that is positive at 4.31E6 IU/mL. The patient has Genotype 1a. His Fibroscan shows a result of 8.7 kPa, which is consistent with F2 (moderate) fibrosis. You start therapy with eight weeks of sofosbuvir and ledipasvir. His ALT declines rapidly on therapy and remains normal, so you do not check his hepatitis B surface antigen. The patient achieves a Sustained Virologic Response. You notify the patient and his primary care provider that the anti-HCV antibody test should not be repeated as it will remain positive, reflecting prior infection. Despite the antibody, he is not immune and can be re-infected if exposed, so you counsel him regarding HCV prevention. HCV PCR should be re-tested if ALT rises in a sustained fashion.

13.4 Hepatitis D

This virus requires hepatitis B virus to complete its life cycle and cause infection. Patients with hepatitis B should be screened for hepatitis D infection if they have low levels of HBV DNA but elevated liver enzymes without another explanation. Some groups recommend that all patients with hepatitis B be screened for infection with hepatitis D [25]. HDV can cause fulminant or more severe progressive disease in those with chronic inactive HBV. Transmission is parenteral or (rarely) sexual. Infection is more common in Southern Italy, Eastern Europe, South America, Africa, and the Middle East. Diagnosis is made through anti-HDV IgG followed by hepatitis D RNA testing. Interferon therapy for 24–96 weeks has been studied in small trials with modest benefits in suppressing viral replication and liver disease activity but without sustained benefits [26].

13.5 Hepatitis E

Hepatitis E is an RNA virus that can cause acute and chronic hepatitis.

Genotypes 1 and 2 cause outbreaks of acute hepatitis in endemic areas (Asia and Africa), are obligate human pathogens, and are spread through the fecal-oral route. These genotypes are associated with a more severe course in pregnancy, with mortality rates of 10–25% in the third trimester [1].

Genotypes 3 and 4 cause sporadic chronic infection in immunocompromised hosts. Most infections are asymptomatic. These genotypes are spread through the consumption of undercooked meat (usually pork) or through blood transfusion.

Hepatitis E infection has been associated with an array of neurologic manifestations, including Guillain–Barré syndrome and neuralgic amyotrophy [27]. Diagnosis is by hepatitis E IgG and IgM as well as HEV PCR of blood and/or feces.

Treatment for acute HEV is supportive. Treatment for chronic HEV includes a reduction of immunosuppression, if possible, and ribavirin monotherapy may be used. This is an active area of research. There is a recombinant vaccine licensed in China.

References

1 Red Book: 2015 Report of the Committee on Infectious Diseases, 30th ed.

2 Miskovsky K. Hepatitis A. Infect Dis Clin North Am. 2000 Sept;14(3): 605–15.

3 Ott JJ, Stevens GA, Groeger J, Wiersma ST. Global epidemiology of hepatitis B virus infection: new estimates of age-specific HBsAg seroprevalence and endemicity. Vaccine. 2012;30(12).

4 Beasley RP, Lin CC, Chien CS, Chen CJ, Hwang LY. Geographic distribution of HBsAg carriers in China. Hepatol. 1982;2(5):553.

5 Terrault NA, Bzowej NH, Chang K-M, Hwang JP, Jonas MM, Murad MH. AASLD guidelines for treatment of chronic hepatitis B. Hepatol. 2016; 63:261–283. doi:10.1002/hep.28156

6 Myers RP, Shah H, Burak KW, Cooper C, Feld JJ. An update on the management of chronic hepatitis C: 2015 Consensus guidelines from the Canadian Association for the Study of the Liver. Can J Gastroenterol Hepatol. 2015;29(1):19–34.

7 Canada, Public Health Agency of Canada, National Advisory Committee on Immunization. (2017). Update on the recommended use of hepatitis B vaccine. Ottawa: Public Health Agency of Canada.

8 T. Calvin Q. Pan, M.D., Zhongping Duan, M.D., Erhei Dai, M.D., Shuqin Zhang, M.D., Guorong Han, M.D., Yuming Wang, M.D., Huaihong Zhang, M.D., Huaibin Zou, M.D., Baoshen Zhu, M.D., Wenjing Zhao, M.D., and Hongxiu Jiang, M.D., for the China Study Group for the Mother-to-Child Transmission of Hepatitis B: Tenofovir to prevent hepatitis B transmission. N Engl J Med. 2016; 374:2324–2334. June 16, 2016DOI: 10.1056/NEJMoa1508660.

9 AASLD-IDSA. Recommendations for testing, managing, and treating hepatitis C. http://www.hcvguidelines.org. 2017.

10 EASL Recommendations on Treatment of Hepatitis C. J Hepatol. 2016;66(1):153–194.

11 Messina et al. Global distribution and prevalence of hepatitis C virus genotypes. Hepatol. 2015 Jan;61(1):77–87. doi: 10.1002/hep.27259. Epub 2014 Jul 28.

12 Centers for Disease Control and Prevention. Hepatitis C FAQs for Health Professionals (2017 January 27). Retrieved June 16, 2017, from https://www.cdc.gov/hepatitis/hcv/hcvfaq.htm

13 Kwong JC et al. Ontario Burden of Infectious Disease Study. Dec 2010. https://www.publichealthontario.ca/en/eRepository/ONBoID_ICES_Report_ma18.pdf

14 Lunel F, Musset, L Cacoub, P, Perrin, M, Frangeul, L, Godeau, P,...Huraux, J. (1994). Cryoglobulinemia in chronic liver diseases: role of hepatitis C virus and liver damage. Gastroenterol. 106(5), 1291–1300.

15 Bonacci M et al. Virologic, clinical, and immune response outcomes of patients with hepatitis C virus—associated cryoglobulinemia treated with direct-acting antivirals. Clin Gastroenterol Hepatol. 2017;15(4):575–583.e1

16 Health Canada. Direct-acting antivirals, used for hepatitis C, may reactivate hepatitis B. (2016, December 1). Retrieved June 16, 2017, from http://healthycanadians.gc.ca/recall-alert-rappel-avis/hc-sc/2016/61274a-eng.php

17 Myers RP, Shah H, Burak KW, Cooper C, Feld JJ. An update on the management of chronic hepatitis C: 2015 Consensus guidelines from the Canadian Association for the Study of the Liver. Can J Gastroenterol Hepatol. 2015;29(1):19–34.

18 Public Health Agency of Canada (2016 September 01). Canadian Immunization Guide. Retrieved June 16, 2017, from https://www.canada.ca/en/public-health/services/canadian-immunization-guide.html

19 World Health Organization. Hepatitis C Fact Sheet. (2017 April). Retrieved June 16, 2017, from http://www.who.int/mediacentre/factsheets/fs164/en/

20 Jacobson IM et al. Gastroenterol. 2017 Mar 23;153(1):113–122.

21 Based on the results of the ION trials — Clinical Trial Results | HCV Treatment Information Project. (n.d.). Retrieved June 16, 2017, from http://www.hepctip.ca/clinical-trial-results/

22 Based on the results of the TURQUOISE/SAPPHIRE/MALACHITE/PEARL trials—Clinical Trial Results | HCV Treatment Information Project. (n.d.). Retrieved June 16, 2017, from http://www.hepctip.ca/clinical-trial-results/

23 Based on the results of the ASTRAL trials—Clinical Trial Results | HCV Treatment Information Project. (n.d.). Retrieved June 16, 2017, from http://www.hepctip.ca/clinical-trial-results/

24 Based on the results of the C-EDGE/C-WORTHY trials—Clinical Trial Results | HCV Treatment Information Project. (n.d.). Retrieved June 16, 2017, from http://www.hepctip.ca/clinical-trial-results/

25 Lok AS, Mcmahon BJ. Chronic hepatitis B: update 2009. Hepatology. 2009;50(3), 661–662. doi:10.1002/hep.23190

26 Abbas Z, Khan MA, Salih M, Jafri W. Interferon alpha for chronic hepatitis D. Cochrane Database Syst Rev. 2011. doi:10.1002/14651858.cd006002.pub2

27 Dalton HR, Kammar N, Van Eijk JJ, Mclean BN, Cintas P, Bendall RP, Jacobs BC. Hepatitis E virus and neurological injury. Nature Rev Neurol. 2016;(12):77–85. doi:10.1038/nrneurol.2015.234.

Chapter 14

Influenza

Ashley Roberts and Joanne M. Langley

Case Presentation 1

A 66-year-old male with type 2 diabetes mellitus presents with a two-day history of fever, cough and myalgia during the month of January. He is having difficulty maintaining his usual tight glucose control during this illness. A retired schoolteacher, he just returned from a visit with his young grandchildren, all of whom had coughs, runny nose, and fever. The patient looks uncomfortable and diaphoretic. His temperature is 38.5 °C, respiratory rate 25 and his heart rate is 90. There is mild increased work of breathing and crackles bilaterally at the lung bases. The chest radiograph reveals non-specific perihilar opacities and streaking bilaterally, but no focal consolidation.

He remembers receiving "a vaccine for pneumonia" last year, but doesn't remember getting an influenza vaccine. You recall getting an e-mail from public health about an influenza virus outbreak in a nearby nursing home, and wonder if you should institute a diagnostic test for influenza in this patient. You also wonder if antiviral treatment might help this patient.

14.1 Diagnosis

Influenza, an acute respiratory tract illness caused by influenza A or B viruses, occurs in epidemics of variable severity every winter in temperate climates, affecting up to 20% of the general population [1]. Diagnostic accuracy is highest when influenza is circulating in the community since the pretest likelihood (prevalence) will be higher. The methods for diagnosis of influenza are clinical and laboratory testing of respiratory tract specimens. Laboratory confirmation of influenza virus infection through detection of virus from a respiratory tract specimen remains the most accurate diagnostic tool. Diagnostic imaging is not useful for influenza diagnosis.

14.1.1 Clinical Diagnosis

Influenza is an acute viral infection of the respiratory tract, which is accompanied by non-specific systemic symptoms. Cough, sore throat, rhinorrhea, tachypnea, and sneezing suggest respiratory illness, while fever, malaise, anorexia, chills, myalgia, and headache are non-specific. In a systematic review of literature from 1962–2010 reporting combinations of signs and symptoms, and clinical decision rules for the diagnosis of influenza, no combination of findings was diagnostic [2]. In the 12 studies reviewed, the sensitivity and specificity of the combinations "fever and cough," and "fever, cough, and acute onset" were the most accurate, but considered only of moderate accuracy (area under the Receiver Operating

Evidence-Based Infectious Diseases, Third Edition. Edited by Dominik Mertz, Fiona Smaill, and Nick Daneman.
© 2018 John Wiley & Sons Ltd. Published 2018 by John Wiley & Sons Ltd.

Curve 0.70 and 0.79, respectively) [2]. Accuracy increased during the influenza season, and decreased during the "shoulder" season before and after the onset of influenza in the community [2].

14.1.2 Laboratory Diagnosis

Human influenza is caused by antigenic types, A and B, based on proteins in the nucleocapsid and matrix. Influenza A is further subtyped according to membrane glycoproteins H (hemagglutinin) and N (neuraminidase). There are 18 known H subtypes and 9N subtypes of influenza A. Influenza B has two major lineages but no subtypes. Influenza C is an uncommon cause of human infection. Influenza viruses undergo small antigenic changes or "drift" over time, which results in yearly epidemics. Major antigenic changes, or "shifts," in influenza A virus, with emergence of a new subtype may result in influenza pandemics such as the most recent pandemic in 2009 with the H1N1 strain. Pandemic influenza is not discussed here; instead, the discussion focuses on seasonal influenza.

Laboratory tests for the timely diagnosis of influenza are conducted on specimens procured from the respiratory tract that are obtained by nasal aspirate, swab, or wash, or a throat swab or wash, which detect the virus. Specimens from the nasopharynx are more useful than those from the throat or nares. Sputum is not a useful specimen in the diagnosis of influenza. Specimens obtained within the first three to five days of illness are more likely to be positive as viral shedding decreases quickly in the immunocompetent host. Viral culture and serological testing for influenza are not useful for the diagnosis of influenza in the clinical setting due to the inherent delay in receipt of test results relative to clinical decision making [3].

In order for an influenza test to be useful in clinical management, it should be available in a timely manner to affect decision-making (e.g., treatment, prophylaxis of contacts, outbreak management). Of the tests with a same-day turnaround time, nucleic acid amplification tests (NAAT) are the most accurate: Reverse Transcription (RT)-Polymerase Chain Reaction (PCR), conventional PCR, and multiplex PCR [4]. NAAT can be done within hours or on the same day, is highly sensitive and specific, and can differentiate between influenza types and subtypes [4]. Rapid antigen and immunofluorescence assays can yield results quickly, but are less sensitive than RT-PCR. A meta-analysis of 159 studies evaluating rapid influenza antigen tests found the pooled sensitivity to be 62.3% (95% CI 57.9–66.6) and the pooled specificity to be 98.2% (95% CI 97.5–98.7) [5], compared to a gold standard of RT-PCR, or where RT-PCR was not available, viral culture. The sensitivity was lower in adults versus children (53.9% vs. 66.6%) and was higher for influenza A than influenza B (64.6% vs. 52.2%) [5].

We recommend the use of NAAT to diagnose influenza due to its high accuracy and rapid turnaround time in clinical settings.

14.1.3 Diagnostic Imaging

Although imaging can confirm involvement of the lungs, findings are not specific for influenza virus infection. The most commonly used diagnostic imaging test for pneumonia is the chest radiograph [6]. Pulmonary infiltrates associated with viral pneumonia appear less confluent and homogenous than those of bacterial pneumonia. The picture in viral infection may be one of air-space nodules (of 4–10 mm), patchy peri-bronchial ground glass opacity, or air-space consolidation [6]. Hyperinflation is more likely in viral than bacterial pneumonia because of the associated bronchiolitis.

14.2 Treatment

Treatment of influenza includes antiviral therapies, alternative therapies, symptomatic supportive measures, and treatment of complications of influenza.

The neuraminidase inhibitors (NIs) are the only antiviral drugs currently available for treatment of influenza. Viral resistance to the M2 ion channel inhibitors, amantadine, and rimantadine has precluded their use in recent years.

NIs interfere with the influenza virus enzyme neuraminidase, which cleaves terminal sialic acid from sialic-acid-containing cell surface glycoproteins during replication. Neuraminidase enables release of virions from infected cells by preventing them from self-aggregating and binding to the surface of infected cells [7]. Oseltamivir is administered twice daily by mouth, while zanamivir is administered by inhalation. Peramivir is an intravenous NI administered once daily [8].

Evidence for the efficacy of NIs has been under intense scrutiny, and multiple systematic reviews have been completed. A Cochrane collaboration meta-analysis of 46 randomized, controlled clinical trials (RCT), found early NI treatment decreased the duration of influenza symptoms by 29 hours in children and 17 hours in adults [7]. Summary estimates from a systematic review of observational studies indicated that oseltamivir may reduce mortality, hospitalization, and duration of symptoms compared to no treatment, but the low quality of the evidence limited confidence in the effect size of those benefits [9]. An individual patient meta-analysis of RCTs of oseltamivir for treatment of influenza in adults found that compared to placebo, oseltamivir accelerated time to symptom resolution (97.5 hours vs. 122.7 hours), reduced risk of lower respiratory tract symptoms (4.9% vs. 8.7%) and admission to hospital for any cause (0.6% vs. 1.7%) [10]. The most common adverse effect associated with oseltamivir and peramivir use is gastrointestinal (nausea, vomiting) [8]. Zanamivir is not recommended in individuals with underlying airway disease (such as asthma or chronic obstructive pulmonary disease) because of the risk of airway irritation leading to bronchospasm.

Corticosteroid therapy is not recommended as adjunctive therapy for influenza; low quality evidence suggests it may increase mortality [11]. There is insufficient evidence to support or reject use of various complementary therapies [12,13]. Supportive care for influenza consists of adequate hydration and symptomatic therapy for discomfort and fever with non-steroidal inflammatory medications or acetaminophen. Patients who are unable to maintain fluid intake or develop respiratory distress may require care in the hospital setting.

In healthy people, influenza is usually an acute febrile illness that lasts for about one week. However, influenza can lead to serious complications, including pneumonia (secondary bacterial or primary viral pneumonia) or exacerbation of preexisting lung, cardiac, or other chronic disease [10]. Other complications of influenza virus infection include myositis, encephalitis and other neurologic disorders, pericarditis, and myocarditis.

We suggest that NIs be used for treatment of confirmed influenza in healthy persons if it can be recognized early in its course, and for treatment in persons with co-morbidities.

14.3 Prognosis

In healthy persons, influenza manifests with various combinations of fever, cough, rigors, myalgia, and headache of about one week's duration often severe enough to result in workplace absenteeism [14]. Complicated influenza can occur in previously healthy persons, but is more likely to occur in persons with certain risk factors. The most striking risk factor for complicated influenza requiring hospital care or influenza-associated death is age. Children under 2 years of age and adults over 65 have admission rates to hospital near 100 per 100,000 age-specific population [15,16]. Certain pre-existing conditions, such as cardiac or pulmonary disease, diabetes, obesity (BMI ≥40), and renal failure have been found in studies with varying methodological rigor as being associated with higher incidence of influenza-associated hospital admission. In a systematic literature review of risk factors for severe or complicated influenza, which included assessment of bias and the quality of the evidence, the level of evidence for these risk factors was assessed as limited to absent [17].The presence of any "any risk factor" was associated with death (odds ratio 2.04, 95% CI 1.74–2.39); estimates for various conditions are provided in that review [17]. Pregnant women with seasonal influenza are more likely than non-pregnant women to be admitted to hospital in several studies, but do not appear to be at increased risk of adverse fetal outcomes or maternal death [18].

14.4 Prevention

Three categories of interventions exist for the prevention of influenza: vaccination, infection prevention and control measures, and antiviral drugs.

Immunization is the cornerstone of public health influenza control programs, and in almost all developed countries, is recommended on an annual basis for persons at high risk of complicated influenza or of being hospitalized for care of influenza (Table14.1), which vary by jurisdiction [19,20] [17,20]. Pregnant women have been identified by the World Health Organization as the highest

Table 14.1 Persons for whom annual influenza immunization may be recommended because of increased risk of hospitalization, complicated influenza, or death.

Children 6–23 months or 6–59 months of age, or all children 6 months to 18 years months of age [22]

Pregnant women

Older person (>65 years or >50 years of age)

Persons with immunosuppression, primary or secondary cardiovascular, renal, metabolic, or hematologic disorders

Persons with obesity (BMI ≥40)

Residents of nursing homes or other chronic care facilities

priority for annual influenza vaccine [21]. Annual influenza immunization is routinely recommended for those who care for, or are in regular contact with, persons at high risk of influenza such as household contacts or healthcare providers. This strategy seeks to interrupt spread to vulnerable persons, especially those who cannot be immunized (e.g., children <6 months of age) or are less likely to respond to the vaccine (e.g., elderly or immune-compromised people).

Commercial influenza vaccines were first introduced in 1945, and multiple vaccine types are available, including injectable inactivated or subunit vaccines, adjuvanted and high dose vaccines, and nasally administered live attenuated products. As recommendations and vaccine availability vary across jurisdictions and time, annual guidance should be determined from national public health bodies.

The efficacy of influenza vaccines in preventing influenza has been evaluated in thousands of patients in RCTs, and many systematic reviews summarizing these studies are available, sometimes with varying conclusions. Vaccine effectiveness (VE) is also assessed annually by many national public health programs in observational studies. Estimates of influenza vaccine efficacy in a particular season vary according to the degree of match of the circulating strains with the vaccine strain, the age of the recipient and their previous experience with infection or immunization, and the type of influenza vaccine. Two types of outcome measures have been used to assess vaccine efficacy and effectiveness: clinical definitions of respiratory illness and laboratory confirmed influenza. Use of the latter incur more accurate outcome results in higher estimates of vaccine efficacy than does a measure of clinical outcome. In a review of 34 RCTs in 47 influenza seasons with 94,821 participants, the VE of trivalent inactivated influenza vaccine in seasons when vaccine antigens matched circulating strains, was 65% (95% CI 54–73), and 52% (95% CI 37–63) when there was mismatch [23]. In children 6 to 36 months, the live attenuated influenza vaccine VE in matched seasons was 83% (95% CI 75–88) and 54% (95% CI 28–21) in mismatched seasons [23]. In a meta-analysis of PCR-diagnosed influenza, vaccine efficacy of inactivated influenza vaccine was 59% (95% CI 51–67) in adults 18 to 64 years of age, and 83% (95% CI 69–91) for the live attenuated vaccine in children 6 months to 7 years [24]. In the most recent Cochrane systematic review the overall efficacy of inactivated vaccines in preventing laboratory confirmed influenza was 60% (95% CI 53–66), and was 62% when the vaccine antigens matched the circulating strain (95% CI 52–69) [25].

We recommend that immunization be used for all persons who wish to reduce their risk of influenza based on RCTs and lower level evidence.

Antiviral drugs have also been approved for the prevention of seasonal influenza as well as for treatment of established illness. Chemoprophylaxis may be used to prevent infection in institutional settings during outbreaks (community or in a facility), or as post-exposure prophylaxis for high-risk persons. The neuraminidase inhibitors are effective in prevention of influenza subtypes A and B, and have been used as seasonal prophylaxis (e.g., for 6 to 8 weeks when influenza is in the community) or as a post-exposure measure in household or other close contacts. A Cochrane review concluded that prophylactic use of either drug reduces the risk of symptomatic influenza [7].

We suggest that antivirals be used for prophylaxis of influenza in institutional settings, and for persons at risk for severe influenza when exposed.

Infection prevention and control measures consist of behaviors and use of personal protective equipment that will interrupt transmission of influenza virus from infected persons or influenza-contaminated articles to susceptible persons. Influenza virus is transmitted predominately through droplets from the respiratory tract which are expelled during coughing or sneezing, or transmitted during direct contact. Hand hygiene using soap or antimicrobial agents (e.g., waterless hand rubs, antimicrobial soap) is effective at eliminating virus from the hands. In addition to Standard Precautions, Additional (transmission-based) Precautions, typically consisting of contact and droplet precautions, are recommended for the care of a hospitalized patient with influenza as is placement in a single room when available [26]. Evidence for the use of these measures include direct evidence of reduced transmission of respiratory infections from RCTs and observational studies [27] as well as indirect evidence from various studies of other infections.

We recommend that routine infection and control measures to prevent influenza transmission be used in health care settings.

References

1 Fiore AE, Bridges CB, Katz JM, Cox NJ. Inactivated influenza vaccines. In: Stanley Plotkin WO, Offit P, editors. Vaccines. 6th ed. China: Elsevier Inc.; 2013.

2 Ebell MH, Afonso A. A systematic review of clinical decision rules for the diagnosis of influenza. Ann Fam Med. 2011;9(1):69–77.

3 Harper SA, Bradley JS, Englund JA, File TM, Gravenstein S, Hayden FG, et al. Seasonal influenza in adults and children—diagnosis, treatment, chemoprophylaxis, and institutional outbreak management: clinical practice guidelines of the Infectious Diseases Society of America. Clin Infect Dis. 2009;48(8):1003–32.

4 Peaper DR, Landry ML. Rapid diagnosis of influenza: state of the art. Clin Lab Med. 2014;34(2):365–85.

5 Chartrand C, Leeflang MM, Minion J, Brewer T, Pai M. Accuracy of rapid influenza diagnostic tests: a meta-analysis. Ann Intern Med. 2012;156(7):500–11.

6 Sharma S, Maycher B, Eschun G. Radiological imaging in pneumonia: recent innovations. Curr Opin Pulm Med. 2007;13(3):159–69.

7 Jefferson T, Jones MA, Doshi P, Del Mar CB, Hama R, Thompson MJ, et al. Neuraminidase inhibitors for preventing and treating influenza in healthy adults and children. Cochrane Database Syst Rev. 2014(4):CD008965.

8 Wester A, Shetty AK. Peramivir injection in the treatment of acute influenza: a review of the literature. Infect Drug Resist. 2016;9:201–14.

9 Santesso N, Hsu J, Mustafa R, Brozek J, Chen YL, Hopkins JP, et al. Antivirals for influenza: a summary of a systematic review and meta-analysis of observational studies. Influenza Other Respir Viruses. 2013;7 Suppl 2:76–81.

10 Dobson J, Whitley RJ, Pocock S, Monto AS. Oseltamivir treatment for influenza in adults: a meta-analysis of randomised controlled trials. Lancet. 2015;385(9979):1729–37.

11 Rodrigo C, Leonardi-Bee J, Nguyen-Van-Tam J, Lim WS. Corticosteroids as adjunctive therapy in the treatment of influenza. Cochrane Database Syst Rev. 2016;3:CD010406.

12 Mathie RT, Frye J, Fisher P. Homeopathic Oscillococcinum(R) for preventing and treating influenza and influenza-like illness. Cochrane Database Syst Rev. 2015;1:CD001957.

13 Jiang L, Deng L, Wu T. Chinese medicinal herbs for influenza. Cochrane Database Syst Rev. 2013(3):CD004559.

14 Nichol KL. Cost-benefit analysis of a strategy to vaccinate healthy working adults against influenza. Arch Intern Med. 2001;161(5):749–59.

15 Schanzer DL, Langley JM, Tam TW. Hospitalization attributable to influenza and other viral respiratory illnesses in Canadian children. Pediatr Infect Dis J. 2006;25(9):795–800.

16 Schanzer DL, Langley JM, Tam TW. Co-morbidities associated with influenza-attributed mortality, 1994–2000, Canada. Vaccine. 2008;26(36):4697–703.

17 Mertz D, Kim TH, Johnstone J, Lam PP, Science M, Kuster SP, et al. Populations at risk for severe or complicated influenza illness: systematic review and meta-analysis. BMJ. 2013;347:f5061.

18 Mertz D, Geraci J, Winkup J, Gessner BD, Ortiz JR, Loeb M. Pregnancy as a risk factor for severe outcomes from influenza virus infection: a systematic review and meta-analysis of observational studies. Vaccine. 2017;35(4):521–8.

19 Grohskopf LA, Sokolow LZ, Broder KR, Olsen SJ, Karron RA, Jernigan DB, et al. Prevention and Control of Seasonal Influenza with Vaccines. MMWR Recomm Rep. 2016;65(5):1–54.

20 National Advisory Committee on Immunization. Canadian Immunization Guide Chapter on Influenza and Statement on Seasonal Influenza Vaccine for 2016–2017 An Advisory Committee Statement. In: Health M, editor. Ottawa: Government of Canada; 2016. p. 64.

21 World Health Organization. Vaccines against influenza WHO position paper—November 2012. Wkly Epidemiol Record. 2012;47(87):461–76.

22 England. PH. Flu vaccination: who should have it this winter and why. London, UK: Public Health England; 2016. p. 12.

23 Tricco AC, Chit A, Soobiah C, Hallett D, Meier G, Chen MH, et al. Comparing influenza vaccine efficacy against mismatched and matched strains: a systematic review and meta-analysis. BMC Med. 2013;11:153.

24 Osterholm MT, Kelley NS, Sommer A, Belongia EA. Efficacy and effectiveness of influenza vaccines: a systematic review and meta-analysis. Lancet Infect Dis. 2012;12(1):36–44.

25 Demicheli V, Jefferson T, Al-Ansary LA, Ferroni E, Rivetti A, Di Pietrantonj C. Vaccines for preventing influenza in healthy adults. Cochrane Database Syst Rev. 2014(3):CD001269.

26 Siegel JD, Rhinehart E, Jackson M, Chiarello L, Health Care Infection Control Practices Advisory C. 2007 Guideline for Isolation Precautions: Preventing Transmission of Infectious Agents in Health Care Settings. Am J Infect Control. 2007;35(10 Suppl 2):S65–164.

27 Jefferson T, Del Mar CB, Dooley L, Ferroni E, Al-Ansary LA, Bawazeer GA, van Driel ML, Nair S, Jones MA, Thorning S, Conly JM. Physical interventions to interrupt or reduce the spread of respiratory viruses. Cochrane Database Syst Rev. 2011 Jul 6;(7):CD006207. doi: 10.1002/14651858. CD006207.pub4

Chapter 15

Critical Care

Bram Rochwerg and Jocelyn A. Srigley

Infection represents a major source of morbidity and mortality in the intensive care unit (ICU). Whether infection is the principal cause of critical illness or a secondary complication, the prevention, surveillance, diagnosis, and treatment of infection in the ICU pose unique challenges and require vigilant care.

Case Presentation 1

Mr. KW is a 56-year-old obese man presenting to the emergency room with fever, abdominal pain, and lightheadedness. Three weeks ago, he underwent an umbilical hernia repair including mesh placement. His temperature is 39.4 °C, heart rate 128 bpm, supine blood pressure 88/60 mmHg, and respiratory rate 34 bpm. The abdominal incision is healed and non-tender. His leukocyte count is 34 with toxic granulation. His chest radiograph shows patchy airspace disease, and a CT scan reveals an infected mesh.

15.1 Sepsis

15.1.1 Epidemiology

Although challenging to quantify, the incidence of severe sepsis varies from 900,000 to 3 million cases in the United States per year depending on methodology used [1]. In-hospital mortality of severe sepsis ranges from 14.7%–30% [1]. While hospital mortality rates from sepsis are declining over the last 20 years, the incidence of sepsis is on the rise [2].

15.1.2 Definitions

Sepsis is defined as life-threatening organ dysfunction caused by a dysregulated host response to infection [3]. Overactivation of the inflammatory cascade and upregulation of related cytokines are primarily implicated. Hemodynamic instability secondary to peripheral vasodilation and dysregulation of coagulation and fibrinolysis are key contributors to tissue hypoxia and vital organ injury [4]. Multiple organ failure is a hallmark of septic shock and the most common cause of death.

In 1992, the American College of Chest Physicians and the Society of Critical Care Medicine published definitions of sepsis-related syndromes [5]. The cornerstone of these definitions was the systemic inflammatory response syndrome (SIRS), characterized by two or more of: hyper- or hypothermia, tachycardia, tachypnea, leukocytosis, or leucopenia. As SIRS may be precipitated by non-infectious events, the diagnosis of sepsis required both SIRS and a confirmed or presumed source of infection.

Evidence-Based Infectious Diseases, Third Edition. Edited by Dominik Mertz, Fiona Smaill, and Nick Daneman.
© 2018 John Wiley & Sons Ltd. Published 2018 by John Wiley & Sons Ltd.

In 2016, the same organizations put forth new definitions of sepsis syndromes [3]. This update removed SIRS from the sepsis taxonomy as the syndrome was felt to lack specificity for infection. The new operational definition for sepsis includes evidence of organ dysfunction as identified by an acute change in total Sequential Organ Failure Assessment (SOFA) score of greater than or equal to 2 points as a consequence of infection (Table 15.1) [3]. The more abbreviated quick SOFA (qSOFA) may be used at the bedside to identify patients with suspected infection who are likely to have a prolonged ICU stay or die, and includes the following criteria: respiratory rate greater than or equal to 22, altered mentation, or systolic blood pressure less than or equal to 100 mmHg.

The updated definitions eliminated the severe sepsis designation, and defined *septic shock* as those with persisting hypotension requiring vasopressors or having a serum lactate level >2mmol/L despite adequate volume resuscitation [3]. Given these definitions are relatively new, it remains to be seen how they will perform with widespread utilization and more prospective study across clinical and geographical settings.

15.1.3 Management

Management of the septic patient involves a multi-faceted approach directed against the complex underlying pathophysiology. Early identification, appropriate fluid resuscitation and prompt administration of antibiotics are

Table 15.1 SOFA score variables.

Organ System	0	1	2	3	4
Respiratory PaO_2 / FiO_2 (mmHg)	>400	301–400	201–300 (with or without respiratory support) <201 (without respiratory support)	101–200 (with respiratory support)	≤100 (with respiratory support)
Coagulation Platelets (x 10^9/L)	>150	101–150	51–100	21–50	≤20
Bilirubin (μmol/L)	<20	20–32	33–101	102–204	>204
Cardiovascular	MAP ≥70 mmHg	MAP <70 mmHg	Dopamine ≤5.0 (μg/kg/min) or any dose of: Dobutamine Milrinone Levosimendan	Dopamine 5.1-15.0 (μg/kg/min) or Epinephrine ≤0.1 or Norepinephrine ≤0.1 or any dose of: Vasopressin Phenylephrine	Dopamine >15.0 (μg/kg/min) or Epinephrine >0.1 or Norepinephrine >0.1
Renal creatinine (μmol/L) OR urine output (mL/day)	<110	110–170	171–299	300–440 OR <500	>440 OR <00

PaO_2: partial pressure of arterial oxygen, FiO_2: fraction of inspiratory oxygen, L: liter, μmol: micromole, mmHg: millimeters of mercury, MAP: mean arterial pressure, kg: kilogram, μg: microgram, min: minute, ml: milliliter.

the mainstays of therapy. Thereafter, consideration of source control, and close, clinical follow-up are crucial.

15.1.3.1 Hemodynamic Resuscitation
The aim of resuscitative therapy in sepsis is the correction of hemodynamic disturbances that contribute to tissue hypoxia through impaired delivery of oxygenated blood to essential organs. Historically, goal-directed therapy referred to specific interventions aimed to achieve supraphysiologic values of cardiac index and oxygen delivery administered sometime in the first few days of sepsis management. The 2001 Rivers trial was one of the first to define clear resuscitative targets that were to be met within the first six hours after sepsis identification (called the "golden hours") rather than waiting until tissue damage had already occurred. The trial randomly allocated 263 septic patients at the time of presentation to the emergency department, to early goal-directed therapy (EGDT) versus standard care prior to ICU admission [6]. The experimental intervention involved an iterative assessment of hemodynamic parameters with specific actions targeted to precise physiologic goals. First intravenous fluids were administered to achieve a central venous pressure (CVP) measurement of 8 to 12 mmHg. At that point, vasopressors were administered to target a mean arterial pressure of at least 65 mmHg. Thereafter, if central venous oxygen saturation was less than 70%, red blood cells were transfused to achieve a hematocrit of at least 30, and if unsuccessful, dobutamine was initiated. With this intervention, 28-day mortality rates decreased from 46.5% to 30.5%, corresponding to a relative risk [RR] of 0.58 ($p = 0.009$) and a number-needed-to-treat of six. EGDT also reduced the duration of vasopressor therapy, mechanical ventilation, and hospital stay. The largest difference in treatment between groups was the amount of fluid administered within the first six hours of the intervention; 5 L in the EGDT group and 3.5 L in the comparator group ($p < 0.001$).

However, three recently completed randomized controlled trials (RCTs) (total of 4,201 patients) re-examined this effect of protocolized EGDT therapy on patients with septic shock and found no difference between the intervention and standard of care groups in any of the three studies [7–9]. Given mortality rates in both arms of the new studies are similar to that of the intervention group of the original trial, this finding may represent a shift in standard of care rather than inefficacy of EGDT. Critical care physicians now recognize the importance of early identification of sepsis, close monitoring, early and aggressive fluids, and vasopressors (when required) in the early management of sepsis. The importance of the other components of the original EGDT protocol, including the specific monitoring thresholds, remains less clear.

Although well recognized that patients with sepsis require fluid resuscitation, observational data suggest that over-zealous administration and hypervolemia in the post-resuscitative period is also associated with poor outcomes [10]. In light of these newer EGDT trials, the physiologic targets used to guide hemodynamic resuscitation remain controversial. CVP demonstrates very poor diagnostic characteristics when used for assessing whether a patient will be fluid responsive [11]. Pulmonary artery catheters have never been shown to improve patient outcomes in sepsis and are also associated with mechanical complications related to placement [12]. As opposed to these static indices (single measurement in time), newer measures such as ultrasound assessment of the inferior vena cava or pulse pressure variation with respiration offer dynamic measurements of volume status; however, evidence and applicability of these modalities is still limited [13]. As such, practically speaking, physicians use a host of bedside indicators for guiding resuscitation in sepsis. These include clinical signs of organ perfusion (mentation, skin mottling, urine output), biochemical indices including lactate level and lactate clearance, and hemodynamic response to fluid therapy [4].

15.1.3.2 Antimicrobial Therapy

Another pillar of sepsis management is the prompt administration of appropriate antimicrobial therapy. The importance of early antimicrobials was highlighted by a five-year retrospective study of 2,700 patients with septic shock [14]. Among patients who received antimicrobial therapy that was adequate to treat subsequently identified pathogens, delays in antimicrobial therapy clearly correlated with mortality (Fig. 15.1). Patients receiving appropriate coverage within the first hour of hypotension had a survival rate of 79.9%, and survival decreased by approximately 8% for each hour of delay.

The choice of empiric antimicrobial therapy is paramount. Among 5,715 critically ill patients with septic shock, hospital mortality when initial antimicrobial therapy was inadequate to treat the pathogen was 52%, far exceeding the 10.3% mortality rate among patients receiving adequate antimicrobial therapy [15]. Regression modeling determined that inadequate antimicrobial treatment was the strongest determinant of hospital mortality, with an adjusted odds ratio (OR) of 9.0 (95% CI 6.6–12.2).

Initial antimicrobial therapy depends on the presumed source of infection. Empiric therapy should cover any pathogens commonly associated with the particular infection, and should account for local ecology and antibiotic resistance rates, as well as patient-specific risk factors for multidrug resistant (MDR) organisms. An evidence-based review determined that acceptable empiric regimens in septic patients with an unclear source include a β-lactam in combination with an aminoglycoside, or monotherapy with a third- or fourth-generation cephalosporin, carbapenem, or extended-spectrum carboxypenicillin, or alternatively, ureidopenicillin with a β-lactamase inhibitor [16]. The prompt administration of broad-spectrum empiric agents should be followed by culture-directed tailoring of therapy as soon as possible [17].

15.1.3.3 Source Control

A persisting collection of microorganisms will continue to trigger the inflammatory response of sepsis [18]. When a source of infection cannot be eradicated solely with antibiotics, consider source control [19]. Percutaneous or surgical drainage is indicated for infection within a closed space, including abscess, empyema, or cholangitis. Debridement involves the removal of infected or necrotic tissue, either surgically, with irrigation, or using wet-to-dry dressings.

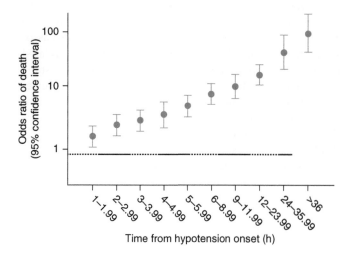

Figure 15.1 Mortality risk (expressed as adjusted odds ratio of death) with increasing delays in initiation of effective antimicrobial therapy. Bars represent 95% confidence interval. Reproduced from reference [14].

Device removal is important in patients with an infected foreign body, such as a central venous catheter, urinary catheter, or prosthetic joint. Other definitive source control measures include amputation of a gangrenous limb and resection of ischemic bowel.

15.1.3.4 Corticosteroid Therapy

Understanding that a dysregulated and over-activated host immune response is a significant inciting factor for end-organ damage in sepsis, steroids seem an attractive therapeutic option; however, the role for systemic corticosteroids in the management of sepsis remains unclear.

A Cochrane review of 27 trials (3,176 patients) demonstrated improved 28-day survival in those receiving corticosteroids compared with placebo (RR 0.87, 95% CI 0.76–1.00); however, the certainty in evidence was limited by inconsistency, imprecision, and the potential for publication bias [20]. Patients treated with steroids did experience higher rates of hyperglycemia and hypernatremia. Those with septic shock and those receiving low dose steroids for a longer course of therapy seemed to benefit most in subgroup analysis compared to those without signs of shock and those receiving a higher dose and shorter course of treatment. There was no significant subgroup effect in patients with critical illness-related corticosteroid insufficiency diagnosed with ACTH-stimulation testing. Since the Cochrane review, a more recent trial of 380 patients with sepsis without signs of shock, demonstrated no difference in mortality or development of subsequent shock with corticosteroid therapy [21].

Two additional trials of corticosteroids in patients with sepsis are underway [22,23]. For now, whether steroids benefit any critically ill septic patients remains uncertain. Refraining from steroid use altogether, administering only to the most ill, and administering to a wider group of septic patients all remain justifiable courses of action. Other immunomodulatory interventions targeting the dysfunctional host response, such as activated protein C or directed cytokine inhibitors have proven either ineffective [24] or harmful [25].

> **Case Presentation 1 (continued)**
>
> In the ER, Mr. KW promptly receives intravenous piperacillin-tazobactam and the mesh is surgically removed that day. Post-operatively, he is transferred to the intensive care unit on vasopressors. His leukocyte count is 36; his lactate level 3.5. His chest radiograph reveals diffuse airspace disease.
>
> Upon ICU admission, 2L of intravenous crystalloid are given, with an improvement in urine output seen. Fluid collected during surgery shows Gram-negative bacilli, as do two blood cultures. Later, *E. coli* sensitive to cefazolin is identified from all three cultures. The clinical team discontinues piperacillin-tazobactam and initiates cefazolin and metronidazole therapy. While his acute lung injury progresses, his blood pressure improves over six hours, no longer requiring vasopressor support.
>
> Later, with his lung injury slowly resolving, Mr. KW develops signs of a new infection: fever, tachycardia, increased respiratory rate, and recurrent leukocytosis with band cells.

15.2 Ventilator-associated Pneumonia

15.2.1 Epidemiology

Ventilator-associated pneumonia (VAP) refers to pneumonia arising more than 48 hours after endotracheal intubation [26]. Incidence and mortality estimates vary depending on the population, diagnostic techniques, and other variables. A meta-analysis estimated an incidence rate of 1.33 cases per 1,000 device days in the United States, with an increase in hospital length of stay (LOS) by 13 days per case and total attributable financial impact of over U.S.$3 billion per year [27].

15.2.2 Pathophysiology and Microbiology

Bacterial colonization of the upper airways and aspiration are the two main factors contributing to VAP [28]. Critically ill patients become colonized with bacteria originating from their own gastrointestinal tract and from the hospital environment, facilitated by patients' inability to clear secretions and by catheters that breach the skin and mucosal barriers. Colonizing bacteria infect the lower airways via aspiration of secretions from the upper respiratory tract.

The microbiology of VAP differs from community-acquired pneumonia, with Gram-negative and MDR organisms accounting for a significant proportion of cases. Surveillance data from the United States reveal that over half of reported VAP cases were caused by Gram-negative bacilli, most commonly *P. aeruginosa*, *Klebsiella* species, and *Enterobacter* species. The most common Gram-positive organism causing VAP was *S. aureus*, in 24.1% of cases [29].

15.2.3 Diagnosis

The diagnosis of VAP presents unique challenges. Clinical manifestations typically consist of new or progressive infiltrates on chest radiography, purulent tracheal secretions, fever, and leukocytosis. However, a variety of alternative pathologies, alone or in combination, can lead to a similar constellation of findings, including acute lung injury, atelectasis, congestive heart failure, and non-pulmonary infections [30]. A study of 84 ICU patients with new infiltrates and purulent secretions demonstrated the limited utility of clinical features in the diagnosis of VAP [31]. A team of physicians predicted whether patients had VAP based on all available clinical information, and the diagnosis was made based on histopathology, pleural fluid culture, or computed tomography criteria. Only 62% of patients with confirmed VAP were correctly diagnosed, as were 84% of patients without pneumonia.

Since clinical criteria alone are insufficiently accurate to diagnose VAP, airway sampling for Gram stain and culture is used to confirm the diagnosis. Samples may be obtained non-invasively via endotracheal aspirate, or alternatively, during bronchoscopy using either a protected specimen brush or bronchoalveolar lavage. A meta-analysis of RCTs of invasive versus non-invasive diagnosis found no difference in clinical outcomes, including mortality, duration of ventilation, and ICU LOS, suggesting that non-invasive tracheal aspiration should be used for diagnosis of VAP in most patients [32].

15.2.4 Management

Patients with suspected VAP require empiric antibiotic therapy to cover potential pathogens while awaiting the results of microbiologic testing. The initial choice of antibiotics will depend on local antibiotic resistance data and the patient's risk of colonization with MDR organisms. Risk factors include duration of hospitalization five or more days, intravenous antibiotic therapy within preceding three months, septic shock at the time of VAP, acute respiratory distress syndrome preceding VAP, or acute renal replacement therapy prior to VAP onset [26].

Prompt initiation of appropriate antibiotic therapy is important. A study of 107 ICU patients with suspected VAP determined that a delay in antibiotic administration of greater than 24 hours was an independent risk factor for hospital mortality, with an adjusted OR of 7.7 (95% CI 4.5–13.1, $p < 0.001$) [33]. Furthermore, a meta-analysis found that inappropriate antibiotics significantly increased the risk of mortality (adjusted OR 3.03, 95% CI 1.12–8.19) [34].

Based on the microbiology of VAP, experts in the field recommend an empiric regimen that includes coverage for *P. aeruginosa* and other Gram negative organisms as well as *S. aureus*. Addition of coverage for methicillin-resistant *S. aureus* or a second antipseudomonal agent may be considered when patients have risk factors for MDR organisms or local resistance rates are high [26].

The duration of antibiotic therapy should be limited to seven or eight days based on a systematic review showing no difference in mortality between 7–8 day courses compared to 10–15 day courses and a possible reduction in emergence of MDR organisms. Two studies reported higher rates of recurrence with shorter courses for VAP caused by *P. aeruginosa* or other non-fermenting gram negative bacilli, so a longer duration may be considered in that setting [35].

15.2.5 Prevention

Several preventive strategies are recommended based on current evidence, broadly categorized as those that prevent aspiration and those that reduce bacterial colonization.

Prevention of aspiration can be achieved through patient positioning and drainage of subglottic secretions. The head of the bed may be elevated to 30°–45°, based on a meta-analysis that showed a significant decrease in clinically diagnosed VAP compared to supine positioning (OR = 0.47, 95% confidence interval, 0.27–0.82) and non-significant decreases in microbiologically confirmed VAP and mortality [36]. Endotracheal tubes with subglottic drainage are recommended based on a meta-analysis demonstrating a statistically significant risk ratio of 0.55 for VAP, along with decreases in duration of mechanical ventilation and ICU LOS [37].

Oropharyngeal decontamination may be considered to reduce bacterial colonization of the oropharynx. A meta analysis of 18 RCTs found a reduction in VAP rates with chlorhexidine oral hygiene compared to placebo or usual care (RR 0.74, 95% CI 0.61–0.89) [38]. However, the safety of this technique has recently been called into question because of a possible signal towards increased mortality.

Case Presentation 1 (continued)

Investigating for a nosocomial infection, the clinical team performs a bronchoscopy (because there are scant secretions on endotracheal aspiration), a urine analysis (which is negative and not sent for culture), and paired quantitative blood cultures. They remove the subclavian catheter that Mr. KW no longer requires. Tenacious secretions are detected on bronchoscopy, and the chest radiograph shows a subtle new opacification in the right middle lobe; Mr. KW is started empirically on piperacillin-tazobactam. However, four days later, with resolution of his fever and leukocytosis, no organisms cultured, and persistent subtle opacification of the right middle lobe, empiric antibiotics are discontinued.

15.3 Central line-Associated Bloodstream Infections

15.3.1 Epidemiology

ICU patients require intravascular catheters for monitoring and treatment purposes, and central line-associated bloodstream infections (CLABSI) are one of the potential complications. Rates of CLABSI differ depending on the type of catheter and site of insertion [39]. A meta-analysis estimated an overall incidence rate of 1.27 cases per 1,000 line days among adult inpatients in the United States, with an attributable increase in hospital LOS by 10 days per case and total cost of over U.S.$1.8 billion per year [27].

15.3.2 Etiology

The pathogenesis of CLABSI involves bacterial colonization of the central venous catheter (CVC), both in biofilms and in free forms [40]. Virtually all intravascular catheters become colonized, but the likelihood of developing a CLABSI is related to bacterial load, surface properties of the catheter, and host immunity. Colonizing organisms commonly originate from the skin and migrate along the extraluminal surface of the catheter into the bloodstream. Organisms may also enter the bloodstream intraluminally through the catheter hub, often via the hands of healthcare workers.

National surveillance in the United States found the most common pathogens causing CLABSI are coagulase-negative staphylococci (20.5%), enteric gram negative bacilli (19.7%), *Enterococcus* species (18.1%), *Candida* species (14.6%), and *S. aureus* (12.3%) [29].

15.3.3 Diagnosis

The surveillance definition of a laboratory-confirmed bloodstream infection requires at least one of the following criteria: isolation of a pathogen from one or more blood cultures that is not related to infection at any other site, or isolation of a common skin commensal from two or more blood cultures drawn on separate occasions with at least one systemic manifestation of infection (e.g., fever, chills, hypotension) and no other suspected source of infection. CLABSI is present if a patient with a bloodstream infection has had a CVC in use during the 48 hours prior to the onset of infection [41].

Clinical features of infection have limited utility in the diagnosis of CLABSI but may warrant further microbiologic evaluation, including two blood cultures with at least one taken from a peripheral venipuncture site. Positive blood cultures drawn from a line can be difficult to interpret because they may represent catheter colonization rather than bloodstream infection. A retrospective study of 271 ICU patients compared the utility of blood cultures drawn from central catheters and peripheral venipuncture [42]. Negative predictive values were similar (97% and 95%, respectively); however, positive predictive values were significantly higher for peripheral samples (82%) than central catheters (61%), suggesting their utility in differentiating CLABSI from colonization.

Once bacteremia is established, several techniques may help to confirm whether a CVC is the source. If the line is removed, the tip can be cultured to confirm colonization. Alternative diagnostic approaches in the absence of line removal include paired quantitative blood cultures and differential time to positivity [43]. Both methods involve obtaining two blood cultures drawn simultaneously from the CVC and a peripheral vein and are based on the principle that the bacterial load will be inversely proportional to the distance from an infected CVC. A five times greater colony count from the CVC than the peripheral sample or a time to positivity from the CVC at least two hours earlier than the peripheral sample is considered diagnostic of CLABSI. A meta-analysis of 51 studies compared the diagnostic properties of qualitative, semi-quantitative, and quantitative catheter segment cultures, qualitative and quantitative catheter-drawn cultures, paired quantitative cultures, differential time to positivity, and acridine orange leukocyte cytospin [44]. Paired quantitative blood culture was most accurate, with an overall sensitivity of 89% and specificity of 98%, although most methods showed acceptable test characteristics and negative predictive values >99%.

Case Presentation 1 (continued)

Among the investigations for nosocomial infection, the blood culture from Mr. KW's central venous catheter identified coagulase-negative staphylococci and the peripheral blood culture was negative, consistent with contamination of the central catheter specimen or colonization of the catheter itself.

15.3.4 Management

Management of CLABSI in patients with short-term CVCs includes antimicrobial therapy and consideration of catheter removal. Experts generally recommend vancomycin for empiric therapy to cover coagulase-negative staphylococci and

S. aureus. Empiric Gram-negative coverage based on local susceptibility data may be considered if the patient is demonstrating signs of sepsis or has a femoral CVC. Empiric therapy for candidemia may be considered if patients have risk factors such as hematologic malignancy, solid organ or bone marrow transplant, or total parenteral nutrition [45].

Identification of the causative organism will guide subsequent management. For coagulase-negative staphylococcal infection, a retrospective study of 70 patients found recurrence in 20% of patients with retained catheters versus 3% of patients whose catheters were removed ($p < 0.05$) [46]. Vancomycin therapy is indicated for 5–7 days if the catheter is removed, versus 10–14 days if the catheter remains in place. Some experts suggest that patients without endovascular or orthopedic hardware may be observed without antibiotic therapy if the CVC is removed [45].

CLABSI caused by *S. aureus* requires removal of the catheter; failure to do so significantly increases the risk for infection recurrence and mortality [47]. *S. aureus* bacteremia is also commonly associated with metastatic infections, including infective endocarditis; therefore, transesophageal echocardiography may be considered to identify cases of *S. aureus* endocarditis, which requires prolonged antibiotic therapy [45,48]. The recommended duration of therapy for patients with no evidence of infective endocarditis is a minimum of 14 days. If the *S. aureus* is susceptible, β-lactam antibiotics or a first-generation cephalosporin are optimal therapy [45].

CLABSI due to Gram-negative bacilli are less common, but CVC removal may be considered based on a small retrospective study which found that catheter removal significantly reduced the likelihood of recurrence (OR 0.13, 95% CI 0.02–0.75) [49]. Experts recommend a 14-day course of antibiotic therapy following CVC removal [45], but level 1 evidence to guide treatment duration is lacking.

CVC removal may also be considered in CLABSI caused by *Candida* species. A prospective study of 145 patients with catheter-related candidemia found that failure to remove the catheter was significantly associated with mortality (OR 4.8) [50]. Experts recommend repeating blood cultures routinely, performing a retinal examination to rule out chorioretinitis, and continuing antifungal treatment for 14 days after the first negative blood culture [45].

15.3.5 Prevention

Preventive measures for CLABSI should be implemented at the time of CVC insertion and during ongoing maintenance.

Key factors related to CVC insertion include site selection, barrier precautions, and skin preparation. A RCT comparing subclavian, jugular, and femoral sites demonstrated a significantly reduced infection rate with subclavian lines, although other factors including experience of the operator will also impact site selection [51]. Sterile technique and full barrier precautions, including cap, mask, sterile gown, and gloves, and large drape should be used for CVC insertion. A systematic review found one RCT and two other studies of maximal barrier precautions showing significant reductions in CLABSI [52]. An alcoholic chlorhexidine preparation should be used for skin antisepsis at the insertion site based on a meta-analysis showing significant reductions in CVC colonization and CLABSI compared to povidone-iodine [53].

Maintenance of the CVC is another important consideration in preventing infection. Chlorhexidine-based solutions should be used for skin disinfection at the insertion site to reduce bacterial colonization. A meta-analysis of studies comparing chlorhexidine and povidone-iodine demonstrated a RR of 0.49 (95% CI 0.28–0.88) for CLABSI [54]. Cleaning catheter hubs with antiseptic prior to accessing the ports will reduce the risk of introducing microbes directly into the catheter lumen. Solutions containing 70% ethanol have been shown to be more effective than chlorhexidine at reducing bacterial contamination of catheter hubs [55].

Insertion and maintenance bundles for CLABSI prevention have been extensively studied and should be implemented based on a meta-analysis of 79 studies showing a significant decrease in CLABSI from a median of 6.4 per 1,000 catheter days to 2.5 per 1,000 catheter days [56]. Insertion bundles consist of at least maximum sterile barrier precautions and chlorhexidine antisepsis. Maintenance bundles consist of at least hand hygiene, daily evaluation of need for a central line, and disinfection prior to accessing the line.

References

1 Gaieski DF, Edwards JM, Kallan MJ, Carr BG. Benchmarking the incidence and mortality of severe sepsis in the United States. Crit Care Med. 2013;41:1167–74.

2 Stevenson EK, Rubenstein AR, Radin GT, Wiener RS, Walkey AJ. Two decades of mortality trends among patients with severe sepsis: a comparative meta-analysis.* Crit Care Med. 2014;42:625–31.

3 Singer M, Deutschman CS, Seymour CW, et al. The Third International Consensus Definitions for Sepsis and Septic Shock (Sepsis-3). JAMA. 2016;315:801–10.

4 Vincent JL, De Backer D. Circulatory shock. N Engl J Med. 2014;370:583.

5 American College of Chest Physicians/ Society of Critical Care Medicine Consensus Conference: definitions for sepsis and organ failure and guidelines for the use of innovative therapies in sepsis. Crit Care Med. 1992;20:864–74.

6 Rivers E, Nguyen B, Havstad S, et al. Early goal-directed therapy in the treatment of severe sepsis and septic shock. N Engl J Med. 2001;345:1368–77.

7 Yealy DM, Kellum JA, Huang DT, et al. A randomized trial of protocol-based care for early septic shock. N Engl J Med. 2014;370:1683–93.

8 Peake SL, Delaney A, Bailey M, et al. Goal-directed resuscitation for patients with early septic shock. N Engl J Med. 2014;371:1496–506.

9 Mouncey PR, Osborn TM, Power GS, et al. Trial of early, goal-directed resuscitation for septic shock. N Engl J Med. 2015;372:1301–11.

10 Bouchard J, Soroko SB, Chertow GM, et al. Fluid accumulation, survival and recovery of kidney function in critically ill patients with acute kidney injury. Kidney Int. 2009;76:422–7.

11 Marik PE, Cavallazzi R. Does the central venous pressure predict fluid responsiveness? an updated meta-analysis and a plea for some common sense. Crit Care Med. 2013;41:1774–81.

12 Rajaram SS, Desai NK, Kalra A, et al. Pulmonary artery catheters for adult patients in intensive care. Cochrane Database Syst Rev. 2013:CD003408.

13 Marik PE, Lemson J. Fluid responsiveness: an evolution of our understanding. Brit J Anaesthesia. 2014;112:617–20.

14 Kumar A, Roberts D, Wood KE, et al. Duration of hypotension before initiation of effective antimicrobial therapy is the critical determinant of survival in human septic shock. Crit Care Med. 2006;34:1589–96.

15 Kumar A, Ellis P, Arabi Y, et al. Initiation of inappropriate antimicrobial therapy results in a fivefold reduction of survival in human septic shock. Chest. 2009;136:1237–48.

16 Bochud PY, Bonten M, Marchetti O, Calandra T. Antimicrobial therapy for patients with severe sepsis and septic shock: an evidence-based review. Crit Care Med. 2004;32:S495–512.

17 Rivers EP, McIntyre L, Morro DC, Rivers KK. Early and innovative interventions for severe sepsis and septic shock: taking advantage of a window of opportunity. CMAJ. 2005;173:1054–65.

18 Martinez ML, Ferrer R, Torrents E, et al. Impact of source control in patients with severe Sepsis and septic shock. Crit Care Med. 2016.

19 Dellinger RP, Levy MM, Rhodes A, et al. Surviving sepsis campaign: international guidelines for management of severe sepsis and septic shock: 2012. Crit Care Med. 2013;41:580–637.

20 Annane D, Bellissant E, Bollaert PE, Briegel J, Keh D, Kupfer Y. Corticosteroids for treating sepsis. Cochrane Database Syst Rev. 2015:CD002243.

21 Keh D, Trips E, Marx G, et al. Effect of hydrocortisone on development of shock among patients with severe sepsis: The HYPRESS Randomized Clinical Trial. JAMA. 2016;316:1775–85.

22 Venkatesh B, Myburgh J, Finfer S, et al. The ADRENAL study protocol: adjunctive corticosteroid treatment in critically ill patients with septic shock. Crit Care Resusc. 2013;15:83–8.

23 Annane D, Buisson CB, Cariou A, et al. Design and conduct of the activated protein C and corticosteroids for human septic shock (APROCCHSS) trial. Ann Intensive Care. 2016;6:43.

24 Bernard GR, Francois B, Mira JP, et al. Evaluating the efficacy and safety of two doses of the polyclonal anti-tumor necrosis factor-alpha fragment antibody AZD9773 in adult patients with severe sepsis and/or septic shock: randomized, double-blind, placebo-controlled phase IIb study.* Crit Care Med. 2014;42:504–11.

25 Marti-Carvajal AJ, Sola I, Gluud C, Lathyris D, Cardona AF. Human recombinant protein C for severe sepsis and septic shock in adult and paediatric patients. Cochrane Database Syst Rev. 2012;12:CD004388.

26 Kalil AC, Metersky ML, Klompas M, et al. Management of adults with hospital-acquired and ventilator-associated pneumonia: 2016 Clinical Practice Guidelines by the Infectious Diseases Society of America and the American Thoracic Society. Clin Infect Dis. 2016;63:e61–e111.

27 Zimlichman E, Henderson D, Tamir O, et al. Health care-associated infections: a meta-analysis of costs and financial impact on the US health care system. JAMA Intern Med. 2013;173:2039–46.

28 Kollef MH. The prevention of ventilator-associated pneumonia. N Engl J Med. 1999;340:627–34.

29 Sievert DM, Ricks P, Edwards JR, et al. Antimicrobial-resistant pathogens associated with healthcare-associated infections: summary of data reported to the National Healthcare Safety Network at the Centers for Disease Control and Prevention, 2009–2010. Infect Control Hosp Epidemiol. 2013;34:1–14.

30 Meduri GU, Mauldin GL, Wunderink RG, et al. Causes of fever and pulmonary densities in patients with clinical manifestations of ventilator-associated pneumonia. Chest. 1994;106:221–35.

31 Fagon JY, Chastre J, Hance AJ, Domart Y, Trouillet JL, Gibert C. Evaluation of clinical judgment in the identification and treatment of nosocomial pneumonia in ventilated patients. Chest. 1993;103:547–53.

32 Berton DC, Kalil AC, Teixeira PJ. Quantitative versus qualitative cultures of respiratory secretions for clinical outcomes in patients with ventilator-associated pneumonia. Cochrane Database Syst Rev. 2014:CD006482.

33 Iregui M, Ward S, Sherman G, Fraser VJ, Kollef MH. Clinical importance of delays in the initiation of appropriate antibiotic treatment for ventilator-associated pneumonia. Chest. 2002;122:262–8.

34 Kuti EL, Patel AA, Coleman CI. Impact of inappropriate antibiotic therapy on mortality in patients with ventilator-associated pneumonia and blood stream infection: a meta-analysis. J Crit Care. 2008;23:91–100.

35 Pugh R, Grant C, Cooke RP, Dempsey G. Short-course versus prolonged-course antibiotic therapy for hospital-acquired pneumonia in critically ill adults. Cochrane Database Syst Rev. 2015:CD007577.

36 Alexiou VG, Ierodiakonou V, Dimopoulos G, Falagas ME. Impact of patient position on the incidence of ventilator-associated pneumonia: a meta-analysis of randomized controlled trials. J Crit Care. 2009;24:515–22.

37 Muscedere J, Rewa O, McKechnie K, Jiang X, Laporta D, Heyland DK. Subglottic secretion drainage for the prevention of ventilator-associated pneumonia: a systematic review and meta-analysis. Crit Care Med. 2011;39:1985–91.

38 Hua F, Xie H, Worthington HV, Furness S, Zhang Q, Li C. Oral hygiene care for critically ill patients to prevent ventilator-associated pneumonia. Cochrane Database Syst Rev. 2016;10:CD008367.

39 Maki DG, Kluger DM, Crnich CJ. The risk of bloodstream infection in adults with different intravascular devices: a systematic review of 200 published prospective studies. Mayo Clinic Proc. 2006;81:1159–71.

40 Raad I. Intravascular-catheter-related infections. Lancet. 1998;351:893–8.

41 The National Healthcare Safety Network (NHSN) Manual: Patient Safety Component Protocol, January 2017. 2017. [cited 2015 November 23]. Available from http://www.cdc.gov/nhsn/pdfs/ pscmanual/4psc_clabscurrent.pdf.

42 Martinez JA, DesJardin JA, Aronoff M, Supran S, Nasraway SA, Snydman DR. Clinical utility of blood cultures drawn from central venous or arterial catheters in critically ill surgical patients. Crit Care Med. 2002;30:7–13.

43 Raad I, Hanna H, Maki D. Intravascular catheter-related infections: advances in diagnosis, prevention, and management. Lancet Infect Dis. 2007;7:645–57.

44 Safdar N, Fine JP, Maki DG. Meta-analysis: methods for diagnosing intravascular device-related bloodstream infection. Anns Internal Med. 2005;142:451–66.

45 Mermel LA, Allon M, Bouza E, et al. Clinical practice guidelines for the diagnosis and management of intravascular catheter-related infection: 2009 Update by the Infectious Diseases Society of America. Clin Infect Dis. 2009;49:1–45.

46 Raad I, Davis S, Khan A, Tarrand J, Elting L, Bodey GP. Impact of central venous catheter removal on the recurrence of catheter-related coagulase-negative staphylococcal bacteremia. Infect Control Hosp Epidemiol. 1992;13:215–21.

47 Fowler VG, Jr., Sanders LL, Sexton DJ, et al. Outcome of Staphylococcus aureus bacteremia according to compliance with recommendations of infectious diseases specialists: experience with 244 patients. Clin Infect Dis. 1998;27:478–86.

48 Fowler VG, Jr., Li J, Corey GR, et al. Role of echocardiography in evaluation of patients with Staphylococcus aureus bacteremia: experience in 103 patients. J Am Coll Cardiol. 1997;30:1072–8.

49 Hanna H, Afif C, Alakech B, et al. Central venous catheter-related bacteremia due to gram-negative bacilli: significance of catheter removal in preventing relapse. Infect Control Hosp Epidemiol. 2004;25:646–9.

50 Nucci M, Colombo AL, Silveira F, et al. Risk factors for death in patients with candidemia. Infect Control Hosp Epidemiol. 1998;19:846–50.

51 Parienti JJ, Mongardon N, Megarbane B, et al. Intravascular complications of central venous catheterization by insertion site. New Engl J Med. 2015;373:1220–9.

52 Hu KK, Lipsky BA, Veenstra DL, Saint S. Using maximal sterile barriers to prevent central venous catheter-related infection: a systematic evidence-based review. Am J Infect Control. 2004;32:142–6.

53 Maiwald M, Chan ES. The forgotten role of alcohol: a systematic review and meta-analysis of the clinical efficacy and perceived role of chlorhexidine in skin antisepsis. PloS One. 2012;7:e44277.

54 Chaiyakunapruk N, Veenstra DL, Lipsky BA, Saint S. Chlorhexidine compared with povidone-iodine solution for vascular

catheter-site care: a meta-analysis. Ann of Intern Med. 2002;136:792–801.

55 Salzman MB, Isenberg HD, Rubin LG. Use of disinfectants to reduce microbial contamination of hubs of vascular catheters. J Clin Microbiol. 1993;31:475–9.

56 Ista E, van der Hoven B, Kornelisse RF, et al. Effectiveness of insertion and maintenance bundles to prevent central-line-associated bloodstream infections in critically ill patients of all ages: a systematic review and meta-analysis. Lancet Infect Dis. 2016;16:724–34.

Part 2

Special Populations

Chapter 16

Infection Prevention and Control

Graham M. Snyder and Eli N. Perencevich

16.1 Preventing Transmission of Multidrug-Resistant Organisms

---

Case Presentation 1

As the Medical Director of an inpatient Internal Medicine unit, you are approached by an infectious diseases colleague with a concern. She has just been consulted regarding three patients over several weeks with a clinical culture positive for a *Klebsiella pneumoniae* resistant to carbapenem antimicrobials. Your colleague is concerned because she has not frequently encountered carbapenem-resistant organisms before at your hospital, yet the patients had unique sites of infection. You call a meeting with the Nurse Manager of the unit, the Infection Control Practitioner who covers that unit, and the Microbiology Director.

In 2013, the Centers for Disease Control and Prevention (CDC) published a report outlining the most important infectious disease threats demonstrating significant antimicrobial-resistance [1]. While foodborne enteric pathogens and other pathogens typically transmitted in a non-healthcare setting were also members of the list, the ignominious "who's who" of nosocomial pathogens were held to account for an estimated 400,000 infections and 30,000 deaths: carbapenem-resistant Enterobacteriaceae (CRE), multidrug-resistant *Acinetobacter*, extended-spectrum β-lactamase producing Enterobacteriaceae (ESBLs), vancomycin-resistant *Enterococcus* (VRE), multidrug-resistant *Pseudomonas aeruginosa*, methicillin-resistant *Staphylococcus aureus* (MRSA), vancomycin-resistant *Staphylococcus aureus* (VRSA) as well as the antimicrobial-associated pathogen *Clostridium difficile* [1].

These are organisms most readily transmitted to patients by direct contact, either following contact with an individual such as a healthcare worker (HCW) or with inanimate objects such as the surfaces in an inpatient room. Therefore, in addition to surveillance for these multidrug-resistant organisms (MDRO) paired with prudent antimicrobial use, key elements of preventing transmission of MDRO in the healthcare setting include hand hygiene, the use of personal protective equipment, and attention to environmental contamination.

16.1.1 Hand Hygiene

Case Presentation 1 (continued)

The microbiology lab is testing the saved isolates to confirm the antimicrobial susceptibility results, and will submit the isolates to a reference laboratory to confirm genetic relatedness. The Infection Preventionist is developing a line list comprising the three

---

Evidence-Based Infectious Diseases, Third Edition. Edited by Dominik Mertz, Fiona Smaill, and Nick Daneman.
© 2018 John Wiley & Sons Ltd. Published 2018 by John Wiley & Sons Ltd.

patients to determine if any epidemiological connections exist to suggest a mechanism of transmission. As a team, you begin to discuss ways the organism may be transmitted on the unit. The Nurse Manager mentions that when the Nurse Champion on the unit performed hand hygiene adherence observations last month, HCW adherence was 55%.

Among Infection Control interventions to prevent transmission of multidrug-resistant organisms, hand hygiene reigns supreme as the most valued intervention due to the simplicity of the intervention, it's efficacy against a broad range of organisms transmitted by direct contact and the ability to observe, measure, and improve the intervention in any healthcare setting. The evidentiary basis for hand hygiene as an effective intervention begins with data supporting the frequency of HCW hand contamination: Pittet and colleagues demonstrated that 89% of hands were culture positive, 10% with *S. aureus* and 13% with Gram-negative pathogens. Factors most strongly associated with contamination included the degree and nature of patient contact and not performing hand hygiene (particularly without an antiseptic agent) [2]. In a real-world setting with standardized interactions, the frequency of HCW hand contamination with *S. aureus* in the absence of performing hand hygiene ranged from approximately 5% to 60%, commensurate with the frequency of positive patient skin and environment cultures [3]. In a study of 22 VRE-positive inpatients, HCWs acquired and transmitted to a new patient or environmental location a genetically indistinguishable VRE isolate in over 10% of contact opportunities [4]. Concisely summarized, the frequency of HCW hand contamination during routine care likely depends on the nature of the care provided, patient factors, and organism characteristics, but is a frequent event.

The *relative* effectiveness of hand hygiene with soap and water, antimicrobial soap and water, and alcohol-based hand rub remains a subject of debate and is likely dependent on the organism and testing conditions. However, there is little debate of the effectiveness of hand hygiene methods in reducing the burden of organisms on hands when performed effectively. A randomized controlled trial (RCT) performed in 2002 compared hand hygiene with alcohol-based hand rub, a non-antiseptic soap and water, and an antiseptic soap and water. While the reduction in bacterial contamination was greatest after using alcohol-based hand rub followed by handwashing with antiseptic soap, all methods reduced bacterial contamination significantly [5]. The relative effectiveness of alcohol-based hand rub against most viral, bacterial, and fungal nosocomial organisms (bacterial spores excepted), as well as the ease of use and lack of known development of resistance, have made its use widely adopted.

Evidence in support of the effectiveness of hand hygiene in reducing transmission is by no means novel. In a seminal quality improvement intervention, Semmelweis observed in 1847 that the use of chlorinated lime among doctors and medical students (who also engaged in the bare-handed dissection of corpses) providing obstetrical care to peri-partum women dramatically reduced the rate of puerperal fever and death [6]. In a more modern setting, Mortimer and colleagues presented in 1962 the results of a RCT with a singular and persuasive design: In a newborn nursery, infants were randomized to one of two bassinet groupings (A and B) and an "index" infant with known *S. aureus* carriage was placed in a central bassinet. Nurses, assigned to care only for infants in a specific group (A or B), were required on entry to the nursery to first handle the *S. aureus*-colonized index infant. "A" group nurses would perform a routine 10-second handwashing with hexachlorophene prior to subsequent patient care while "B" group nurses would proceed directly to patient care without handwashing. Strikingly, the rate ratio for infant acquisition of *S. aureus* between the hand hygiene (A) group and the direct care (B) group was 0.58 (95% confidence interval [95% CI] 0.41–0.81), and the incidence rate ratio for the same was 0.26 (95% CI 0.14–0.47), suggesting an approximately 50–75% reduction in the transmission of *S. aureus* through hand hygiene alone [7].

Although it is the very unlikely that a RCT comparing hand hygiene to no hand hygiene will ever again be performed, contemporary data, including ecological data, supports the association between adherence to hand hygiene and the nosocomial acquisition of MDRO and healthcare-associated infections. A systematic review conducted by the World Health Organization (WHO) in 2014 identified 37 observational studies in which "hand hygiene was the key intervention implemented in the study period and hand hygiene indicators…were measured along with MDRO infection and/or transmission rates" [8]. These studies, most commonly designed with only a few exceptions as before/after intervention studies or time-series analyses, demonstrated an inverse association between hand hygiene adherence and MDRO frequency; the relationship was most frequently studied for MRSA.

Despite the evidence in support of hand hygiene, adherence in many healthcare settings remains dismal, often struggling to approach 50%, although some small- and large-scale campaigns have demonstrated greater success. Clinical role (typically physician) and excessive workload are most often identified as associated with poor adherence, although product availability and acceptability, education and beliefs, and other sociological factors may also play a significant role [9].

One of the standard mechanisms for quality improvement is audit-and-feedback. Several methods for measuring hand hygiene compliance exist, including: direct observation by trained observers, with or without utilization of electronic devices to facilitate data collection or with the use of video to allow remote observation; quantification of product usage as a surrogate; and automated monitoring using remote video monitoring or radio frequency identification technology. While direct observation is considered the gold standard, there are potential shortcomings to all methods, and an optimal method of observing hand hygiene adherence has not been established. A recent systematic review outlined the limitations of current electronic systems to directly observe or enhance hand hygiene compliance, and identified a need for more studies reporting accuracy and effectiveness of these systems [10]. Self-observation and observations by patients have not been demonstrated to be reliable compared to direct observation [11].

While there is some debate on the optimal hand hygiene surveillance method, there is even less conclusive evidence supporting interventions that result in sustainable improvements in hand hygiene compliance. A systematic review of studies conducted in 2015 demonstrated 6 RCTs, 1 non-randomized trial, 2 controlled before/after studies, and 32 interrupted time series analyses. The components of interventions included availability infrastructure, institutional safety climate, education and training, goal setting, feedback on adherence, workplace reminders, reward incentives, and HCW accountability. Importantly, single interventions (system change or education) demonstrated a smaller and non-significant impact than a multimodal strategy promoted by the World Health Organization comprising five components (WHO-5): system change, training and education, observation and feedback, workplace reminders, and institution safety climate. Interventions utilizing WHO-5 *plus* goal setting or accountability demonstrated the greatest effectiveness [8,12].

Hand hygiene is highly recommended as a simple intervention broadly effective at preventing the transmission of many pathogens. Absent conclusive data on best approaches, institutions may choose from various methods of observation and a spectrum of intervention types to improve hand hygiene adherence.

16.1.2   Contact Precautions

> ### Case Presentation 1 (continued)
>
> While observing workflow on the unit with the Nurse Manager, you observe a nurse with a handful of dressing change supplies enter a room of a patient assigned to contact precautions for methicillin-resistant *Staphylococcus aureus*. After dropping off supplies at the bedside, he exits the room to collect medications from the medication room. On return to the patient room the second time, he dons a disposable isolation gown, performs hand hygiene, dons gloves, and enters the room to administer medications and perform a dressing change.

Contact precautions entail the use of personal protective equipment, namely, disposable or washable gowns and disposable non-sterile gloves. In theory, contact precautions serve as a physical barrier between the HCW and both the patient and the patient's environment to prevent the translocation of pathogens from patient carriage or environmental contamination to the HCW, and subsequently, to other patients through direct contact or fomites. While contact precautions are used for a broad array of specific pathogens and situations, we focus this discussion on their role in the acute care setting for MDRO including MRSA, VRE, and resistant Gram-negative pathogens including CRE. Current guidelines recommend the use of contact precautions for MDRO, although areas of uncertainty remain, including the duration of contact precautions and the role of active surveillance and pre-emptive use of contact precautions [13,14].

In practice, the effectiveness of contact precautions for MDRO remains a subject of ongoing debate, particularly in the case of MRSA and VRE. There are two important high-quality cluster-randomized trials focusing specifically on contact precautions as an intervention. In the Strategies to Reduce Transmission of Antimicrobial Resistant Bacteria in Intensive Care Units (STAR*ICU)

trial, Huskins and colleagues randomized 18 intensive care units to an intervention of active surveillance cultures for MRSA and VRE on admission with subsequent contact precautions if positive as well as universal gloving until surveillance cultures results were available, or to a control arm of isolation precautions per usual protocols (in both arms contact precautions were used for patients previously identified as colonized or infected with MRSA or VRE) [15]. While a substantial portion of patients were identified as colonized or infected with MRSA or VRE and the use of contact precautions doubled in the intervention arm, the incidence of MRSA or VRE colonization or infection among the 9,139 admissions did not significantly change with the intervention. The interpretation of this study has been influenced by the suboptimal rate of adherence to contact precautions and hand hygiene, reduced adherence to hand hygiene among providers using gown and gloves, and the long turn-around time of screening results. Additionally, the study design tested the effect of active surveillance, universal gloving (in part), and increased use of contact precautions, rather than a specific focus on standard versus contact precautions for patients with MRSA and VRE. The second and more recent trial—Benefits of Universal Glove and Gown (BUGG) trial—sought to address some of these shortcomings by randomizing 20 intensive care units to either universal gown and glove use (intervention group) or the usual standard of care, including the use of contact precautions for patients with a history of colonization or infection with MRSA or VRE [16]. For the primary outcome—the composite of acquisition of MRSA or VRE—there was no difference between intervention and control arms. Although there was a significant reduction in MRSA acquisition, VRE acquisition and other secondary outcomes, including hospital-acquired infections and mortality in the intensive care unit did not differ between the two groups.

Several other noteworthy studies may help shed light on the potential benefit of contact precautions. The Mastering Hospital Antimicrobial Resistance in Intensive Care Units (MOSAR-ICU) trial utilized an interrupted time series and cluster-randomized design to investigate two sequential interventions: universal chlorhexidine body washing and enhanced hand hygiene, and in a subsequent phase, rapid versus conventional screening for MRSA, VRE, and highly-resistant Enterobacteriaceae with the use of contact precautions if positive. The initial body washing and hand hygiene interventions resulted in a decrease in the acquisition of MDRO (driven by changes in MRSA acquisition), and in the rapid screening group the assignment of contact precaution was increased (although the adherence was not audited), but the acquisition of MDRO was not significantly improved compared to the conventional screening group [17]. The REDUCE-MRSA trial was a cluster-randomized trial of three interventions: active surveillance and isolation with contact precautions; active surveillance, contact precautions, and decolonization; and universal decolonization alone. The use of contact precautions was reduced in the universal decolonization arm, and for the primary outcome of MRSA acquisition, the hazard ratio was lower for universal decolonization (HR 0.63, 95% CI 0.52–0.75) than for targeted decolonization (HR 0.75, 95% CI 0.63–0.89) or active surveillance and isolation (HR 0.92, 95% CI 0.77–1.10, $p = 0.01$ for comparison of all three groups) [18]. Last, a nationwide initiative among all Veterans Affairs hospitals starting in 2007 using a "MRSA bundle" consisting of institutional culture change, enhanced hand hygiene interventions, universal active surveillance on admission and discharge, and contact precautions for all MRSA carriers. The intervention demonstrated a remarkable improvement in MRSA acquisition and specific healthcare-associated infections in both intensive care unit and non-intensive care unit settings, though the relative contribution of contact precautions to this improvement is not known given the bundle approach [19].

Taking these studies in context, it is notable that "perfect" data remains elusive to quantify the independent benefit of contact precautions and the benefit of contact precautions as part of a bundle of MDRO interventions. In particular, no RCT has investigated only the role of contact precautions, without being part of a bundle, universal use of gloves with or without gowns, and the role of screening. A contemporaneous systematic review of recent (10 years) studies that investigated the "placement of the infected or colonized patient in a single room or in a cohort facility, [and] application of standard precautions and disposable gown and glove use for close patient contact" concluded that five of six identified studies identified no change in colonization or infection rates with various MDRO, and the sixth demonstrated a decrease in colonization rates of the target MDRO, *Acinetobacter baumannii* [20].

While the use of contact precautions is an intuitive intervention, the relative lack of high-quality evidence supporting these measures must be balanced against potential harms associated with the use of contact precautions. These potential harms include reductions in the frequency of patient care/contact, an increase in patient adverse events, negative psychological effects on patients, and diminished patient satisfaction. A systematic review from 2009 found that among 15 studies investigating adverse outcomes associated with contact precautions, there was a suggestion that HCW contact, adverse events, patient perception of care, and patient symptoms of depression and anxiety were potentially worse among patients on contact precautions, though significant methodological limitations were common [21]. Hand hygiene may be worse when providers are using contact precautions though this finding has not been replicated. Moreover, subsequent studies investigating the frequency of adverse events and the psychological effects of contact precautions have demonstrated conflicting results with the highest quality studies, such as the BUGG trial, which do not find an increase in harm related to contact precautions [22].

Last, it could be noted that decision-making among infection control and healthcare leaders may be demonstrating a shift in the perceived impact of contact precautions for MRSA and VRE. A survey of Society for Healthcare Epidemiology of America Research Network members published in 2015 found that although greater than 90% of responding institutions use contact precautions for MRSA and VRE, a strong majority felt contact precautions caused harm, only a minority of respondents felt the routine use of surveillance cultures and contact precautions was helpful (in a variety of situations), over 60% would consider alternative strategies that exclude contact precautions, and over 30 hospitals in the United States either never implemented contact precautions or have discontinued precautions for MRSA or VRE [23].

In summary, published data suggests uncertainty about the benefits of contact precautions in preventing the transmission of MDRO, and further research is necessary to clarify the potential risk of contact precautions on patient care. When deciding on the role of contact precautions in a comprehensive infection control program, we suggest institutions consider factors such as MDRO infection rate and colonization density, HCW adherence to other infection control interventions such as hand hygiene, and patient safety outcomes.

16.1.3 Environmental Sources

Case Presentation 1 (continued)

With the Director of Environmental Services and the Housekeeper for your unit, you walk through the common areas and several unoccupied patient rooms. When asked about wall-mounted computer stations recently installed for a new electronic medication administration record system, the housekeeper reports Information Technology does not permit cleaning the computer stations with the standard quaternary ammonium-based cleaning product used in the hospital.

The environment almost certainly plays a role in the transmission of MDRO in the acute care setting, though the relative importance of the environment is difficult to quantify [24]. For example, in a mathematical modeling study varying hand hygiene adherence and thoroughness of environmental cleaning on the transmission of MRSA, VRE, and multidrug-resistant *A. baumannii*, hand hygiene was found to be approximately twice as efficient as environmental cleaning although both play significant roles in reducing transmission [25].

Nosocomial bacterial pathogens may survive up to months on environmental surfaces, and there are innumerable studies demonstrating contamination of common inanimate objects in the healthcare setting [26]. Despite the findings of positive cultures from a broad array of fomites, any direct relationship between culture-positive fomites or non-invasive medical equipment and patient acquisition of MDRO is difficult to study, and therefore, not well established [27]. A prospective study by Koganti and colleagues stands out as worthy of closer consideration [28]. By inoculating a 30 x 30 cm area of floor adjacent to the bed of 10 ambulatory patients with *C. difficile* infection or MRSA carriage with a bacteriophage preparation, they were able to demonstrate that despite high-quality room cleaning (85% of surfaces were cleaned as assessed using fluorescent marker) there was rapid dissemination *within one day* of the bacteriophage to the hands of patients, high-touch surfaces inside the patient room, portable equipment, and the unit nursing station.

Several studies have characterized the risk of MDRO acquisition during admission to an inpatient room following the discharge of a patient with colonization or infection with that same MDRO. In a first-of-its-kind study, Huang and colleagues used a retrospective dataset of over 11,000 intensive care unit admissions over 20 months, including over 10,000 patients at risk for acquiring MRSA and VRE. Patients at risk had a 1.4 times higher odds of acquiring MRSA or VRE if the prior room occupant was colonized or infected with that MDRO than if the prior occupation was MDRO-negative. While this circumstantial evidence suggests the environment may play a role in transmission, this association only accounted for approximately 5–7% of the acquisition events for both organisms [29]. A recent systematic review published in 2015 identified seven studies characterizing the risk of MDRO acquisition from a prior room occupant. While the meta-analysis demonstrated a combined odds ratio of 2.14 (95% CI 1.65–2.77) for the acquisition of an MDRO from a prior room occupant, the systematic review highlighted missing information that raises a question about the validity of these studies; antimicrobial use, hand hygiene compliance, and indwelling devices were not considered in most analyses [30]. Taken together, these studies make a compelling case, albeit a very circumstantial one, that MDRO environmental contamination has a small but significant role in the acquisition of MDRO in intensive care units in an endemic setting.

Environmental contamination has also been associated with MDRO-associated outbreaks. This relationship may be most strongly seen in the case of *Acinetobacter spp.*, for which multiple investigators have described the role of environmental cleaning in the control of the outbreak. Among the intensive care unit rooms of patients with infection or recent or remote history of colonization with multidrug-resistant *A. baumannii* infections, researchers in Maryland identified environmental contamination in 48% of rooms on a very broad range of surfaces in the room. Thorough post-discharge cleaning markedly improved contamination rates, but low levels of contamination persisted [31]. In another rigorous study of nine acute care facilities and two long-term care facilities, investigators describe several novel findings: While post-discharge room cleaning resulted in reduced concentrations of environmental contamination with MDRO, contamination during patient admission in the setting of daily room cleaning was

severalfold higher; MDRO were recovered from 44% of routine cleaned room samples and 30% of post-discharge samples; the frequency of specific MDRO identified on routine and post-discharge cleaning varied, though VRE was most common and the concordance between MDRO for which the patient was isolated and the MDRO identified on cultures was highest for MRSA [32].

There are several options to assess the effectiveness of patient room cleaning, particularly post-discharge room cleaning: direct observation (either of the cleaning process or visual examination of the cleaned surfaces); cultures of the surfaces, arguably the gold standard; the placement of a low-visibility fluorescent marker either prior to patient admission or just prior to post-discharge cleaning, with re-assessment after room cleaning for physical removal; and quantification of adenosine triphosphate (ATP) contamination of surfaces [33]. There is a paucity of data making a direct comparison of these methods, however, the few published studies making a meaningful comparison of visual inspection, fluorescent marker, and/or ATP quantification with bacterial contamination have shown a poor correlation between the non-microbiologic methods with the culture results [34]. Numerous studies have demonstrated that the use of ATP measurement or fluorescent marker with education and feedback to Environmental Services staff can improve the frequency of positive sampling events [35]. Whether or not these interventions can decrease the frequency of MDRO acquisition from the environment remains to be proven.

Last, there is currently a brisk interest in the use of "no-touch" disinfection technology that entails either the exposure of surfaces to ultraviolet (UV) light or exposure to hydrogen peroxide. Each of these systems have pragmatic advantages and disadvantages, and both systems have demonstrated effectiveness in decreasing microbial contamination though clinical trials have been limited to trial designs other than controlled trials [36]. Preliminary results from a cluster-randomized clinical trial comparing UV disinfection, bleach, and UV disinfection with bleach compared to a quaternary ammonium standard suggest that the frequency of patient MDRO acquisition in rooms assigned to all intervention arms were similar and lower than the quaternary ammonium reference [37]. The impact of these systems (including cost-effectiveness assessments) in reducing patient acquisition and infection with MDRO requires further study; therefore, we cannot recommend the routine use of these non-touch technologies at this time.

16.2   Surgical Site Infections

Case Presentation 2

A new Chief of Surgery, who happens to be a cardio-thoracic surgeon, arrives at your hospital. She calls you and says that she is concerned that the risk-adjusted surgical site infection rates at your hospital might be higher than the rates at her previous hospital. She wants to set up a meeting with you to discuss ways to minimize the risk of surgical site infection in her patients.

16.2.1   Surveillance and Burden of Illness

Surgical site infections (SSIs) are defined as either incisional or organ/organ space infections occurring within 30 to 90 days of the procedure (depending on the procedure type). Incisional SSIs are then divided into superficial, involving the skin and subcutaneous tissue, and deep, involving the muscle and fascia. SSI rates vary by procedure; however, as estimated by a survey of a sample of facilities reporting to the National Healthcare Safety Network (NHSN), SSIs are the most common type of healthcare-associated infections in the United States. From this sample, it is estimated that there are 157,500 (95% CI 50,800–281,400) SSIs

annually, comprising 22% of healthcare associated infections [38].

16.2.2   Risk Factors

The incidence of SSIs varies depending on the surgeon, the hospital, procedure type and duration, and individual patient risk factors. However, the identification of risk factors associated with SSIs is most useful when identified risk factors are modifiable. Therefore, we describe the evidence related to modifiable risk factors including RCTs demonstrating improved outcomes with their modification. Furthermore, while it may seem that identifying an individual surgeon as a risk factor could be more disruptive than helpful, it has been shown that one of the most successful ways to reduce SSIs is proper surveillance (i.e., audit) of infection rates and feedback of rates to individual surgeons [39].

16.2.3   Glucose Control

Diabetes is known to increase the risk of developing a SSI. One proposed mechanism includes impaired neutrophil phagocytic function (but not antibody-dependent cell cytotoxicity), as demonstrated in a randomized trial of patients receiving either intensive or standard insulin treatment during surgery [40].

A systemic review and meta-analysis published by Martin and colleagues in 2016 identified 1.53 times higher odds (95% CI 1.11–2.12) of SSI among patients with diabetes compared to those without, independent of SSI class and patient body mass index (BMI) [41]. The magnitude of the effect may be dependent on procedure type: In a subgroup analysis of cardiac surgeries, the pooled odds ratio was 2.03 (95% CI 1.13–4.05), while the relationship was weakest for colorectal surgeries (1.16, 95% CI 0.93–1.44) [41]. In one study of cardiothoracic surgery patients, a post-operative glucose level greater than 200 mg/DL within 48 hours after surgery was shown to increase the odds of developing an SSI by 86% in known diabetic patients and by

114% in patients with no history of diabetes, and these results were largely unchanged with multivariable analysis [42].

Despite the strength of this association, it is not clear that intensive peri-operative management of blood glucose can impact the risk of surgical outcomes. A Cochrane review identified 12 RCTs comprising 694 diabetic patients randomized to intensive glucose management versus standard care. There was not a significant association with any outcome including death, infectious complications and cardiovascular events, although the intensive management arm did have a substantially higher risk of hypoglycemic episodes [43]. Optimal glucose management protocols may be complex including procedure- and patient-dependent components; further investigation is warranted, and its routine implementation cannot be recommended yet.

16.2.4 Peri-operative Warming

Un-warmed patients in surgery lose heat until their core temperature falls about 2 °C, after which core temperature is stabilized by peripheral vasoconstriction and altered heat distribution [44]. Hypothermia is thought to increase a patient's risk of developing a SSI through thermoregulatory vasoconstriction and resultant reduced tissue oxygen levels, and impairment of the immune function [45].

A Cochrane review identified 67 RCTs investigating a variety of active warming strategies during surgery in order to avoid complications and increase patient comfort after surgery. Only two studies, both of low quality, were identified that provided data for their meta-analysis: The risk for surgical site infection (risk ratio 0.36 [95% CI 0.20–0.66]) was significantly lower when warming the patients [46]. One of these two RCTs was conducted in patients undergoing colorectal surgery. Kurz et al. demonstrated an approximately threefold reduction in SSI rates in patients actively warmed approximately 2 °C to the desired temperature of 36.6 °C by intravenous fluid warming and forced-air warming in the intra-operative period [47].

The second RCT, by Melling et al., found that warming patients before surgery reduced post-operative SSIs in patients undergoing breast, varicose vein, or hernia surgery. The study found that both systemic warming (absolute risk reduction 7.9%, 95% CI 1.0–14.8) and local warming (10.1%, 95% CI 3.6–16.6) were associated with reduced SSIs compared to standard non-warmed treatment [48].

The evidence is limited and these two studies were undertaken for a limited number of procedure types. Therefore, no firm recommendations can be made on the use of peri-operative warming to prevent SSI. Furthermore, a broad recommendation across all types of surgery cannot be given since patients who undergo certain procedures may benefit from peri-operative hypothermia. For example, mild hypothermia has a documented cerebro-protective effect in neurosurgery patients and core temperatures are lowered in cardiac surgery to protect the myocardium and central nervous system.

16.2.5 Supplemental Oxygen

Neutrophilic bactericidal activity is mediated by superoxide radical dependent oxidative killing, which is linked to the partial pressure of oxygen in the tissue [49]. A cohort study of patients at high risk for SSI found that the oxygen tension of the subcutaneous tissue measured peri-operatively was a very strong predictor of subsequent development of SSI [50]. The infection rate was 43% (6 of 14 patients) in those with maximum oxygen tension between 40 to 50 mmHg and 0% (0 of 15 patients) in those with maximum oxygen tension above 90 mmHg.

Greif et al. performed a RCT in patients undergoing colorectal surgery comparing patients who received 30% versus 80% inspired oxygen intra-operatively and in the two hours after surgery [49]. Even though arterial oxygen saturation was normal in both groups, the subcutaneous partial pressure of oxygen was significantly higher in those that received 80% inspired oxygen.

The infection rate was significantly lower in the 80% inspired oxygen group (5.2 vs. 11.2%, absolute risk reduction 6.0%, 95% CI 7.3–15.1%) [49].

Subsequently, a double-blind RCT among 165 patients undergoing major intra-abdominal surgery compared SSIs within 14 days of surgery among 160 patients receiving either 80% or 35% inspired oxygen intra-operatively and two hours post-operatively [51]. Twenty patients in the 80% inspired oxygen group (25.0%) and nine patients in the 35% inspired oxygen group (11.3%) had SSIs ($p = 0.02$). Significant limitations to this study include the small sample size, analysis of infection rates by retrospective chart review, inadequate assessment of tissue perfusion and possibly oxygenation, and imbalance of several potentially confounding variables [51].

Prompted by the discrepancy between these two trials, another RCT similar in methodology to Greif et al. [49] compared rates of SSI in 291 patients undergoing elective colorectal resection who received either 30% or 80% inspired oxygen intra-operatively and six hours post-operatively [52]. Again, the 80% inspired oxygen group had a lower SSI risk (14.9 vs. 24.4%, RR 0.61, 95% CI 0.38–0.98). In multivariate analysis, only 30% inspired oxygen and coexisting respiratory disease significantly increased risk of SSI [52].

A Cochrane review published in 2016 has identified a total of 15 RCTs, including the representative studies described, comparing a high fraction of inspired oxygen (60–90%) with a usual care fraction of inspired oxygen (30–40%). The pooled relative risk demonstrated no significant difference in the risk of infection 14 to 30 days post-operatively (relative risk 0.87, 95% CI 0.71–1.07), including when restricted to five trials with an overall low risk of bias (relative risk 0.86, 95% CI 0.63–1.17) [53]. On the balance, while some data suggest a possible benefit of high fraction of inspired oxygen in the prevention of SSIs, debate regarding limitations of study methodology highlights residual uncertainty in the efficacy of this intervention. Thus, no recommendation can be made on the routine use of supplemental oxygen to prevent SSIs.

16.2.6 Hair Removal

Hair removal as part of the preparation of the surgical site has long been a practice of surgeons to improve exposure to the surgical site. Three methods of hair removal are commonly practiced: shaving, clipping, and depilatory creams. Shaving may change the normal skin flora, remove the hairs' natural protective effect, and cause minor trauma that may allow for an entry site for bacteria or produce exudates that support bacterial growth—all factors which may increase the risk of infection.

The most comprehensive and recent review of the evidence for hair removal in reducing SSI rates is a network meta-analysis comparing no hair removal, clipping, shaving, and chemical depilation [54]. Nineteen clinical trials were included in the analysis. Compared to shaving, clipping (relative risk 0.55, 95% CI 0.38–0.79), chemical depilation (0.60, 95% CI 0.36–0.97), and no hair removal (relative risk 0.56, 95% CI 0.34–0.96) conferred a lower risk of surgical site infection. There was not a significant difference in pairwise comparisons of the non-shaving methods [54].

Based on this data, we recommend that hair removal should be limited to situations where hair will impede the operation, and if necessary, hair should be removed with clippers or depilatory cream and not by shaving. Issues without definitive data include optimal timing of hair removal in proximity to surgery and optimal location to perform hair removal (i.e., ward, pre-operative suite, or operating room).

16.2.7 Smoking Cessation

Smoking likely affects the risk of SSI in mechanisms similar to hypoxemia, including inhibiting immune response, promoting peripheral vasoconstriction, disruption of endothelial function, and superoxide radical ion production [55].

Several cohort studies have demonstrated a positive association between smoking and SSI, including the following two particularly large study cohorts. Recently, a study of 47,574 patients undergoing colorectal resections demonstrated a 1.32 (95% CI 1.22–1.42) and 1.27 (95% CI 1.17–1.37) times higher adjusted odds of incisional infections among current and ex-smokers, respectively, compared to never smokers [56]. A study of 393,794 patients undergoing various surgical procedures in Veterans Affairs facilities demonstrated similar relationships between tobacco smoking and surgical site infection: Researchers found a 1.11 times higher adjusted odds for SSIs for prior smokers and 1.18 (95% CI 1.13–1.24) for current smokers compared to never smokers [57].

RCTs of smoking cessation intervention have demonstrated a decrease in SSI risk among smokers who quit prior to surgery. Among three small RCTs randomizing patients to pre-operative smoking cessation versus usual care, one study in 60 patients demonstrated no significant difference in post-operative complications, including wound infection (33% [95% CI 17–54%] in the intervention group versus 27% [95% CI 12–46] in the control groups), [58] while two trials (78 and 120 patients, respectively) demonstrated a significant decrease in post-operative wound infections in patients randomized to smoking cessation interventions [59,60]. It should be noted that the smoking cessation intervention in the trial demonstrating no difference was undertaken only two to three weeks pre-operatively, a time period potentially too short for effects of tobacco exposure to be mitigated.

While the magnitude of effect and optimal time for cessation is not fully characterized, there is strong evidence that smoking contributes to SSI risk and that cessation prior to surgery decreases this risk. Due to SSI and other peri-operative risk, as well as non-surgical, non-infectious health risks, we highly recommend counseling patients on smoking cessation prior to surgery.

16.2.8 *Staphylococcus Aureus* Elimination with Mupirocin Ointment and Chlorhexidine Scrub

S. aureus is a frequent cause of SSIs, and *S. aureus* carriage has been found to be a risk factor for SSIs. In 75–80% of instances, the *S. aureus* strain implied in SSI had been indistinguishable from the strain colonizing the patients prior to surgery [61]. Mupirocin ointment can be used to eliminate nasal carriage of *S. aureus* and chlorhexidine body wash to reduce carriage and bacterial density at the surgical site and body sites remote to the surgery. The risks of these agents include topical adverse effects and the development of antimicrobial resistance [62]. Therefore, the optimal strategy is of interest to providers and infection preventionists. Two strategies are commonly employed: pre-operative surveillance for *S. aureus*, including MRSA with subsequent use of topical agent(s), or universal use of the topical agent(s) without screening for colonization.

A recent systematic review and meta-analysis identified 39 controlled trials or observational studies with a control group reporting SSI outcomes with Gram-positive bacteria including *S. aureus* among patients undergoing cardiac or orthopedic procedures [63]. The 17 studies (10 in cardiac and 7 in orthopedic surgery; 5 RCTs) investigating nasal decolonization demonstrated a pooled relative risk of 0.41 (95% CI 0.30–0.55) for prevention of Gram-positive SSI and 0.39 (95% CI 0.31–0.5) for *S. aureus* SSI. As would be expected, the relative risk among RCT was less pronounced, and in fact, did not demonstrate a significant reduction for Gram-positive SSI (RR 0.63, 95% CI 0.36–1.13), but did for S. aureus SSI (RR 0.46, 95% CI 0.29–0.73). Whether the studies performed universal decolonization (11) or selectively decolonized *S. aureus* nasal carriers (6), the relative risk reduction of *S. aureus* SSI remained significant. Last, the relative risk of *S. aureus* SSI was lower among the six studies pairing nasal decolonization with topical chlorhexidine or triclosan (RR 0.29, 95% CI 0.19–0.44) than among the 11 studies investigating nasal decolonization alone (RR 0.70, 95% CI 0.50–0.97) [63]. Clinical trials investigating the use of mupirocin in surgical procedure types other than cardiac or orthopedic surgery have not demonstrated a significant decrease in SSIs among patients receiving mupirocin compared to controls.

The use of pre-operative chlorhexidine to prevent surgical site infections has been reviewed by the Cochrane group, which identified seven trials using 4% chlorhexidine gluconate. The studies did not demonstrate a significant reduction in SSI, whether chlorhexidine was compared to placebo (3 RCTs, RR 0.91, 95% CI 0.80–1.04), compared to bar soap (3 RCTs, RR 1.02, 95% CI 0.57–1.84), or compared to no wash (3 RCTs, RR 0.82, 95% CI 0.26–2.62). Surgical procedure types varied among the studies included in this research, including general surgery, clean surgery, vascular surgery, vasectomy, and plastic surgery.

Notably, a recent prospective quasi-experimental trial among 20 U.S. hospitals implemented a bundle of interventions including pre-operative *S. aureus* nares screening, nasal mupirocin, and chlorhexidine bathing for five pre-operative days in *S. aureus* colonized patients, chlorhexidine bathing the night before and morning of surgery in non-colonized patients, and among MRSA-colonized patients, vancomycin in addition to cefazolin or cefuroxime for peri-operative prophylaxis [64]. Surgical procedure types included cardiac operations, hip arthroplasties, and knee arthroplasties. Bundle adherence was 83% after the phase-in period. After adjusting for age, diabetes, Charlson comorbidity index, and MRSA history, the implementation of the bundle was associated with a 40% reduction in complex *S. aureus* SSIs among individual patients (OR 0.60, 95% CI 0.37–0.98) and the hospital-level analysis estimated that the SSI rate decreased significantly after implementation of the bundle (RR 0.58, 95% CI 0.37–0.92) [64].

In a recent cost-effectiveness analysis assuming a baseline prevalence of MRSA carriage of 5.1% (surgical type unspecified), investigators found that universal screening (using PCR) reduced SSI risk, but was associated with a higher cost compared to no screening; using risk factors to guide screening was not cost-effective [65]. An earlier decision analysis study of MRSA screening for vascular surgical procedures suggested that screening would be cost-effective when MRSA prevalence is at least 1% and decolonization was at least successful in 25% of attempts [66]. Further studies may establish a clear role for mupirocin and/or chlorhexidine in populations of *S. aureus* carriers or specific surgeries, particularly surgeries other than cardiac or orthopedic.

Taking the data in its entirety, we suggest that—depending on the baseline rate of SSIs as well as the colonization prevalence of *S. aureus* generally and MRSA specifically—decolonization using mupirocin and chlorhexidine universally or among identified *S. aureus* carriers may be considered. Chlorhexidine alone is unlikely effective at reducing SSI rates.

16.2.9 Peri-operative Antimicrobial Prophylaxis

Not all surgeries require antibiotic prophylaxis. The initial step in deciding whether antimicrobial prophylaxis is indicated in a particular surgery is to determine which type of procedure will be performed. Table 16.1 lists the surgical wound classification scheme. This classification allows the surgeon to estimate preoperatively the wound class of a given operation, although, the classification is by definition a post-operative assessment of intra-operative wound contamination, since breaks in sterile technique and other intra-operative findings cannot be predicted preoperatively. Antimicrobial prophylaxis is considered indicated for clean-contaminated wounds (Class II), and in clean wounds (Class I) if the SSI might be a clinical catastrophe (e.g., intravascular or joint prosthesis implantations). Antimicrobial prophylaxis is not indicated in Class III or IV

Table 16.1 Surgical Wound Classification.

Class I/Clean: Uninfected operative wound with no inflammation and the respiratory, alimentary, genital, or uninfected urinary tract is not entered. Cleans wounds are primarily closed and necessary drains are closed.

Class II/Clean-Contaminated: Operative wound with controlled entry into the respiratory, alimentary, genital, or urinary tract. Specifically, operations of the biliary tract, appendix, vagina, and oropharynx are included if no evidence of infection or break in sterile technique.

Class III/Contaminated: Open, fresh accidental wounds or ones with breaks in sterile technique, gastrointestinal spillage, or incisions in which non-purulent inflammation is encountered are contaminated.

Class IV/Dirty-Infected: Presence of old traumatic wounds with devitalized tissue or ones with existing clinical infection or perforated viscera suggesting pre-existing organisms prior to the operation.

Mangram et al. [67].

operations since these would involve specific antimicrobial treatment.

There are several issues surrounding the use of prophylactic antibiotics during the peri-operative period, including the timing of antibiotic initiation and the duration of dosing in the post-operative period. Classen et al. in a large prospective cohort study determined the effect of prophylactic antibiotic timing (based on the start of antimicrobial infusion) on the rate of SSI in 2,847 patients who had clean (Class I) or clean-contaminated (Class II) operations [68]. Patients who received antibiotics preoperatively, defined as zero to two hours prior to incision, had the lowest rate of SSI (0.6%). Higher rates of SSI were seen for peri-operative administration, within three hours after incision (1.4%), and in those that received antibiotics more than two hours before (3.8% SSI rate) and more than three hours after (3.3% SSI rate) the incision [68]. One recent large study investigating the timing of antimicrobial prophylaxis in 32,459 operations of various surgical procedure types demonstrated a higher risk of SSI among patients receiving prophylaxis >60 minutes prior to incision

(unadjusted OR 1.34, 95% CI 1.08–1.66) and after incision (unadjusted OR 1.26, 95% CI 0.92–1.72) compared to patients receiving prophylaxis within the 60 minute pre-operative window. After adjustment for confounders, the relationship between appropriate timing of antimicrobial administration and SSI was no longer significant. Other studies have also suggested an association between timing and risk. Although the ideal timing has not been determined and may depend on the half-life of the drug administered, professional guidelines continue to recommend antimicrobial administration within 60–120 minutes of the first surgical incision [69,70].

To minimize the risk of adverse drug reaction and the development of *C. difficile* infection, the post-operative duration of antimicrobial prophylaxis should be less than 24 hours (for cardiothoracic procedures a 48-hour duration is commonly accepted but not based on clinical trial data) [69]. A meta-analysis of 28 RCTs with 9,478 patients compared single versus multiple dose antimicrobial prophylaxis in a broad range of surgical procedure types and found no difference between the two groups (OR 1.04, 95% CI 0.86–1.25) [71]. A more contemporary meta-analysis of 12 RCTs comparing <24 and ≥24 hours of antimicrobial prophylaxis following cardiac surgery highlights ongoing uncertainty on this issue: Although 11 of 12 trials were at high risk for bias, antimicrobial prophylaxis ≥24 hours post-operatively was associated with a lower risk of SSI (RR 1.38, 95% CI 1.13–1.69) though no significant difference in overall infections [72].

In summary, based on expert opinion, antimicrobial prophylaxis (when indicated) may most optimally be administered within 60–120 minutes of the first surgical incision and continued no more than 24 hours after the end of surgery.

16.2.10 Comprehensive "Bundled" Interventions

Ultimately, no single intervention should be relied on to improve SSI rates. A partnership between surgical and infection control services focusing on the strategies described will have the greatest benefit through additive independent mechanisms and a combined effect. Multiple studies have nearly universally demonstrated that a multidisciplinary team-based approach to incorporate a "bundle" of interventions targeting SSI reduction improves process measures such as adherence to antimicrobial selection, timing, and duration, and does result in a reduction of SSI [73].

The National Surgical Infection Prevention Collaborative (later developed into the Surgical Care Improvement Project) was begun in 2002 with an aim to improve several process measures related to SSI prevention. An early report of 44 collaborative hospitals showed improvement among various surgical procedure types in several measures: antibiotic timing within one hour of surgery, appropriate antibiotic selection, discontinuation of antibiotic within 24 hours of surgery, normothermia (intra-operative temperature >36 °C), avoiding shaving surgical site, high fraction inspired oxygen (FIO2 >80%), and glucose control (≤200 mg/dL). Among 35,543 surgical cases over a 12-month period, the overall SSI rate fell significantly from 2.28% in the first quarter to 1.65% in the final quarter, though the month-to-month trends were not significant by Poisson regression analysis [74].

Single-center studies have generally showed improvement in SSI rates following implementation of a bundle of interventions. For example, a four-year observational study of a cardiothoracic surgery service after the initiation of a comprehensive infection control program that included surveillance, feedback to the surgeons, chlorhexidine showers the night before and morning of surgery, hair clipping if necessary, antibiotic prophylaxis in the holding area 30–120 minutes prior to

surgery, and elimination of iced cardioplegia solutions along with other changes was found to significantly reduce the rate of SSIs (OR 0.37, 95% CI 0.22–0.63) [75]. Conversely, in a three-year study at a Veteran's Administration facility, 211 patients undergoing transabdominal colorectal surgery were randomized to either usual practice or a bundle intervention including: omission of mechanical bowel preparation, pre-operative and intra-operative warming, supplemental oxygen during and following surgery, intra-operative intravenous fluid restriction, and use of surgical wound protector. The rate of SSI was 45% in the intervention arm and 24% in the control arm, primarily attributed to superficial incisional SSIs, and corresponding to a 2.49 times higher risk (95% CI 1.36–4.56) of SSI in the intervention arm even after controlling for SSI risk factors [76]. Although the authors cite evidentiary basis for each of their individual interventions, it should be noted that for several of the interventions, either the data in support of the intervention is conflicting or limited to one or two RCTs.

In conclusion, an optimal infection control program to limit SSIs in surgical patients depends on surveillance for SSIs in the inpatient setting, and if possible, tracking of SSIs that manifest after hospital discharge, with consideration of reporting SSI rates to individual surgeons. Modifiable risk factors and peri-operative interventions have variable strength of evidence to support their implementation. Institutions embarking on SSI reduction efforts should consider limitations to bundling multiple interventions, as bundled interventions have shown mixed success in improving SSI rates and individual elements of bundles may have weak evidence to support their use.

References

1 Centers for Disease Control and Prevention. Antibiotic resistance threats in the United States, 2013: Centers for Disease Control and Prevention; 2013.

2 Pittet D, Dharan S, Touveneau S, Sauvan V, Perneger TV. Bacterial contamination of the hands of hospital staff during routine patient care. Arch Intern Med. 1999;159:821–6.

3 Bhalla A, Aron DC, Donskey CJ. Staphylococcus aureus intestinal colonization is associated with increased frequency of S. aureus on skin of hospitalized patients. BMC Infect Dis. 2007;7:105.

4 Duckro AN, Blom DW, Lyle EA, Weinstein RA, Hayden MK. Transfer of vancomycin-resistant enterococci via health care worker hands. Arch Intern Med. 2005;165:302–7.

5 Lucet JC, Rigaud MP, Mentre F, et al. Hand contamination before and after different hand hygiene techniques: a randomized clinical trial. J Hosp Infect. 2002;50:276–80.

6 Classics in infectious diseases. Childbed fever by Ignaz Philipp Semmelweis. Rev Infect Dis. 1981;3:808–11.

7 Mortimer EA, Jr., Lipsitz PJ, Wolinsky E, Gonzaga AJ, Rammelkamp CH, Jr. Transmission of staphylococci between newborns. Importance of the hands to personnel. Am J Dis Child. 1962;104:289–95.

8 World Health Organization. Evidence of hand hygiene to reduce transmission and infections by multidrug resistant organisms in health-care settings. 2014.

9 Smiddy MP, R OC, Creedon SA. Systematic qualitative literature review of health care workers' compliance with hand hygiene guidelines. Am J Infect Control. 2015;43: 269–74.

10 Ward MA, Schweizer ML, Polgreen PM, Gupta K, Reisinger HS, Perencevich EN. Automated and electronically assisted hand hygiene monitoring systems: a systematic review. Am J Infect Control. 2014;42:472–8.

11 Ellingson K, Haas JP, Aiello AE, et al. Strategies to prevent healthcare-associated infections through hand hygiene. Infect Control Hosp Epidemiol. 2014;35:937–60.

12 Luangasanatip N, Hongsuwan M, Limmathurotsakul D, et al. Comparative efficacy of interventions to promote hand hygiene in hospital: systematic review and network meta-analysis. BMJ. 2015;351:h3728.

13 Siegel JD, Rhinehart E, Jackson M, Chiarello L. Management of multidrug-resistant organisms in health care settings, 2006. Am J Infect Control. 2007;35:S165–93.

14 Banach D, Bearman G, Barnden M, Hanrahan J, Leekha S, Morgan D, et al. Duration of Contact Precautions for Acute-Care Settings. Infect Control Hosp Epidemiol. 2018;39(2):127–144. doi:10.1017/ice.2017.245.

15 Huskins WC, Huckabee CM, O'Grady NP, et al. Intervention to reduce transmission of resistant bacteria in intensive care. N Engl J Med. 2011;364:1407–18.

16 Harris AD, Pineles L, Belton B, et al. Universal glove and gown use and acquisition of antibiotic-resistant bacteria in the ICU: a randomized trial. JAMA. 2013;310:1571–80.

17 Derde LP, Cooper BS, Goossens H, et al. Interventions to reduce colonisation and transmission of antimicrobial-resistant bacteria in intensive care units: an interrupted time series study and cluster randomised trial. Lancet Infect Dis. 2014;14:31–9.

18 Huang SS, Septimus E, Kleinman K, et al. Targeted versus universal decolonization to prevent ICU infection. N Engl J Med. 2013;368:2255–65.

19 Jain R, Kralovic SM, Evans ME, et al. Veterans Affairs initiative to prevent methicillin-resistant Staphylococcus aureus infections. N Engl J Med. 2011;364:1419–30.

20 Cohen CC, Cohen B, Shang J. Effectiveness of contact precautions against multidrug-resistant organism transmission in acute care: a systematic review of the literature. J Hosp Infect. 2015;90:275–84.

21 Morgan DJ, Diekema DJ, Sepkowitz K, Perencevich EN. Adverse outcomes associated with Contact Precautions: a review of the literature. Am J Infect Control. 2009;37:85–93.

22 Kullar R, Vassallo A, Turkel S, Chopra T, Kaye KS, Dhar S. Degowning the

controversies of contact precautions for methicillin-resistant Staphylococcus aureus: a review. Am J Infect Control. 2016;44:97–103.

23 Morgan DJ, Murthy R, Munoz-Price LS, et al. Reconsidering contact precautions for endemic methicillin-resistant Staphylococcus aureus and vancomycin-resistant Enterococcus. Infect Control Hosp Epidemiol. 2015;36:1163–72.

24 Otter JA, Yezli S, Salkeld JA, French GL. Evidence that contaminated surfaces contribute to the transmission of hospital pathogens and an overview of strategies to address contaminated surfaces in hospital settings. Am J Infect Control. 2013;41:S6–11.

25 Barnes SL, Morgan DJ, Harris AD, Carling PC, Thom KA. Preventing the transmission of multidrug-resistant organisms: modeling the relative importance of hand hygiene and environmental cleaning interventions. Infect Control Hosp Epidemiol. 2014;35:1156–62.

26 Russotto V, Cortegiani A, Raineri SM, Giarratano A. Bacterial contamination of inanimate surfaces and equipment in the intensive care unit. J Intensive Care. 2015;3:54.

27 Haun N, Hooper-Lane C, Safdar N. Healthcare personnel attire and devices as fomites: a systematic review. Infect Control Hosp Epidemiol. 2016:1–7.

28 Koganti S, Alhmidi H, Tomas ME, Cadnum JL, Jencson A, Donskey CJ. Evaluation of hospital floors as a potential source of pathogen dissemination using a nonpathogenic virus as a surrogate marker. Infect Control Hosp Epidemiol. 2016: 1–4.

29 Huang SS, Datta R, Platt R. Risk of acquiring antibiotic-resistant bacteria from prior room occupants. Arch Intern Med. 2006;166:1945–51.

30 Mitchell BG, Dancer SJ, Anderson M, Dehn E. Risk of organism acquisition from prior room occupants: a systematic review and meta-analysis. J Hosp Infect. 2015;91:211–7.

31 Strassle P, Thom KA, Johnson JK, et al. The effect of terminal cleaning on environmental contamination rates of multidrug-resistant Acinetobacter baumannii. Am J Infect Control. 2012;40:1005–7.

32 Shams AM, Rose LJ, Edwards JR, et al. Assessment of the overall and multidrug-resistant organism bioburden on rnvironmental surfaces in healthcare facilities. Infect Control Hosp Epidemiol. 2016:1–7.

33 Han JH, Sullivan N, Leas BF, Pegues DA, Kaczmarek JL, Umscheid CA. Cleaning hospital room surfaces to prevent health care-associated infections: a technical brief. Ann Intern Med. 2015;163:598–607.

34 Snyder GM, Holyoak AD, Leary KE, Sullivan BF, Davis RB, Wright SB. Effectiveness of visual inspection compared with non-microbiologic methods to determine the thoroughness of post-discharge cleaning. Antimicrob Resist Infect Control. 2013;2:26.

35 Leas BF, Sullivan N, Han JH, Pegues DA, Kaczmarek JL, Umscheid CA. Environmental cleaning for the prevention of healthcare-associated infections. Agency for Healthcare Research and Quality. Rockville (MD); 2015.

36 Non-Manual Techniques for Room Disinfection in Healthcare Facilities: A Review of Clinical Effectiveness and Guidelines. Canadian Agency for Drugs and Technologies in Health. Ottawa (ON); 2014.

37 Anderson D, Knelson L, Moehring R, Lewis S, Weber D, Chen L, et al. Implementation Lessons Learned From the Benefits of Enhanced Terminal Room (BETR) Disinfection Study: Process and Perceptions of Enhanced Disinfection with Ultraviolet Disinfection Devices. Infect Control Hosp Epidemiol. 2018;39(2): 157–163. doi:10.1017/ice.2017.268.

38 Magill SS, Edwards JR, Bamberg W, et al. Multistate point-prevalence survey of health care-associated infections. N Engl J Med. 2014;370:1198–208.

39 Gaynes RP, Culver DH, Horan TC, Edwards JR, Richards C, Tolson JS. Surgical site infection (SSI) rates in the United States, 1992–1998: the National Nosocomial Infections Surveillance System basic SSI risk index. Clin Infect Dis. 2001;33 Suppl 2:S69–77.

40 Rassias AJ, Marrin CA, Arruda J, Whalen PK, Beach M, Yeager MP. Insulin infusion improves neutrophil function in diabetic cardiac surgery patients. Anesth Analg. 1999;88:1011–6.

41 Muratore S, Statz C, Glover JJ, Kwaan M, Beilman G. Risk adjustment for determining surgical site infection in colon surgery: are all models created equal? Surg Infect. 2016;17: 173-8.

42 Latham R, Lancaster AD, Covington JF, Pirolo JS, Thomas CS. The association of diabetes and glucose control with surgical-site infections among cardiothoracic surgery patients. Infect Control Hosp Epidemiol. 2001;22:607–12.

43 Buchleitner AM, Martinez-Alonso M, Hernandez M, Sola I, Mauricio D. Perioperative glycaemic control for diabetic patients undergoing surgery. Cochrane Database Syst Rev. 2012:CD007315.

44 Sessler DI. Mild perioperative hypothermia. N Engl J Med. 1997;336:1730–7.

45 Sessler DI. Non-pharmacologic prevention of surgical wound infection. Anesthesiol Clin. 2006;24:279–97.

46 Madrid E, Urrutia G, Roque i Figuls M, et al. Active body surface warming systems for preventing complications caused by inadvertent perioperative hypothermia in adults. Cochrane Database Syst Rev. 2016;4:CD009016.

47 Kurz A, Sessler DI, Lenhardt R. Perioperative normothermia to reduce the incidence of surgical-wound infection and shorten hospitalization. Study of Wound Infection and Temperature Group. N Engl J Med. 1996;334:1209–15.

48 Melling AC, Ali B, Scott EM, Leaper DJ. Effects of preoperative warming on the incidence of wound infection after clean surgery: a randomised controlled trial. Lancet. 2001;358:876–80.

49 Greif R, Akca O, Horn EP, Kurz A, Sessler DI. Supplemental perioperative oxygen to reduce the incidence of surgical-wound infection. Outcomes Research Group. N Engl J Med. 2000;342:161–7.

50 Hopf HW, Hunt TK, West JM, et al. Wound tissue oxygen tension predicts the risk of wound infection in surgical patients. Arch Surg. 1997;132:997–1004; discussion 5.

51 Pryor KO, Fahey TJ, 3rd, Lien CA, Goldstein PA. Surgical site infection and the routine use of perioperative hyperoxia in a general surgical population: a randomized controlled trial. JAMA. 2004;291:79–87.

52 Belda FJ, Aguilera L, Garcia de la Asuncion J, et al. Supplemental perioperative oxygen and the risk of surgical wound infection: a randomized controlled trial. JAMA. 2005;294:2035–42.

53 Wetterslev J, Meyhoff CS, Jorgensen LN, Gluud C, Lindschou J, Rasmussen LS. The effects of high perioperative inspiratory oxygen fraction for adult surgical patients. Cochrane Database Syst Rev. 2015:CD008884.

54 Lefebvre A, Saliou P, Lucet JC, et al. Preoperative hair removal and surgical site infections: network meta-analysis of randomized controlled trials. J Hosp Infect. 2015;91:100–8.

55 Sopori M. Effects of cigarette smoke on the immune system. Nat Rev Immunol. 2002;2:372–7.

56 Sharma A, Deeb AP, Iannuzzi JC, Rickles AS, Monson JR, Fleming FJ. Tobacco smoking and postoperative outcomes after colorectal surgery. Ann Surg. 2013;258:296–300.

57 Hawn MT, Houston TK, Campagna EJ, et al. The attributable risk of smoking on surgical complications. Ann Surg. 2011;254:914–20.

58 Sorensen LT, Jorgensen T. Short-term pre-operative smoking cessation intervention does not affect postoperative complications in colorectal surgery: a

randomized clinical trial. Colorectal Dis. 2003;5:347–52.

59 Sorensen LT, Karlsmark T, Gottrup F. Abstinence from smoking reduces incisional wound infection: a randomized controlled trial. Ann Surg. 2003;238: 1–5.

60 Moller AM, Villebro N, Pedersen T, Tonnesen H. Effect of preoperative smoking intervention on postoperative complications: a randomised clinical trial. Lancet. 2002;359:114–7.

61 Wenzel RP, Perl TM. The significance of nasal carriage of Staphylococcus aureus and the incidence of postoperative wound infection. J Hosp Infect. 1995;31:13–24.

62 Poovelikunnel T, Gethin G, Humphreys H. Mupirocin resistance: clinical implications and potential alternatives for the eradication of MRSA. J Antimicrob Chemother. 2015;70:2681–92.

63 Schweizer M, Perencevich E, McDanel J, et al. Effectiveness of a bundled intervention of decolonization and prophylaxis to decrease Gram positive surgical site infections after cardiac or orthopedic surgery: systematic review and meta-analysis. BMJ. 2013;346:f2743.

64 Schweizer ML, Chiang HY, Septimus E, et al. Association of a bundled intervention with surgical site infections among patients undergoing cardiac, hip, or knee surgery. JAMA. 2015;313:2162–71.

65 Murthy A, De Angelis G, Pittet D, Schrenzel J, Uckay I, Harbarth S. Cost-effectiveness of universal MRSA screening on admission to surgery. Clin Microbiol Infect. 2010;16:1747–53.

66 Lee BY, Tsui BY, Bailey RR, et al. Should vascular surgery patients be screened preoperatively for methicillin-resistant Staphylococcus aureus? Infect Control Hosp Epidemiol. 2009;30:1158–65.

67 Mangram AJ, Horan TC, Pearson ML, Silver LC, Jarvis WR. Guideline for prevention of surgical site infection, 1999.

Hospital Infection Control Practices Advisory Committee. Infect Control Hosp Epidemiol. 1999;20:250-78; quiz 79–80.

68 Classen DC, Evans RS, Pestotnik SL, Horn SD, Menlove RL, Burke JP. The timing of prophylactic administration of antibiotics and the risk of surgical-wound infection. N Engl J Med. 1992;326:281–6.

69 Bratzler DW, Dellinger EP, Olsen KM, et al. Clinical practice guidelines for antimicrobial prophylaxis in surgery. Am J Health Syst Pharm. 2013;70:195–283.

70 World Health Organization. Global Guidelines for the Prevention of Surgical Site Infection. Geneva; 2016.

71 McDonald M, Grabsch E, Marshall C, Forbes A. Single- versus multiple-dose antimicrobial prophylaxis for major surgery: a systematic review. Aust N Z J Surg. 1998;68:388–96.

72 Mertz D, Johnstone J, Loeb M. Does duration of perioperative antibiotic prophylaxis matter in cardiac surgery? A systematic review and meta-analysis. Ann Surg 2011;254:48-54.

73 Gillespie BM, Kang E, Roberts S, et al. Reducing the risk of surgical site infection using a multidisciplinary approach: an integrative review. J Multidiscip Healthc 2015;8:473–87.

74 Dellinger EP, Hausmann SM, Bratzler DW, et al. Hospitals collaborate to decrease surgical site infections. Am J Surg 2005;190:9–15.

75 McConkey SJ, L'Ecuyer PB, Murphy DM, Leet TL, Sundt TM, Fraser VJ. Results of a comprehensive infection control program for reducing surgical-site infections in coronary artery bypass surgery. Infect Control Hosp Epidemiol 1999;20:533–8.

76 Anthony T, Murray BW, Sum-Ping JT, et al. Evaluating an evidence-based bundle for preventing surgical site infection: a randomized trial. Arch Surg 2011;146:263–9.

Chapter 17

Antimicrobial Stewardship

Alainna J. Jamal and Andrew M. Morris

17.1 Antimicrobial Stewardship

Antimicrobial resistance (AMR) is a major global health threat associated with significant morbidity, mortality, and cost [1]. Up to 50% of antimicrobial use in humans has been labelled inappropriate, which is believed to contribute to AMR [2–4].* McGowan and Gerding coined the term *antimicrobial stewardship* in 1996 to describe the notion that the appropriate use of antimicrobials could slow or even reverse AMR [5]. Judicious use of antimicrobials is one strategy emphasized to address AMR given the lack of new antimicrobials in development to replenish our depleting armamentarium [6].

The definition of *antimicrobial stewardship* has been refined to refer to "coordinated interventions designed to improve and measure the appropriate use of antimicrobial agents by promoting the selection of the optimal antimicrobial drug regimen including dosing, duration of therapy, and route of administration" [7]. The aims of antimicrobial stewardship include achieving clinical cure or prevention of infection while simultaneously minimizing costs, adverse drug events (e.g., allergy and toxicity), and emergence of AMR, including *Clostridium difficile* infection (CDI) [8].

---

* Although the inappropriate use of antimicrobials in humans is not the sole driver of AMR (use of antimicrobials in agriculture and pollution of the environment with antimicrobials are significant contributors), it is the focus of this chapter.

Hospital antimicrobial stewardship programs (ASPs) have been implemented globally in attempts to improve antimicrobial use. This chapter discusses the key issues that ASPs face; the methodological challenges associated with evaluating ASPs and their interventions; and the advantages, disadvantages, and evidence for interventions most commonly used to improve prescribing in the healthcare setting.

17.2 Issues in Prescribing: What it Means to get it Right

Judicious prescribing involves avoiding (a) *effective but unnecessary treatment* (i.e., antimicrobials that are too broad in spectrum and/or too long in duration), (b) *undertreatment* (i.e., not treating a serious infection or using antimicrobials that have insufficient activity to treat the identified/presumed organism(s) and/or are too short in duration), and (c) *inappropriate treatment* (i.e., antimicrobials that are not indicated altogether, such as when there is no infection).

17.2.1 Studies on Effective but Unnecessary Antimicrobial Use: A Focus on Duration and Spectrum of Activity

Several studies in recent years have investigated whether antimicrobial durations for a variety of infectious syndromes could be

Evidence-Based Infectious Diseases, Third Edition. Edited by Dominik Mertz, Fiona Smaill, and Nick Daneman.
© 2018 John Wiley & Sons Ltd. Published 2018 by John Wiley & Sons Ltd.

shortened without compromising efficacy and safety. The multi-center STOP-IT trial randomized 518 adults with complicated intra-abdominal infection and adequate source control to either four days of antimicrobial therapy or to antimicrobial therapy until two days following resolution of sepsis signs/symptoms [9]. Primary and secondary outcomes were similar in both groups [9]. Similarly, Sandberg et al. randomized 248 adults with acute pyelonephritis to either 7 days or 14 days of ciprofloxacin, and found that 7 days was not inferior to 14 days at both short- and long-term follow-up. Other trials that have found short-course antimicrobial therapy to be just as effective as long-course therapy have been summarized elsewhere [10]. However, it is worth mentioning that a shorter duration of therapy is not always preferred. For example, outcomes are less favorable with a shorter duration of therapy in children aged 6 to 23 months with acute otitis media [11].

Studies in recent years have also investigated whether monotherapy could be used instead of combination therapy for a variety of infectious syndromes. A multi-center trial randomized 600 patients with severe sepsis or septic shock to either meropenem alone or meropenem and moxifloxacin [12]. Degree of organ failure and 28- and 90-day all-cause mortality did not differ significantly between groups. A multi-center trial that randomized 739 critically ill patients with suspected late-onset ventilator-associated pneumonia to either meropenem alone or meropenem and ciprofloxacin found no statistically significant difference in all-cause 28-day mortality and organ function between groups [13].

Studies in a non-intensive care unit (ICU) setting have had similar findings. Monotherapy was found to be non-inferior to combination therapy in a cluster-randomized crossover trial including 656 patients with clinically suspected community-acquired pneumonia admitted to non-ICU hospital wards [14].

A systematic review that included 47 trials with 7,807 patients concluded that there was no significant difference in all-cause mortality in patients with febrile neutropenia treated with β lactam monotherapy versus β lactam-aminoglycoside combination therapy [15]. Furthermore, rates of superinfection were similar between groups and adverse events were significantly more likely in the combination versus monotherapy group [15].

17.2.2 Studies on Under-treatment

There is a paucity of literature on under-treatment because it is challenging to study. Patients most likely to be undertreated probably have antibiotic-resistant organisms, meaning that these patients probably also have a number of risk factors for worse outcomes. For example, it is difficult to determine the impact of delays in therapy when factors that impact outcomes, such as underlying comorbidities, cannot be adequately accounted for [16].

Research in this area mainly involves cohort studies focused on the association between inadequate or delayed treatment and mortality. A large multi-center retrospective cohort study including 2,731 patients showed that delays in effective antimicrobial therapy led to a significantly higher risk of death in recurrent/persistent hypotension of septic shock [17]. Similarly, in a systematic review that included 70 prospective studies, appropriate empiric antibiotic treatment was found to have a significant association with reduced all-cause mortality among adult inpatients with sepsis [18].

17.2.3 Studies on Inappropriate Antimicrobial Use

Some studies have examined whether no antibiotic treatment is sufficient for a variety of infectious syndromes. A Cochrane systematic review has assessed whether antibiotics influence outcomes for patients with acute respiratory tract infections (common colds) and acute purulent rhinitis [19]. When six double-blinded randomized controlled trials were pooled, antibiotics were no better than placebo in terms of cure and symptoms among 1,047 patients with the common cold [19]. Additionally, among adults the risk of adverse events was significantly greater in the antibiotic group as compared to the placebo group [19]. This lack of benefit for antibiotics was also observed in acute purulent rhinitis, when four double-blinded randomized controlled trials were pooled [19]. Additionally, Cochrane systematic reviews assessing the impact of antibiotics on outcomes in acute bronchitis [20] and laryngitis [21] have found no substantial benefit of antibiotics as compared to placebo.

17.3 The Assessment of ASPS and Antimicrobial Stewardship Interventions

A number of reviews have detailed the challenges associated with assessing ASPs and antimicrobial stewardship interventions [8,22–25]. These challenges are related to outcome measures and study design, and are largely a consequence of antimicrobial stewardship research being in its infancy. Although there has been a recent surge in the amount of research in the field, at the time of writing, there are only approximately 2,500 articles that pertain to antimicrobial stewardship on PubMed (Figure 17.1). For comparison, there are approximately 40,000 articles that pertain to infection prevention and control on PubMed.

17.3.1 Outcomes Measured in the Assessment of ASPs and Their Interventions

McGowan highlights that much of the literature evaluating ASPs and associated interventions has focused on assessing process measures [22]. Specifically, authors tend to describe whether ASPs and their interventions have improved adherence to recommendations, ensured that interventions

occurred, or altered routine changes in antimicrobial choice [22]. Although process measures relate to factors that theoretically lead to better prescribing, they do not necessarily affect patient-centered or public health outcomes (e.g., mortality, resistance rates, etc.) [8].

Outcomes that have been measured in studies assessing ASPs and their interventions can be divided into three broad categories: antimicrobial utilization measures, microbe outcomes, and clinical outcomes [8,24]. *Antimicrobial utilization measures* refer to antibiotic consumption and costs; *microbe outcomes* refer to resistance patterns or species epidemiology, and *clinical outcomes* refer to mortality, length of stay, readmission to hospital, adverse events, quality of life, and cure (clinical or microbiologic) [8,24]. Most of these outcomes are not entirely objective, with drawbacks that are summarized in Table 17.1 and further detailed elsewhere [8].

ASP research has mainly used antimicrobial utilization measures as an outcome (i.e., reducing overall antimicrobial use, including duration and how broad-spectrum). These studies have not clearly demonstrated that ASPs and their interventions improve antimicrobial resistance and other meaningful outcomes. It will be critical to define and measure the best outcomes to directly demonstrate the effectiveness and value of ASPs. Work to overcome this challenge has begun [26], but much more is needed before antimicrobial stewardship research can progress significantly.

17.3.2 Study Designs Employed in the Assessment of ASPs and Their Interventions

Appropriate study design and analytic methods must be employed to adjust for confounding factors, and thereby, properly assess the impact of an ASP or intervention on the outcome(s) of interest. Unfortunately, the quality of antimicrobial stewardship research remains poor overall, consisting

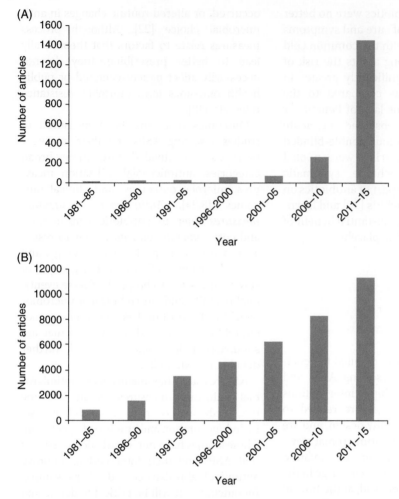

Figure 17.1 Number of articles pertaining to antimicrobial stewardship (**A**) and infection prevention and control (**B**) on PubMed. Search terms: ("antimicrobial stewardship" OR "antibiotic stewardship" OR "antibiotic management") (**A**); ("infection prevention" OR "infection control" OR "infection prevention and control") (**B**).

primarily of quasi-experimental studies (e.g., "uncontrolled before-and-after studies") [23,27]. Such study designs are inherently weak, failing to adequately adjust for secular trends or confounders, and thereby preventing definitive attribution of the change to the intervention. The reason ASP research consists primarily of uncontrolled before-and-after studies may be that antimicrobial stewardship interventions are often implemented in the context of an outbreak, where using stronger research methodology might be viewed as unethical and impractical [22]. Additionally, independent investigator-driven,

antimicrobial-related research has been historically sparse.

The emphasis on "care bundles," which are a group of interventions implemented concurrently, poses another challenge in ASP research [22,28]. When several interventions are implemented simultaneously, it is difficult to determine the contribution of each individual intervention to the effect observed.

Future research should involve multi-center studies to increase statistical power and randomized (especially cluster-randomized) study designs for high priority research questions.

Table 17.1 Outcome measures reported in the literature and their associated disadvantages.

Outcome measure	Disadvantages
Antimicrobial Utilization	
Defined Daily Dose (DDD)	• Biases against combination therapy even if combination therapy is narrower in spectrum. • Assumes routine dosing, so using higher doses when appropriate (e.g., in obesity or central nervous system infections) is "penalizing." Using lower doses when appropriate (e.g. in kidney dysfunction) underestimates antimicrobial exposure. • Based on adult dosing, so uninterpretable in paediatrics.
Days of Therapy (DOT)	• Challenging for smaller hospitals to calculate with ease and accuracy. • Incentivizes use of broad-spectrum monotherapy.
Length of Therapy (LOT)	• Cannot be used to compare use of specific drugs.
Cost of Therapy (COT)	• Varies by institution and country and over time. • Dependent on whether drug is brand name or generic.
Appropriateness of Therapy	• Subjective, and labor-intensive to assess. • No standard definitions (often assumes that guidelines are best practices) [80].
Microbe	
Antimicrobial-resistant Organisms	• Difficult to compare between institutions because screening (and thus, "prevalence") may differ between institutions. • Antimicrobial use alone may not significantly impact prevalence of antimicrobial-resistant organisms. • Included organisms may vary over time. • No standard definitions.
Antibiograms	• Minimal data demonstrating that antimicrobial use impacts antibiograms. • Few aggregate measures in the literature [81,82].
Clinical	
Mortality	• Vulnerable to secular trends. • Many factors influence mortality. • Often insensitive to important changes in quality of care.
Length of Stay	• Vulnerable to secular trends. • Many factors influence length of stay.
Cure	• Difficult to measure reliably and consistently. • Unclear if microbiologic, clinical, or radiographic cure is best to measure.

17.4 Interventions Aimed to Impact Prescribing Behavior

17.4.1 Prospective Audit and Feedback

There are many types of interventions that may be employed to impact behavior [29].

Prospective audit and feedback and academic detailing are commonly used core enabling strategies that aim to improve prescribing in hospital inpatient settings. In prospective audit and feedback, a trained person (usually an infectious diseases physician or pharmacist) assesses (audits) the antimicrobial therapy prescribed and provides recommendations (feedback) to prescribers based on an accepted standard (e.g., guideline) [28,30,31]. There is variability in the personnel conducting audit and feedback, the frequency with which audit and feedback is performed, and the patient population whose antimicrobial therapy undergoes audit and feedback [28,31]. For example, physicians, pharmacists, or nurses may provide the audit and feedback, and interventions may be selected on the basis of infectious condition, ward, antimicrobial agent, or duration of therapy [31].

Prospective audit and feedback is similar to academic detailing; they are both personalized, educational interventions that require active participation from the clinician receiving the intervention. However, academic detailing simply refers to individualized educational outreach. The clinician's prescribing habits are not necessarily compared against a standard (e.g., guidelines or norms), and this is the key feature that distinguishes it from prospective audit and feedback. Unfortunately, academic detailing and prospective audit and feedback are sometimes used interchangeably and/or incorrectly in the literature.

Given that the prescriber's acceptance of recommendations provided is voluntary, the main advantage of prospective audit and feedback is the prescriber's preserved sense of autonomy [28,30–32]. Other advantages include the opportunity to provide education to prescribers as part of the feedback component [28,30,32], adapt the implementation of this strategy to the specific institution's resources [28,30,31], and individualize therapy to the patient's unique clinical situation [28]. Furthermore, this strategy carries no risk of delay in therapy initiation because audit and feedback occurs after the antimicrobial is already prescribed [30,31]. Finally, this strategy can incorporate multiple facets of optimal prescribing, including duration, de-escalation, and parenteral to oral conversion [31,32].

Disadvantages of prospective audit and feedback include its intense dependence on healthcare human resources, requiring staff who are providing prospective audit and feedback to be adequately trained [28,31]. Furthermore, this strategy may not yield immediate results given that time may be required for prescribers to trust the recommendations of stewardship personnel [28]. Acceptance of recommendations may also be dependent on who provides them; prescribers are more likely to accept recommendations when they know the steward or when the steward is also a physician as opposed to a pharmacist [31].

The evidence for prospective audit and feedback has been examined in numerous reviews [23,30,32–37]. Prospective audit and feedback has been labeled the gold standard antimicrobial stewardship intervention to reduce inappropriate antimicrobial use [36]. This label is likely the result of this intervention's A-1 grading in the original IDSA guidelines [33] based on two small RCTs [38,39] (200–300 patients each RCT) and two observational studies [40,41]. Since the publication of the original IDSA guidelines, three additional RCTs [42–44] (two [43,44] with approximately 800 patients, and one [42] with approximately 300 patients) assessing prospective audit and feedback have been performed and reviewed [35]. Much like the RCTs cited in the IDSA guidelines, these studies reported improved prescribing outcomes (reduced antibiotic utilization [42,43] and increased antibiotic appropriateness [44]). None of these studies reported significant changes in patient outcomes (length of stay and mortality) or in rates of resistance and CDI.

Although prospective audit and feedback has never been assessed using RCTs in the ICU setting specifically, a recent systematic review [36] supported the use of this strategy in the ICU based on several methodologically rigorous quasi-experimental studies [45–47] that used a time-series analysis and/or a control group. These studies reported improved antibiotic utilization [45–47], costs [45–47], resistance [45], and CDI rates [45], but unchanged patient outcomes (length of stay and mortality).

17.4.2 Education

Didactic education on antimicrobial stewardship in the form of lectures or pamphlets is another commonly used persuasive strategy [32]. Education may focus on antimicrobial stewardship principles, appropriate prescribing for different types of infections, and activities supporting ASPs (such as culture and susceptibility interpretation and antibiogram interpretation) [48].

When surveyed, the vast majority of fourth-year medical students at three American medical schools indicated that they wanted more education on the appropriate use of antimicrobials and that they did not feel adequately prepared in the fundamental principles of antimicrobial use [49]. Similar results have been reported in the United Kingdom [50]. These data suggest that education efforts should target not only prescribers, but also future health care professionals who typically receive no formal education in antimicrobial stewardship. An antimicrobial stewardship curriculum developed at the University of California, San Francisco, for pharmacy and medical students was shown to positively impact knowledge and attitudes toward antimicrobial stewardship and its interprofessional nature [51].

The evidence for didactic education has been summarized in a Cochrane systematic review by Davey et al. [23]. There were five studies whose main intervention was dissemination of educational materials or educational meetings. All but one of these studies showed a positive effect on antimicrobial use. This Cochrane systematic review also found that educational strategies were most effective when combined with other interventions, such as prospective audit and feedback. Another study has shown that education is only effective for as long as it is maintained [52]. Similarly, systematic reviews examining the effects of education interventions on behavior change in health care more broadly have shown that didactic education alone does not impact clinician behavior [53,54].

17.4.3 Formulary Restriction and Preauthorization

Formulary restriction, preauthorization, and post-prescription review is a commonly used core restrictive strategy that aims to improve antimicrobial prescribing in hospital settings. In this strategy, restrictions are placed on specific antimicrobials within a hospital formulary, and before one of these restricted agents is dispensed (preauthorization) or after a first dose is dispensed (post-prescription review), the appropriateness of its use is approved by a trained person (usually an infectious diseases physician and/or pharmacist) [30,33,55]. Prior to inclusion in a hospital formulary, the efficacy, toxicity, and cost of antimicrobials are assessed; care is also taken to ensure that there is no redundancy between agents [33].

The main advantage of formulary restriction and preauthorization is that it provides direct control over antimicrobial use and can result in significant decreases in antimicrobial use and cost [30,32–34]. Other advantages of formulary restriction and preauthorization include the opportunity to provide education to prescribers when they request drugs and the optimization of empiric choices (especially because this strategy prompts the review of clinical and microbiologic data prior to treatment initiation) [32,55]. It also enables limiting the use of specific antimicrobials [32,55]. Finally, restricted antimicrobial requests can be recorded and summarized to determine the extent to which guidelines are followed [55].

Disadvantages of formulary restriction and preauthorization are a loss of prescriber autonomy, the potential for delay in therapy initiation (in preauthorization), and its resource-intensive nature requiring knowledgeable, skilled individuals to be regularly available to approve requests in real time [32,34,55]. Furthermore, this strategy only impacts restricted agents as well as initial empiric therapy; as such, it has minimal impact on reducing effective but unnecessary treatment, under-treatment, and inappropriate treatment [32,55]. Prescribers may also manipulate the system in such a way that their requests for restricted drugs are approved (by exaggerating illness severity or biasing information, for example) [32,55,56]. Finally, restriction of one drug may lead to increased utilization of other drugs ("squeezing the balloon"), which may contribute to additional resistance patterns [32,55,56].

The evidence for formulary restriction and preauthorization has been examined in a number of reviews [30,32–34], some of which have been systematic [23,35,36]. In the recent IDSA guidelines [32], formulary restriction and preauthorization is a strongly recommended intervention to reduce inappropriate antimicrobial use and associated resistance and costs based on five quasi-experimental studies [57–61]. of which none included a control group and two [58,61] employed a time-series analysis. Only two of these studies [57,58] assessed the impact of this strategy on patient outcomes (mortality, length of stay), and reported that clinical outcomes were unchanged. Similarly, two studies included in a recent systematic review [35] (one RCT [62] and one quasi-experimental interrupted time-series [63]) reported reduced antimicrobial use, but unchanged patient outcomes with formulary restriction and preauthorization.

In the ICU setting specifically, a systematic review identified three recent studies related to formulary restriction and preauthorization [36]. Two of these studies employed a quasi-experimental design, and one employed a matched cohort design. These studies showed decreased antimicrobial use [64–66] and resistance [65], but patient outcomes were not reported.

Few studies have directly compared preauthorization and prospective audit and feedback, although a recent quasi-experimental cross-over trial compared these two interventions for adult inpatients in four medical wards at an acute care hospital [67]. This trial found that prospective audit and feedback had more of an impact on decreasing antibiotic days of therapy as compared to preauthorization. These findings differ from those of Mehta et al., who compared antimicrobial use during the 24-month period before and after a change in ASP strategy (i.e., a switch from preauthorization to prospective audit and feedback) [68]. However, this study is particularly vulnerable to confounding given its uncontrolled before-after design.

17.4.4 Nudging Interventions

Antimicrobial prescribing is increasingly being recognized as a complex human behavior [69]. This has motivated some researchers to study and understand the factors that influence the behaviors of prescribers and patients [69]. These factors may be external (related to the prescribing environment) or internal (related to the prescriber's desire to practise good medicine) [69]. It is believed that the field of behavioral science, which includes psychology and behavioral economics, can assist in identifying and targeting specific influences on behavior to ultimately change antimicrobial prescribing [69,70].

There is a growing body of literature on the use of social and cognitive devices to "nudge" prescriber decision-making while preserving prescriber autonomy. A recent RCT in England by Hallsworth et al. randomized general practitioner (GP) practices with prescribing rates in the top 20% for their National Health Services Local Area Team (NHSLAT) to receiving either a letter from England's Chief Medical Officer or no communication [71]. This letter indicated that the practice was prescribing at a rate higher than 80% of the practices in its NHSLAT, and offered three actions that GPs in the practice could easily take to reduce unnecessary antibiotic prescribing. These actions included offering patients advice on self-care, providing delayed prescriptions, and discussing issues with colleagues. The rate of antibiotic prescribing was significantly lower in the intervention group as compared to the control group. These data suggest that social norm feedback/peer comparison and a high-profile messenger (concepts from behavioral science) could reduce antibiotic prescribing on a national scale and at a low cost.

A cluster RCT by Meeker et al. included 47 primary care practices in Boston and Los Angeles and assessed the impact of three behavioral interventions on the rate of inappropriate antibiotic prescribing for acute respiratory tract infections [72]. These interventions were implemented either alone or in combination, and included (a) *suggested alternatives*, where electronic order sets suggested non-antibiotic treatments; (b) *accountable justification*, where clinicians entered a free-text justification in the patient's electronic health record for each antibiotic prescription; and (c) *peer comparison*, where clinicians received emails comparing their antibiotic prescribing rates to those of clinicians with the lowest inappropriate antibiotic prescribing rates. The use of accountable justification and peer comparison significantly decreased the rate of inappropriate antimicrobial prescribing by 7.0% and 5.2%, respectively.

The studies by Hallsworth et al. and Meeker et al. provide high quality evidence for nudging interventions. Although microbial and clinical outcomes were not reported, these studies suggest potential avenues to improve prescribing in the outpatient setting.

17.5 Organization of Antimicrobial Stewardship Programs

The emergence of formal ASPs on the healthcare landscape has been met with considerable challenges, not the least of which are organization and funding. There is very little written about the topic, but optimizing these two aspects for ASPs are essential for leading change [73]. Institutional ASPs are optimally staffed with an inter-professional team that includes physician and pharmacist support—with at least some interest or expertise in infectious diseases—but should also include representation from nursing, the microbiology laboratory, and infection prevention and control/hospital epidemiology, where available. Antimicrobial stewards are increasingly recognized to require specific skill sets [74–77]. Ideally, the program has a designated leadership, and has a manager with administrative support, and includes or aligns itself with decision support and information technology staff wherever possible. ASPs can be situated organizationally in many areas, including within Infection Prevention and Control, Pharmacy, or even Medicine. However, it is likely best suited under the auspices of Quality and Safety, reflecting its primary mandate. Additionally, the program should report to an individual (e.g., Vice-President—Quality and Safety), rather than a committee (e.g., Medical Advisory Committee or Pharmacy & Therapeutics Committee): committees are usually not action-oriented, cannot directly address issues relating to personnel, and have no control over budget.

ASPs need to be adequately funded. These require formal business plans that are presented to hospital executives [78]. Ideally, funding is not tied too closely to cost reductions or avoidance, but rather to quality metrics. (E.g., if a drug-resistant organism becomes endemic, requiring routine use of an expensive antimicrobial, then costs will increase.) How the specific positions are funded will vary, largely dependent on the specific healthcare environment. There are no specific recommendations on the number of funded positions. Recently, the Association of Medical Microbiology and Infectious Diseases Canada posted online recommendations for staffing, based on environmental scan and expert opinion, recommending 1.0 full-time equivalent (FTE) physician, 3.0 FTE Pharmacist, 0.5 FTE Project/Program Administrative and Coordination Support, and 0.4 Data Analyst per 1,000 acute care beds [79].

17.6   Future Directions

Antimicrobial stewardship is a young field with potential for growth. Research in this area has largely occurred in the hospital setting, and study designs have been largely quasi-experimental with inherent vulnerability to bias and confounding. One of the biggest challenges in antimicrobial stewardship research is the development of measurable, moveable, and meaningful outcome measures. Overcoming this challenge would greatly benefit the field, and as such, should be a priority. Future research should also give the outpatient setting greater attention and employ stronger study designs (especially cluster RCTs).

References

1 WHO. Antimicrobial resistance. Bull World Health Organ. 2014;61(3):383–94. doi:10.1007/s13312-014-0374-3

2 Hecker MT, Aron DC, Patel NP, Lehmann MK, Donskey CJ. Unnecessary Use of Antimicrobials in Hospitalized Patients. Arch Intern Med. 2003;163(8):972–8. doi:10.1001/archinte.163.8.972

3 Werner NL, Hecker MT, Sethi AK, Donskey CJ. Unnecessary use of fluoroquinolone antibiotics in hospitalized patients. BMC Infect Dis. 2011;11(1):187. doi:10.1186/1471-2334-11-187

4 Marr JJ, Moffet HL, Kunin CM. Guidelines for improving the use of antimicrobial agents in hospitals: a statement by the Infectious Diseases Society of America. J Infect Dis. 1988;157(5):869–876. http://www.ncbi.nlm.nih.gov/pubmed/3361154.

5 McGowan JJ, Gerding D. Does antibiotic restriction prevent resistance? New Horiz. 1996;4(3):370–6.

6 Boucher HW, Talbot GH, Bradley JS, et al. Bad bugs, no drugs: no ESKAPE! An update from the Infectious Diseases Society of America. Clin Infect Dis. 2009;48(1):1–12. doi:10.1086/595011

7 Society for Healthcare Epidemiology of A, Infectious Diseases Society of A, Society PID, Fishman N. Policy Statement on Antimicrobial Stewardship by the Society for Healthcare Epidemiology of America (SHEA), the Infectious Diseases Society of America (IDSA), and the Pediatric Infectious Diseases Society (PIDS). Infect Control Hosp Epidemiol. 2012;33(4):322–7. doi:10.1086/665010

8 Morris AM. Antimicrobial Stewardship Programs: Appropriate Measures and Metrics to Study their Impact. Curr Treat Options Infect Dis. 2014;6(2):101–12. doi:10.1007/s40506-014-0015-3

9 Sawyer RG, Claridge JA, Nathens AB, et al. Trial of short-course antimicrobial therapy for intraabdominal infection. N Engl J Med. 2015;372(21):1996–2005. doi:10.1056/NEJMoa1411162

10 Spellberg B. The New Antibiotic Mantra—"Shorter Is Better." JAMA Intern Med. 2016;176(9):1–2. doi:10.1001/jamainternmed.2016.3633.4

11 Hoberman A, Paradise JL, Rockette HE, et al. Shortened Antimicrobial Treatment for Acute Otitis Media in Young Children. N Engl J Med. 2016;375(25):2446–56. doi:10.1056/NEJMoa1606043

12 Brunkhorst FM, Oppert M, Marx G, et al. Effect of Empirical Treatment With Moxifloxacin and Meropenem vs Meropenem on Sepsis-Related Organ Dysfunction in Patients With Severe Sepsis: A Randomized Trial. JAMA J Am Med Assoc. 2012:1. doi:10.1001/jama.2012.5833

13 Heyland DK, Dodek P, Muscedere J, Day A, Cook D. Randomized trial of combination versus monotherapy for the empiric treatment of suspected ventilator-associated pneumonia. Crit Care Med. 2008;36(3):737–44. doi:10.1097/01.CCM.0B013E31816203D6

14 Postma D, van Wekhoven C, van Elden L, et al. Antibiotic treatment strategies for community-acquired pneumonia in adults.

N Engl J Med. 2015 April 2;372;14:1312–23. doi:10.1056/NEJMoa1406330

15 Paul M, Soares-Weiser K, Leibovici L. Beta lactam monotherapy versus beta lactam-aminoglycoside combination therapy for fever with neutropenia: systematic review and meta-analysis. BMJ. 2003;326(7399):1111. doi:10.1136/bmj.326.7399.1111

16 Sexton DJ, Miller BA, Anderson DJ. Measuring the effect of inappropriate initial antibiotic therapy on outcomes of patients with Gram-negative sepsis: an imprecise science. Crit Care Med. 2011;39(1):199–200. doi:10.1097/CCM.0b013e318202e68f

17 Kumar A, Roberts D, Wood KE, et al. Duration of hypotension before initiation of effective antimicrobial therapy is the critical determinant of survival in human septic shock. Crit Care Med. 2006;34(0090-3493 (Print)):1589–96. doi:10.1097/01.CCM.0000217961.75225.E9

18 Paul M, Shani V, Muchtar E, Kariv G, Robenshtok E, Leibovici L. Systematic review and meta-analysis of the efficacy of appropriate empiric antibiotic therapy for sepsis. Antimicrob Agents Chemother. 2010;54(11):4851–63. doi:10.1128/AAC.00627-10

19 Kenealy T, Arroll B, Kenealy T. Antibiotics for the common cold and acute purulent rhinitis. Cochrane Database Syst Rev. 2013;6(3):CD000247. doi:10.1002/14651858.CD000247.pub3

20 Smucny J, Fahey T, Becker L, Glazier R. Antibiotics for acute bronchitis. Cochrane Database Syst Rev. 2004;(4):CD000245.

21 Reveiz L, Cardona a F, Ospina EG. Antibiotics for acute laryngitis in adults. Cochrane Database Syst Rev. 2015;(5):CD004783. doi:10.1002/14651858.CD004783.pub5.www.cochranelibrary.com

22 McGowan Jr JE. Antimicrobial Stewardship—the State of the Art in 2011 Focus on Outcome and Methods. Infect Control Hosp Epidemiol. 2012;3321517188(4):331–7. doi:10.1086/664755

23 Davey P, Brown E, Charani E, et al. Interventions to improve antibiotic prescribing practices for hospital inpatients. Cochrane Database Syst Rev. 2013;(4). doi:10.1002/14651858.CD003543.pub3

24 McGregor JC, Furuno JP. Optimizing research methods used for the evaluation of antimicrobial stewardship programs. Clin Infect Dis. 2014;59(Suppl 3):S185–S192. doi:10.1093/cid/ciu540

25 Davey P, Brown E, Charani E, et al. Interventions to improve antibiotic prescribing practices for hospital inpatients. Cochrane Database Syst Rev. 2017. doi:10.1002/14651858.CD003543.pub3

26 Evans SR, Rubin D, Follmann D, et al. Desirability of outcome ranking (DOOR) and response adjusted for duration of antibiotic risk (RADAR). Clin Infect Dis. 2015;61(5):800–6. doi:10.1093/cid/civ495

27 Kaki R, Elligsen M, Walker S, Simor A, Palmay L, Daneman N. Impact of antimicrobial stewardship in critical care: A systematic review. J Antimicrob Chemother. 2011;66(6):1223–30. doi:10.1093/jac/dkr137

28 Chung GW, Wu JE, Yeo CL, Chan D, Hsu LY. Antimicrobial stewardship: a review of prospective audit and feedback systems and an objective evaluation of outcomes. Virulence. 2013;4(2):151–7. doi:10.1016/j.clinthera.2013.05.007

29 Michie S, Richardson M, Johnston M, et al. The behavior change technique taxonomy (v1) of 93 hierarchically clustered techniques: Building an international consensus for the reporting of behavior change interventions. Ann Behav Med. 2013;46(1):81–95. doi:10.1007/s12160-013-9486-6

30 Owens RC. Antimicrobial stewardship: concepts and strategies in the 21st century. Diagn Microbiol Infect Dis. 2008;61(1):110–28. doi:10.1016/j.diagmicrobio.2008.02.012

31 Public Health Ontario. Antimicrobial Stewardship Strategy: Prospective audit with intervention and feedback. 1–12.

http://www.publichealthontario.ca/en/
BrowseByTopic/InfectiousDiseases/
AntimicrobialStewardshipProgram/
Documents/ASP_Strategy_Prospective_
Audit_Intervention_Feedback.pdf.

32 Barlam TF, Cosgrove SE, Abbo LM, et al.
Executive Summary: Implementing an
Antibiotic Stewardship Program:
Guidelines by the Infectious Diseases
Society of America and the Society for
Healthcare Epidemiology of America.
Clin Infect Dis. 2016;62(10):11971202.
doi:10.1093/cid/ciw217

33 Dellit TH, Owens RC, McGowan JE, et al.
Infectious Diseases Society of America and
Society for Healthcare Epidemiology of
America guidelines for developing an
institutional program to enhance
antimicrobial stewardship. Infect Control
Hosp Epidemiol. 2007;44:159–77.
doi:10.1097/IPC.0b013e318068b1c0

34 Griffith M, Postelnick M, Scheetz M.
Antimicrobial stewardship programs:
methods of operation and suggested
outcomes. Expert Rev Anti Infect Ther.
2012;10(1):63–73. doi:10.1586/eri.11.153

35 Wagner B, Filice GA, Drekonja D, et al.
Antimicrobial stewardship programs
in inpatient hospital settings:
a systematic review. Infect Control Hosp
Epidemiol. 2014;35(10):1209–28.
doi:10.1086/678057

36 Mertz D, Brooks A, Irfan N, Sung M.
Antimicrobial stewardship in the intensive
care setting—a review and critical appraisal
of the literature. Swiss Med Wkly.
2015;145(December):w14220. doi:10.4414/
smw.2015.14220

37 Feazel LM, Malhotra A, Perencevich EN,
Kaboli P, Diekema DJ, Schweizer ML.
Effect of antibiotic stewardship
programmes on Clostridium difficile
incidence: a systematic review and meta-
analysis. J Antimicrob Chemother.
2014;69(7):1748–54. doi:10.1093/
jac/dku046

38 Fraser GL, Stogsdill P, Dickens JD,
Wennberg DE, Smith RP, Prato BS.
Antibiotic optimization: an evaluation of
patient safety and economic outcomes.
Arch Intern Med. 1997;157:1689–94.

39 Solomon DH, Van Houten L, Glynn RJ,
et al. Academic detailing to improve use of
broad-spectrum antibiotics at an academic
medical center. Arch Intern Med.
2001;161(15):1897–1902. doi:10.1001/
archinte.161.15.1897

40 LaRocco AJ. Concurrent antibiotic review
programs—a role for infectious diseases
specialists at small community hospitals.
Clin Infect Dis. 2003;37:742–3.

41 Carling P, Fung T, Killion A, Terrin N,
Barza M. Favorable impact of a
multidisciplinary antibiotic management
program conducted during 7 years. Hosp
Epidemiol. 2003;24(9):699–706.

42 Masiá M, Matoses C, Padilla S, et al.
Limited efficacy of a nonrestricted
intervention on antimicrobial prescription
of commonly used antibiotics in the
hospital setting: results of a randomized
controlled trial. Eur J Clin Microbiol Infect
Dis. 2008;27(7):597–605. doi:10.1007/
s10096-008-0482-x

43 Lesprit P, Landelle C, Brun-Buisson C.
Clinical impact of unsolicited post-
prescription antibiotic review in surgical
and medical wards: a randomized
controlled trial. Clin Microbiol Infect.
2013;19(2):E91–E97.
doi:10.1111/1469-0691.12062

44 Camins BC, King MD, Wells JB, Heidi L,
Patel M, Kourbatova E V. The impact of an
antimicrobial utilization program on
antimicrobial use at a large teaching
hospital: a randomized controlled trial.
Control. 2009;30(10):931–8.
doi:10.1086/605924.The

45 Elligsen M, Walker SAN, Pinto R, et al.
Audit and feedback to reduce broad-
spectrum antibiotic use among intensive
care unit patients: a controlled interrupted
time series analysis. Infect Control Hosp
Epidemiol. 2012;33(4):354–61.
doi:10.1086/664757

46 Wang HY, Chiu CH, Huang CT, et al.
Blood culture-guided de-escalation of
empirical antimicrobial regimen for critical

patients in an online antimicrobial stewardship programme. Int J Antimicrob Agents. 2014;44(6):520–7. doi:10.1016/j.ijantimicag.2014.07.025

47 Bornard L, Dellamonica J, Hyvernat H, et al. Impact of an assisted reassessment of antibiotic therapies on the quality of prescriptions in an intensive care unit. Med Mal Infect. 2011;41(9):480–5. doi:10.1016/j.medmal.2010.12.022

48 Public Health Ontario. Antimicrobial Stewardship Strategy: Prescriber education. 2016;(June).

49 Abbo LM, Cosgrove SE, Pottinger PS, et al. Medical students' perceptions and knowledge about antimicrobial stewardship: how are we educating our future prescribers? Clin Infect Dis. 2013;57(5):631–8. doi:10.1093/cid/cit370

50 Heaton A, Webb DJ, Maxwell SRJ. Undergraduate preparation for prescribing: the views of 2413 UK medical students and recent graduates. Br J Clin Pharmacol. 2008;66(1):128–34. doi:10.1111/j.1365-2125.2008.03197.x

51 MacDougall C, Schwartz BS, Kim L, Nanamori M, Shekarchian S, Chin-Hong P V. An Interprofessional Curriculum on Antimicrobial Stewardship Improves Knowledge and Attitudes Toward Appropriate Antimicrobial Use and Collaboration. 2016.

52 Landgren F, Harveky K, Mashford M, Moulds R, Guthrie B, Hemming M. Changing antibiotic prescribing by educational marketing. Med J Aust. 1988;149(11–12):595–9.

53 O'Brien M, Freemantle N, Oxman A, Wolfe F, Davis D, Herrin J. Continuing education meetings and workshops: effects on professional practice and health care outcomes (Review). Cochrane Database Syst Rev. 2001;(2):CD003030.

54 Davis D, O'Brien MAT, Freemantle N, Wolf FM, Mazmanian P, Taylor-Vaisey A. Impact of formal continuing medical education. JAMA J Am Med Assoc. 1999;282(9):867–74. doi:10.1001/jama.282.9.867

55 Public Health Ontario. Antimicrobial Stewardship Strategy : Formulary restriction with preauthorization. :1–6. http://www.publichealthontario.ca/en/BrowseByTopic/InfectiousDiseases/AntimicrobialStewardshipProgram/Documents/ASP_Strategy_Formulary_Restriction_Preauthorization.pdf.

56 Reed EE, Stevenson KB, West JE, Bauer K a, Goff DA. Impact of formulary restriction with prior authorization by an antimicrobial stewardship program. Virulence. 2013;4(2):158–62. doi:10.4161/viru.21657

57 White Jr. AC, Atmar RL, Wilson J, Cate TR, Stager CE, Greenberg SB. Effects of requiring prior authorization for selected antimicrobials: expenditures, susceptibilities, and clinical outcomes. ClinInfectDis. 1997;25(1058–4838 (Print)):230-239. doi:10.1016/S0002-9394(99)80267-0

58 Buising KL, Thursky KA, Robertson MB, et al. Electronic antibiotic stewardship - Reduced consumption of broad-spectrum antibiotics using a computerized antimicrobial approval system in a hospital setting. J Antimicrob Chemother. 2008;62(3):608–16. doi:10.1093/jac/dkn218

59 Pakyz AL, Oinonen M, Polk RE. Relationship of carbapenem restriction in 22 university teaching hospitals to carbapenem use and carbapenem-resistant Pseudomonas aeruginosa. Antimicrob Agents Chemother. 2009;53(5):1983–6. doi:10.1128/AAC.01535-08

60 Metjian T a, Prasad P a, Kogon A, Coffin SE, Zaoutis TE. Evaluation of an antimicrobial stewardship program at a pediatric teaching hospital. Pediatr Infect Dis J. 2008;27(2):106–11. doi:10.1097/INF.0b013e318158603a

61 Lewis GJ, Fang X, Gooch M, Cook PP. Decreased resistance of Pseudomonas aeruginosa with restriction of ciprofloxacin in a large teaching hospital's intensive care and intermediate care units. Infect Control Hosp Epidemiol. 2012;33(4):368–73. doi:10.1086/664763

62 Rattanaumpawan P, Sutha P, Thamlikitkul V. Effectiveness of drug use evaluation and antibiotic authorization on patients' clinical outcomes, antibiotic consumption, and antibiotic expenditures. Am J Infect Control. 2010;38(1):38–43. doi:10.1016/j.ajic.2009.04.288

63 Peto Z, Benko R, Matuz M, Csullog E, Molnar A, Hajdu E. Results of a local antibiotic management program on antibiotic use in a tertiary intensive care unit in hungary. Infection. 2008;36(6): 560–4. doi:10.1007/s15010-008-7377-8

64 Sharma P, Barman P. Antimicrobial consumption and impact of "Reserve antibiotic indent form" in an intensive care unit. Indian J Pharmacol. 2010;42(5):297–300.

65 Sistanizad M, Kouchek M, Miri M, et al. Carbapenem Restriction and its Effect on Bacterial Resistance in an Intensive Care unit of a Teaching Hospital. Iran J Pharm Res IJPR. 2013;12(3):503–9. http://www.pubmedcentral.nih.gov/articlerender.fcgi?artid=3813286&tool=pmcentrez&rendertype=abstract.

66 Guarascio AJ, Slain D, McKnight R, et al. A matched-control evaluation of an antifungal bundle in the intensive care unit at a university teaching hospital. Int J Clin Pharm. 2013;35(1):145–8. doi:10.1007/s11096-012-9712-5

67 Tamma PD, Avdic E, Keenan JF, et al. What is the more effective antibiotic stewardship intervention: pre-prescription authorization or post-prescription review with feedback? Clin Infect Dis. 2016:1–25.

68 Mehta JM, Haynes K, Wileyto EP, et al. Comparison for prior authorization and prospective audit with feedback for antimicrobial stewardship. Infect Control Hosp Epidemiol. 2014;35(9):1092–9. doi:10.1002/dev.21214.Developmental

69 Tonkin-Crine S, Walker AS, Butler CC. Contribution of behavioural science to antibiotic stewardship. BMJ. 2015;350(June):h3413. doi:10.1136/bmj.h3413

70 Loewenstein G, Brennan T, Volpp KG. Asymmetric paternalism to improve health behaviors. JAMA. 2007;298(20):2415–7. doi:10.1001/jama.298.20.2415

71 Hallsworth M, Chadborn T, Sallis A, et al. Provision of social norm feedback to high prescribers of antibiotics in general practice: a pragmatic national randomised controlled trial. Lancet. 2016;387(10029):1743–52. doi:10.1016/S0140-6736(16)00215-4

72 Meeker D, Linder JA, Fox CR, et al. Effect of behavioral interventions on inappropriate antibiotic prescribing among primary vare practices: a randomized clinical trial. J Am Med Assoc. 2016;315(6):562–70. doi:10.1001/jama.2016.0275

73 Morris AM, Stewart TE, Shandling M, McIntaggart S, Liles WC. Establishing an antimicrobial stewardship program. Heal Q. 2010;13(2):64–70.

74 Dyar OJ, Pulcini C, Howard P, et al. European medical students: a first multicentre study of knowledge, attitudes and perceptions of antibiotic prescribing and antibiotic resistance. J Antimicrob Chemother. 2014;69(3):842–6. doi:10.1093/jac/dkt440

75 Ashiru-Oredope D, Cookson B, Fry C, et al. Developing the first national antimicrobial prescribing and stewardship competences. J Antimicrob Chemother. 2014;69(11):2886–8. doi:10.1093/jac/dku350

76 Sneddon J, Gilchrist M, Wickens H. Development of an expert professional curriculum for antimicrobial pharmacists in the UK. J Antimicrob Chemother. 2014;70(5):1277–80. doi:10.1093/jac/dku543

77 Rocha-Pereira N, Lafferty N, Nathwani D. Educating healthcare professionals in antimicrobial stewardship: can online-learning solutions help? J Antimicrob Chemother. 2015;70(12):3175–7. doi:10.1093/jac/dkv336

78 Spellberg B, Bartlett JG, Gilbert DN. How to pitch an antibiotic stewardship program to the hospital C-suite. Open Forum Infect Dis. 2016;3(4):1–5. doi:10.1093/ofid/ofw210

79 Antimicrobial Stewardship. Association of Medical Microbiology and Infectious Disease. https://www.ammi.ca/.

80 Spivak ES, Cosgrove SE, Srinivasan A. Measuring appropriate antimicrobial use: attempts at opening the black box. Clin Infect Dis. 2016;63:1639–44. doi:10.1093/cid/ciw658

81 Laxminarayan R, Klugman KP. Communicating trends in resistance using a drug resistance index. BMJ Open. 2011;1(2):e000135. doi:10.1136/bmjopen-2011-000135

82 Hughes JS, Hurford A, Finley RL, Patrick DM, Wu J, Morris AM. How to measure the impacts of antibiotic resistance and antibiotic development on empiric therapy: new composite indices. BMJ Open. 2016;6(12):e012040. doi:10.1136/bmjopen-2016-012040

Chapter 18

Infections in Neutropenic Hosts

Eric J. Bow

Case Presentation 1

A 34-year-old male was admitted complaining of fever, generalized malaise, and increasing fatigue for four weeks. On examination, he was pale; his blood pressure was 122/78 mmHg, oral temperature 38.2 °C, and pulse 110 per minute. His liver had a 14 cm span in the mid-clavicular line and the spleen tip was 10 cm below the left costal margin. Petechiae were present in the skin of the lower limbs. A complete blood count revealed a total leukocyte count of 35×10^9/L, an absolute neutrophil count (ANC) of 0.824×10^9/L, and a circulating blast count of 33×10^9/L. Bone marrow examination revealed a hypercellular marrow specimen 90% infiltrated by blast cells, some of which contained Auer rods. Acute myeloid leukemia (AML) (French–American–British classification, M2) was diagnosed. A typical AML remission-induction regimen was administered, consisting of a seven-day continuous infusion of cytarabine plus an anthracycline, and daunorubicin, administered daily on days 1, 2, and 3. Beginning on day + 1 of cytotoxic therapy, oral ciprofloxacin 500 mg every 12 hours, acyclovir 800 mg every 12 hours, and fluconazole 400 mg daily were administered. Blood cultures obtained on admission remained sterile and the fever resolved as the cytotoxic therapy was administered. The ANC fell to $< 0.5 \times 10^9$/L on day + 3 of induction therapy and to $< 0.1 \times 10^9$/L on day + 5.

Acute leukemia is a rapidly progressive disease. In the untreated patient, it results in early death owing to hemorrhage or infection—the consequences, respectively, of thrombocytopenia and neutropenia from marrow failure. Historically, infection has been the major contributor to mortality and has been designated as the primary cause of death in over one-third of acute leukemia cases. Notwithstanding advances in cytotoxic chemotherapy for the underlying malignancy and the use of marrow-stimulating growth factors and antimicrobials, infection remains the major contributor to 66% of deaths in patients treated for acute myeloid leukemia (AML) [1]. The early recognition and appropriate treatment of infection remains a priority in the care of these profoundly immunocompromised individuals.

Neutrophils are one of the principal mediators of nonspecific (innate) cellular immunity. A deficiency in either the number or function of neutrophils can predispose an individual to infection, particularly infection due to pyogenic bacterial organisms. Diminished numbers of neutrophils, as opposed to qualitative defects in granulocyte function, are the more common cause of granulocytic immunodeficiency.

Evidence-Based Infectious Diseases, Third Edition. Edited by Dominik Mertz, Fiona Smaill, and Nick Daneman.
© 2018 John Wiley & Sons Ltd. Published 2018 by John Wiley & Sons Ltd.

While a total neutrophil count of $<1.0 \times 10^9/L$ defines neutropenia, the risk of bacterial and fungal sepsis rises exponentially below a level of $0.5 \times 10^9/L$ (2). This profound degree of neutropenia occasionally results from an underlying inflammatory, infectious, or malignant condition, but is more often a consequence of the treatment of these diseases. While there may be subtle differences in the characteristics of neutropenia-related sepsis arising from one disease state to the next, most of what we have learned from hematology and oncology studies can be generalized to other conditions producing neutropenia of similar magnitude and duration.

18.1 The Febrile Neutropenic Episode

Cytotoxic therapy for acute myeloid leukemia will predictably result in neutropenia, with absolute neutrophil counts of $<0.5 \times 10^9/L$ for 10–14 days or longer. The designation of a "febrile neutropenic episode" (FNE) applies when a neutropenic patient's oral temperature exceeds 38 °C for at least one hour [3]. The fever itself arises from the production of pro-inflammatory cytokines [4], most often in response to either infection- or therapy-related cell membrane damage. While fever is generally the first, and frequently the only sign of infection, not all febrile episodes will be the result of infection. Some of the common noninfectious causes of fever in populations being treated for malignancies are outlined in Box 18.1.

Box 18.1 Fever in the Neutropenic Cancer Patient: Non-infectious Causes.

- Underlying malignancy
- Infusion of blood products
- Drugs: cytarabine, cyclophosphamide, hydroxyurea, polyenes (e.g., amphotericin B deoxycholate), filgrastim, certain monoclonal antibody therapies
- Noninfectious inflammatory conditions: phlebitis, hematomas, thromboembolic disease, tumor lysis

---

18.2 Assessment and Management of the Febrile Neutropenic Episode

The majority of neutropenic patients who have an infection present with fever, regardless of whether a definable clinical focus of infection can be identified. Accordingly, the most important component of the clinical assessment of these patients is having an index of suspicion. The time course for a neutropenic episode is referenced from the first day of the current cycle on which the patient received cytotoxic therapy. Most neutropenic fevers occur after the first week at a median of day +14, and coincide with the time of maximal cytotoxic therapy-induced intestinal mucosal damage [5–7]. This understanding can safely guide the clinical approach to triage.

18.2.1 That Guy Looks Septic—The Clock Starts Now

An oncology patient presenting with a history of recent onset of subjective fever and having received anticancer therapy within the preceding six weeks suggests the possibility of a neutropenic fever syndrome. This composite should trigger an algorithmic pathway of assessment and treatment, illustrated in Figure 18.1, resulting in the administration of appropriate initial empirical antibacterial therapy within 60 minutes of triage [8]. The clinician should be able to assess the patient and develop an initial management plan for execution within 60 minutes based on a set of vital signs (including body temperature, heart rate, respiratory rate, arterial oxygen saturation, and blood pressure), history of the current problem and recent chemotherapy, and physical examination focusing on potential anatomical sites of infection, without having the results of laboratory tests available. The likelihood that the patient is neutropenic must be judged from the chemotherapy history and the timing of presentation from the first day of the current cycle of treatment.

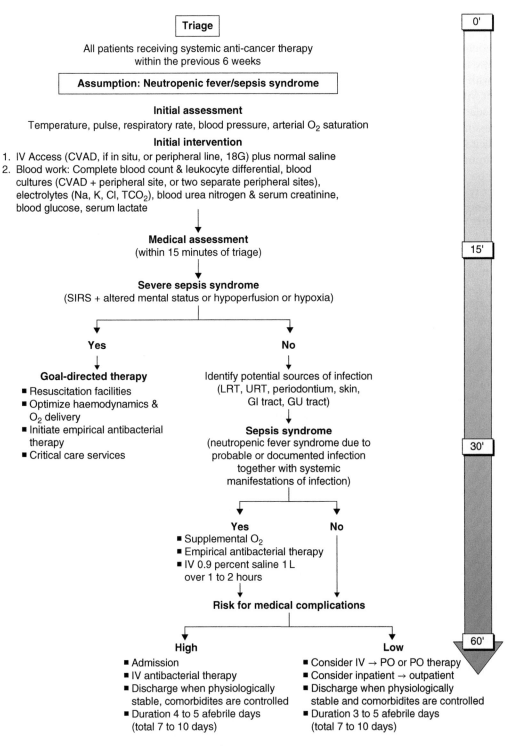

Triage

All patients receiving systemic anti-cancer therapy
within the previous 6 weeks

Assumption: Neutropenic fever/sepsis syndrome

Initial assessment
Temperature, pulse, respiratory rate, blood pressure, arterial O_2 saturation

Initial intervention
1. IV Access (CVAD, if in situ, or peripheral line, 18G) plus normal saline
2. Blood work: Complete blood count & leukocyte differential, blood
   cultures (CVAD + peripheral site, or two separate peripheral sites),
   electrolytes (Na, K, Cl, TCO_2), blood urea nitrogen & serum creatinine,
   blood glucose, serum lactate

Medical assessment
(within 15 minutes of triage)

Severe sepsis syndrome
(SIRS + altered mental status or hypoperfusion or hypoxia)

Yes

Goal-directed therapy
■ Resuscitation facilities
■ Optimize haemodynamics &
  O_2 delivery
■ Initiate empirical antibacterial
  therapy
■ Critical care services

No

Identify potential sources of infection
(LRT, URT, periodontium, skin,
GI tract, GU tract)

Sepsis syndrome
(neutropenic fever syndrome due to
probable or documented infection
together with systemic
manifestations of infection)

Yes
■ Supplemental O_2
■ Empirical antibacterial therapy
■ IV 0.9 percent saline 1 L
  over 1 to 2 hours

No

Risk for medical complications

High
■ Admission
■ IV antibacterial therapy
■ Discharge when physiologically
  stable, comorbidites are controlled
■ Duration 4 to 5 afebrile days
  (total 7 to 10 days)

Low
■ Consider IV → PO or PO therapy
■ Consider inpatient → outpatient
■ Discharge when physiologically
  stable and comorbidites are controlled
■ Duration 3 to 5 afebrile days
  (total 7 to 10 days)

0'

15'

30'

60'

Figure 18.1 Algorithm for the approach to the febrile neutropenic cancer patient in the triage setting,
"time-to-initial empirical antibacterial therapy" [8]. Abbreviations: CTAS, Canadian triage assessment score;
SIRS, systemic inflammatory response syndrome; IV, intravenous; CVAD, central venous access device; Na,
serum sodium; K, serum potassium; Cl, serum chloride, TCO2, serum total CO_2; MASCC, Multinational
Association for Supportive Care in Cancer; IDSA, Infectious Diseases Society of America; ANC, absolute
neutrophil count, x 10^9/L; PO, per os (orally).

Patients satisfying these criteria should be triaged as "emergent" cases by the triage facility with the expectation of physician assessment within 15 minutes of presentation [9]. In Canada, this corresponds to a Canadian Triage Assessment Score (CTAS) of II, emergent [10].

Elicitation of elements of the systemic inflammatory response syndrome (SIRS) [11] can be helpful to the clinician to estimate severity of the process. SIRS is defined by the presence of ≥2 of abnormal body temperature (>38 °C or <36 °C), tachycardia (defined by a heart rate >90 beats per minute), tachypnea (defined by a respiratory rate of >20 breaths per minute) or hyperventilation (defined by a $PaCO_2$ of <32 mmHg), and an alteration in the peripheral leukocyte count (defined by a leukocytosis of >12.0 × 10^9/L or leucopenia of <4.0 × 10^9/L or a "left shift" in the leukocyte differential count with >10% band neutrophils). Febrile neutropenic patients, by this definition, have at least two SIRS criteria.

The SIRS criteria have had prognostic value for the severity of the processes associated with infection. In a retrospective Argentinian cohort of 62 febrile neutropenic patients, the all-cause mortality rates were 0, 11%, 43%, 50%, and 90% for patients with two SIRS criteria, three SIRS criteria, four SIRS criteria, severe sepsis, and septic shock, respectively [12]. The reported 30-day all-cause mortality rates among European patients with bacteremic neutropenic fever syndromes have been 10%, 25%, and 71% for those presenting with two or more SIRS criteria, severe sepsis, and septic shock, respectively [13]. The application of additional SIRS criteria to the febrile neutropenic patient appears to provide a quantitative element to the assessment of the burden of illness that may influence clinical management planning.

18.2.2 The Physical Examination in Febrile Neutropenic Patients may be Misleading

The salient features of a focused history and physical examination in the evaluation of a febrile neutropenic patient are summarized in Table 18.1. The classic signs of inflammation associated with pyogenic infection in an otherwise immunocompetent individual may be absent or diminished in the context of absolute neutropenia. A seminal descriptive analysis of presenting signs and symptoms for neutropenic versus non-neutropenic hosts showed that, with regard to skin and soft-tissue infections, edema was reduced in neutropenic patients, while fluctuance and exudation were for the most part absent [14]. Where pneumonia was ultimately diagnosed, cough and sputum production were less frequent among neutropenic patients but bacteremia was more common. This effect of neutropenia on the presentation of bacterial infection must be taken into account in the evaluation of the patient.

18.2.3 Initial Laboratory Investigations for the Febrile Neutropenic Patient

When a patient with an absolute neutrophil count of <0.5 × 10^9/L meets the temperature criteria for a febrile neutropenic episode, vigorous attempts to document a source and/or to isolate a potential pathogen must be made. This requires a focused physical examination, and a minimum laboratory evaluation consisting of a full blood count, creatinine, liver enzyme tests, serum lactate, and where appropriate, a chest radiographic examination; cultures of urine and sputum if urinary or respiratory symptoms are present; and cultures of blood drawn from each of two sites, including each lumen of any indwelling venous catheter, as well as blood from at least one peripheral site. The latter recommendation derives from a study of neutropenic cancer patients [15], in which a negative culture from either a central or peripheral site had a predictive value for the absence of "true bacteremia" of 98–99%. A positive culture at either site had a substantially lower predictive value for the presence of "true bacteremia" (63% for the central venous catheter; 73% for the peripheral site) owing

Table 18.1 Physical examination of the febrile neutropenic patient.

Region	Examine for
Head and neck	
–fundi	Retinal hemorrhages (bleeding diatheses)
	Retinal exudates (disseminated fungal infection)
–auditory canals/ tympanic membranes	Erythema (otitis externa/media; viral upper respiratory infection)
	Vesicles (herpetic infection)
–anterior nasal mucosa	Ulcerations/vesicular lesions (fungal disease, herpetic infection)
–oropharynx	Mucositis (predisposition to bacteremias/fungemias)
	Ulcerative gingivo-stomatitis (anaerobic bacteria)
	Pseudomembranous pharyngitis (thrush, a risk for candidemia)
Chest	Râles (more consistent than cough/sputum in diagnosis of pneumonia)
	Edema, tenderness, erythema around central venous catheter tunnel and exit sites
Abdomen	Localized tenderness (right lower quadrant: typhlitis; right upper quadrant: hepatobiliary infection; perianal tissues [avoid a digital rectal examination]: cellulitis, abscess or fistula)
Skin	Tenderness, erythema, swelling around intravenous sites
	Ulcerative or necrotic lesions (*Pseudomonas aeruginosa, Staphylococcus aureus*)
	Diffuse pustular/erythematous lesions (metastatic seeding with *Candida* spp.)
	Vesicular lesions (herpes simplex/zoster)
	Hypersensitivity reactions

to the confounding effect of contaminants (e.g., coagulase-negative *Staphylococcus* spp.) as false positives.

Patients who develop a febrile neutropenic episode in the community setting and who present with symptoms that suggest an influenza-like illness including fever, cough, and additional viral infection-like symptoms, particularly in the setting of a community-based outbreak, should be considered for a community-acquired respiratory virus infection. This should include the collection of nasopharyngeal swabs for respiratory virus detection by nucleic acid amplification testing.

18.2.4 Initial Assessment at the Triage Site—For What Should We Look?

The initial triage assessment establishes the likelihood that the patient has a neutropenic fever syndrome based on the history and initial vital signs data. Intravenous access through an existing central venous access device (CVAD) or a peripheral site should be established for intravenous fluids (0.9% saline is recommended initially). Prior to the return of any results of laboratory investigations (including the complete blood count), the initial medical assessment is intended to confirm the presence of SIRS criteria, identify possible clinical foci of infection, and evidence for severe sepsis with organ dysfunction, suspected by documentation of hypotension, hypoxia, acute oliguria, or an acute alteration in mental status. These findings may ultimately be supported by laboratory test results such as an elevated serum lactate, an acutely elevated serum creatinine (>177 umol/L), an elevated serum bilirubin (>34 umol/L), or an elevated International Normalized Ratio (INR) of >1.5. If a working diagnosis of severe sepsis can be sustained, then immediate initial empirical combination antibacterial therapy should be administered, goal-directed resuscitation procedures should be implemented, and admission to hospital should be expedited.

18.2.5 Timing of Antimicrobial Therapy—The Triage-to-Antibiotic Time is Important

The benchmark for the administration of initial empirical broad-spectrum antibacterial therapy in febrile neutropenic cancer patients is a time from triage-to-first dose of antibiotic of less than 60 minutes [3,8,16]. Consensus recommendations also advise that any neutropenic individual with a clinically suspected infection should receive treatment, even in the absence of fever [17], as might be the case among patients receiving concomitant antipyretic therapy or who may be hypothermic. The clinician should be able to make an initial assessment and administer the first dose of initial empirical antibacterial therapy within the 60-minute timeframe without the benefit of laboratory results or diagnostic imaging. The choice of empiric therapy will be influenced by the results of the physical examination and key laboratory tests, by whether or not the individual's circumstances suggest a low risk for medical complications of the neutropenic fever syndrome (see later), and by an understanding of which endogenous microflora cause infections most often in this population.

The timing of antibiotic administration for patients with neutropenic fever syndromes impacts on outcome. Many studies have focused on the time from triage to the administration of the first dose of initial empirical antibiotic in this setting. A Brazilian cohort study of 307 febrile neutropenic cancer patients reported that each hour delay in the time to antibiotic administration increased the 28-day all-cause mortality by 28% [18]. In a single center retrospective cohort study of 1,628 neutropenic fever syndromes in 653 pediatric cancer patients adverse events were observed in 5.2% and 12.6% of patients in whom the time-to-first dose of antibiotic was administered in 60 minutes or less and more than 60 minutes, respectively ($p < .001$) [19]. While other studies have not been able to observe a relationship between time-to-antibiotic administration and complication rates [20,21], an independent direct relationship between time-to-first dose of antibiotic for febrile neutropenia and length of hospital stay has been reported in a Canadian study [22].

These observations support the recommendation from multiple groups that as a standard of practice the first dose of initial empirical antibacterial therapy in the setting of suspected infection or sepsis should be administered in 60 minutes or less from the time of assessment [16,23,24].

18.2.6 What Kinds of Infections Should We Expect?

In 1990, the International Immunocompromised Host Society published a set of case definitions of infections observed in febrile neutropenic patients for the purpose of having a common language to standardize reporting in clinical trials [25]. *Microbiologically documented infections* (MDIs) were defined as those for which a pathogen and a focus could be defined. These infections were sub-classified as bacteremic and non-bacteremic. *Clinically documented infections* (CDIs) were those with a defined clinical focus such as a pulmonary infiltrate or a cellulitis, but no identifiable pathogen. While a diligent search for infection may result in as few as 8% of febrile episodes being classified as "unexplained" [26], contemporary studies suggest that the actual proportion for which no infectious cause can be found may be much higher. An *unexplained fever* (UF) defines a circumstance for a febrile neutropenic patient for whom neither a pathogen nor a clinical focus could be defined.

A Spanish prospective cohort of 1,298 adult patients with solid tissue malignancies who developed chemotherapy-induced neutropenic fever syndromes reported a distribution of sites of infection including respiratory tract in 26% (upper respiratory tract 13%, acute bronchitis 10%, pneumonia 3%), gastrointestinal tract in 21% (oropharyngeal mucositis 10%, enteritis 11%), urinary tract in 5%, primary bloodstream infection in 9%, severe sepsis/septic shock in 9%, and unexplained fevers in 30% [27].

A registry study of 1,001 consecutive febrile neutropenic episodes examined the distribution of infections encountered among 863 patients attending the emergency department of the Asan Medical Center in Seoul, Korea [21]. The majority of these patients had solid tumors (78%) and remainder (22%) had hematological malignancies, the majority (90%) of which were lymphomas. Of the 1,001 episodes, MDIs accounted for 122 (12%) of which bacteremia accounted for 64 (52%) and other foci 58 (48%). There were 69 isolates for the 64 bacteremic infections. The majority (44 of 69, 64%) of isolates were Gram-negative bacteria and the remainder (25 of 69, 36%) were Gram-positive organisms. There were 94 MDIs with clinical foci (associated with secondary bacteremia in 36) that included the respiratory tract in 46 (49%), urinary tract in 21 (22%), skin and soft tissue infection in 10 (11%), gastrointestinal tract in 9 (10%), central venous access site infection in 5 (5%), and other sites in 3 (3%). CDIs accounted for 209 infections (21%). The clinical sites consisted of the respiratory tract in 143 (68%), the gastrointestinal tract in 33 (16%), skin and soft tissue infection in 16 (7%), urinary tract in 5 (2%), and other sites in 12 (6%). UFs accounted for 670 episodes (67%) of these neutropenic fever syndromes. Severe sepsis or septic shock was documented in 67 patients (7%). The overall mortality among the 863 patients was 2.7%.

Viruses may be prominent causes of neutropenic fever syndromes that develop in the community setting. These may represent reactivations of human herpes viruses such as varicella-zoster virus, herpes simplex virus, or human cytomegalovirus, or they may represent upper or lower respiratory tract infections due to community-acquired respiratory viruses (CARVs) [28]. In a prospective Chilean study of 1,044 children with cancer being evaluated for hospital admission for febrile neutropenia, almost half (46%) of the episodes were associated with CARV infections [29].

Antibacterial therapy initiated empirically for the treatment of the febrile neutropenic episode may be safely discontinued once the viral diagnosis is established by isolation of a CARV along with a compatible clinical syndrome and by the exclusion of a bacterial infection. A study by Santolaya and colleagues was designed to examine this question [30]. A cohort of 951 children with cancer admitted to hospital for febrile neutropenia underwent molecular testing for CARVs on admission. In the cohort, 319 patients (33.5%) had a CARV infection without evidence for an associated bacterial infection, and 178 of these who were clinically stable at 48 hours after admission were randomly allocated to either continue the prescribed antibacterial regimen or to discontinue treatment. An uneventful resolution of the neutropenic fever episode was observed in 97% of patients who continued therapy and in 95% of those who discontinued antibacterial therapy (OR 1.48, 95% CI 0.32–6.83, $p = .61$). The use of molecular CARV testing, in season, has implications for antimicrobial stewardship and on length of hospital stay.

18.2.7 Risk Assessment

Patients, for whom the initial medical assessment suggests a working diagnosis of sepsis or SIRS should be evaluated for risk for complications of infection. Such complications include hypotension, respiratory failure, need for critical care services, altered state of consciousness, coagulopathy, clinical bleeding needing transfusion support, dysrhythmia requiring treatment, acute kidney injury, hyperglycemia, congestive heart failure, and poor performance status.

The dichotomization of febrile neutropenic patients into low-risk and high-risk categories for the purposes of empiric antimicrobial therapy and judging prognosis has been advocated by the Multinational Association for Supportive Care in Cancer (MASCC) [31]. A seven-item scoring system has been developed and validated consisting of burden of incident illness (no or mild symptoms, 5 points; moderate symptoms, 3 points), lack of hypotension (5 points), no obstructive airways disease (4 points), solid tumor or no previous history of invasive fungal disease (4 points), no evidence for dehydration (3 points), outpatient status at onset of febrile neutropenia (3 points), and age <60 years (2 points) [31]. Scores of ≥21 have defined a group of patients for whom resolution rates for the neutropenic fever episode were high (90%) and the overall complication rates, including death, were low (overall complications 9.3%; mortality 1.7%) compared to those with scores of <21 (overall complications 37.7%; mortality 12.4%) [32]. MASCC scores between 15 and 21 and less than 15 have identified patients with even poorer outcomes (overall complication rates 32.2% and 66.0%, respectively; and mortality rates 9.1% and 29.2%, respectively). The performance of the MASCC score for identifying those febrile neutropenic patients at low risk for serious medical complications was examined in a recent systematic review [33]). The sensitivity, specificity, and positive and negative predictive values were 85%, 68%, and 83%, and 68%, respectively, which compares closely to the original derivation data set. The misclassification rate for the MASCC score was 0.2 (95% CI 0.1–0.29).

The Infectious Disease Society of America (IDSA) has supplemented the designation of high-risk with additional criteria including the presence of profound neutropenia (absolute neutrophil count of <0.1 x 10^9/L) with an expected duration of >7 days and the presence of a significant co-morbidity, including hemodynamic instability, mucositis that impairs oral intake or causes severe diarrhea, mental status changes, indwelling CVAD infection, new pulmonary infiltrates or hypoxemia, or evidence of acute hepatic or kidney injury [3]. It is recommended that these patients be hospitalized.

The ability to reliably identify patients at low risk for febrile neutropenia-related serious complications has led to the consideration of whether such patients could be safely and effectively managed on an outpatient basis with orally administered rather that intravenously administered initial empirical antibacterial therapy. The safety and efficacy of this approach for low-risk patients has been the subject of several comparative clinical trials. A systematic review with meta-analysis of six trials comparing outpatient and inpatient management of neutropenic fever syndromes in low-risk cancer patients demonstrated no differences in the relative risks for treatment failure and death, 0.81 (95% CI 0.55 to 1.19, $p=.28$) and 1.11 (95% CI 0.41 to 3.05, $p=.83$), respectively [34]. Further, an analysis of treatment failures among febrile neutropenic low-risk patients in eight trials comparing oral and intravenous administration of antibacterial therapy identified no differences in efficacy (RR 0.93, 95% CI 0.65–1.32, $p=.67$) [34].

18.3 Initial Empirical Antibacterial Therapy for the Febrile Neutropenic Patient

18.3.1 Which Regimen Should I Prescribe and For How Long Should I Prescribe It?

The choice of initial empirical antibacterial therapy for the febrile neutropenic patient must be based on the bacterial microorganisms being targeted, and the results of the initial triage and medical assessment described earlier identifying the presenting syndrome as sepsis, severe sepsis, or septic shock, and the potential focus of infection.

The target microorganisms are most commonly bacteria that normally colonize body surfaces on the skin, periodontium, oropharynx, and gastrointestinal tract. Accordingly, the spectrum of antibacterial activity must include microaerophilic cocci such as the viridans group streptococci and methicillin-susceptible *Staphylococcus aureus*, aerobic Gram-negative bacillary members of the facultatively anaerobic family Enterobacteriaceae most commonly *Escherichia coli*, *Klebsiella* spp., and *Enterobacter* spp., and less commonly hospital-acquired afermentative Gram-negative bacilli such as *Pseudomonas aeruginosa*, *Stenotrophomonas maltophilia*, or *Acinetobacter* spp. Also less commonly isolated are obligate anaerobic bacteria such as *Peptostreptococcus* spp., *Prevotella* spp., *Porphyromonas* spp., *Clostridium* spp., or *Bacteroides* spp. Also less common as a cause of a first neutropenic fever syndrome are fungi such as molds (e.g., *Aspergillus* spp.) or yeasts (e.g., *Candida* spp. or *Cryptococcus* spp.). These latter potential pathogens are not usually included in the spectrum of the initial empirical antibacterial regimen. Last, in the setting of a community outbreak of community-acquired respiratory viruses, only influenza is amenable to initial empirical treatment with a neuraminidase inhibitor for a compatible influenza-like illness syndrome as described earlier.

The triage- and medical assessment-based determination of the syndrome largely influences the initial empirical antibacterial regimen choice. A patient with neutropenic fever syndrome associated with several SIRS criteria, perhaps an evident clinical focus, with evidence for organ dysfunction, including mental changes, cardiovascular dysfunction such as documented hypotension, or renal dysfunction, even before the return of the results of initial laboratory testing should be treated with intravenous broad-spectrum antibacterial therapy and early goal-directed therapy within the 60-minute time-line and in accordance with guidelines [8,23].

The term *broad-spectrum* as applied to the antibacterial regimen, refers to spectrum of antibacterial activity to be expected for the candidate potential pathogens assumed to be driving the neutropenic fever syndrome.

The initial empirical antibacterial regimen may be a single agent, such as a carbapenem β-lactam antibiotic, or multi-agent, such as an antipseudomonal β-lactam/β-lactamase inhibitor agent like piperacillin-tazobactam plus an aminoglycoside like tobramycin or a glycopeptide like vancomycin. The addition of the glycopeptide to the β-lactam/β-lactamase inhibitor is intended to extend the spectrum of activity of the regimen; in this example, to include methicillin-resistant *S. aureus*. The addition of the aminoglycoside to the β-lactam/β-lactamase inhibitor is intended to enhance the rate of clearance of target pathogens such as aerobic Gram-negative bacilli through synergistic or additive drug interaction. Among febrile neutropenic patients with Gram-negative infections treatment failure is less common among recipients of β-lactam plus aminoglycoside combination antibacterial therapy than for β-lactam monotherapy recipients (34% and 47%, respectively, RR 0.73, 95% CI 0.54–0.98) [35].

Low-risk patients for whom oral therapy may be appropriate may be treated with a multi-agent regimen consisting of ciprofloxacin and amoxicillin-clavulanate, if the fluoroquinolone agent has not been administered as part of a prophylactic regimen. While vancomycin is not routinely recommended as part of the initial empirical antibacterial regimen, it may be added to an empiric regimen at the start of treatment if infection of an intravascular device is suspected (and coagulase-negative staphylococci are therefore implicated), or if the individual is known to be colonized with a β-lactam-resistant Gram-positive pathogen such as methicillin-resistant *S. aureus* [3,36]. Systematic reviews of published clinical trials have not demonstrated that the early addition of a glycopeptide to the initial empirical antibacterial regimen provides any advantage for outcomes such as time-to-resolution of the febrile episode or mortality [37,38]. Alternatively, it may be added as a modification to the initial empirical antibacterial regimen in the setting of persistent unexplained neutropenic fever after day 4 of antimicrobial treatment in high-risk patients, if the chosen empirical regimen is judged to have suboptimal coverage for *S. aureus* and streptococci (e.g., ceftazidime monotherapy).

Vancomycin use is not without risks. There is an enhanced risk of acute kidney injury among febrile neutropenic patients receiving glycopeptides as part of the initial empirical antibacterial regimen [38]. Similarly, the combination of a ß-lactam plus an aminoglycoside enhances the risk for nephrotoxicity. In a systematic review of 39 studies encompassing 6,608 febrile neutropenic subjects randomly allocated to receive ß-lactam monotherapy or a ß-lactam plus aminoglycoside, the rate of kidney injury was 2.4% and 5.7%, respectively (RR 2.38, 95% CI 1.84–3.08) [35].

The results of a systematic review with meta-analysis suggested that β-lactam monotherapy options were equivalent to dual-therapy regimens in terms of both mortality and other less rigorous endpoints, with two possible exceptions: cefepime monotherapy was associated with higher all-cause mortality in both the systematic review (RR 1.44, 95% CI 1.06–1.94) [39] and a subsequently published randomized controlled trial [40]; and the carbapenems (principally imipenem/cilastatin) were associated with a greater risk of *Clostridium difficile* toxin-mediated diarrhea (RR 1.94, 95% CI 1.24–3.04) [39]. In another recent systematic review with meta-analysis of patients with microbiologically documented neutropenic fever syndromes, meropenem and ceftazidime performed less well than monotherapy [41]. Notwithstanding these distinctions, and acknowledging that individual patient factors such as pre-existing renal impairment and a history of penicillin allergy may also influence the choice of antibacterial agents, the selection of any particular regimen will depend more on institutional practice and local antimicrobial resistance patterns than on a proven survival benefit for any single drug or combination therapy.

The use of a single agent broad-spectrum initial empirical regimen for relatively stable high-risk patients is recommended in a number of international guidelines [3,16,24,42]. In circumstances in which the patient many not be stable and is manifesting evidence of organ dysfunction with a severe sepsis or septic shock syndrome, a combination of an antipseudomonal β-lactam plus an aminoglycoside has been recommended [3,43] based on observed survival advantages in neutropenic as well as non-neutropenic patients [44,45].

18.3.2 When Should I Expect a Treatment Response and For How Long Should I Treat?

Treatment response is judged on the basis of resolution of baseline signs and symptoms. For patients with unexplained neutropenic fever syndrome or primary bacteremia, response is measured largely by defervescence. For those manifesting focal anatomical sites of infection, response must include resolution of signs and symptoms of inflammation at those sites.

The median time-to-defervescence for low-risk patients is two to three days, while for high-risk patients it is four to six days. Given these parameters, and in the absence of a positive culture, a documented source of infection, or clinical deterioration, changes to the empirical regimen are generally not warranted for the first three days of therapy for low-risk patients and five days for high-risk patients. Persistent neutropenic fever in a stable patient without evidence for progression may only require ongoing observation without antibacterial regimen modification [3].

The recommended duration of antibacterial therapy among patients with unexplained neutropenic fever syndromes who had been afebrile for at least two days had been until myeloid reconstitution [3], but the proceedings of the 4th European Conference on Infections in Leukemia (ECIL) have now recommended that empirical intravenous antibacterial therapy may be discontinued after 72 hours or longer of administration if the patient has been hemodynamically stable and afebrile for ≥48 hours independent of the absolute neutrophil count [46].

Recommendations for the duration of initial empirical and subsequent antibacterial therapy among neutropenic patients with clinically and microbiologically documented infections have varied depending on institutional protocol. The duration should be at least seven days, and the patient should have been afebrile for ≥4 days [47]. Patients who remain severely neutropenic at the time designated for antibiotic discontinuance should be observed for another 24–48 hours for signs of recrudescence and the need to re-institute systemic antibacterial therapy, or should have the prophylactic antibacterial therapy regimen restarted at the time of intravenous antibiotic discontinuance. In summary, the duration of antibacterial therapy for low- and high-risk neutropenic fever syndrome patients is recommended as two to three days and four to five days following defervescence, respectively [48].

18.4 Persistent and Recrudescent Neutropenic Fever Syndromes

Patients who are profoundly neutropenic, who remain febrile (without a documented source of infection) despite five to seven days of empirical antibacterial therapy, and for whom neutrophil counts are not expected to recover in the short term define the persistent neutropenic fever syndrome and should be re-assessed for consideration of the need for regimen modification [49].

Such patients, in the past, have been regarded to be at high-risk (approximately 20%) for invasive fungal infection [50–52]. The modification of the initial empirical antibacterial regimen for persistent fever by the addition of empirical antifungal therapy has become accepted standard of practice [3,53,54]. Empirical antifungal therapy may reduce the risk of invasive fungal infection and reduce mortality from fungal infections and may be used in the neutropenic patient who remains febrile on broad-spectrum

antibacterials for >3 days, if the neutrophil counts are not expected to recover in the ensuing five to seven days [3,54].

Circumstances in which febrile neutropenic patients who become afebrile following the institution of empirical antibacterial therapy then become febrile again after remaining afebrile for at least 48 hours define the recrudescent neutropenic fever syndrome. The frequency for this syndrome may be of the order of 15% (95% CI 13%–18%) [55]. These patients must also undergo rigorous reassessment to look for secondary bacterial infections, often associated with central venous catheters and invasive fungal infections, many of which have been invasive mold infections. Accordingly, blood cultures and high-resolution computerized tomographic imaging of the chest constitute some of the most important investigations in this syndrome. Further, the antimicrobial regimen modifications for consideration should include Gram-positive organism coverage and mold-active therapy.

18.5 Management of Patients with Reported Penicillin Hypersensitivity

Cancer patients presenting with a neutropenic fever syndrome should receive initial empirical antibacterial therapy in a timely manner in order to prevent excess morbidity and mortality and β-lactam antibacterial agents form the backbone of effective treatment of neutropenic fever syndromes. Approximately 10% of patients may provide a history of penicillin "allergy" that may result in a delay or modify the effectiveness of timely treatment. In such cases, it is estimated that only a minority, approximately 10% of those reporting a penicillin allergy, will have a potentially life-threatening immune-mediated immediate-type allergic reaction when challenged with a penicillin-type β-lactam agent [56]. Accordingly, high-risk patients presenting with a neutropenic fever syndrome and a history of a possible penicillin allergy may be considered for carbapenem-based initial empirical antibacterial therapy over that of an antipseudomonal cephalosporin-based regimen, particularly if that allergy history is characterized by an immediate- or accelerated-type onset. For those patients providing a history of delayed-type onset penicillin hypersensitivity, either a carbapenem-based or an antipseudomonal cephalosporin-based regimen may be considered.

18.6   Antibacterial Resistance—What If I Choose Incorrectly?

There have been major shifts in the spectrum of bacterial resistance that influence the choice of the initial empirical therapy of febrile neutropenic patients. As the prevalence of antibacterial resistant microorganisms increases in both the hospital and community settings, the probability that the clinician may choose an antibacterial regimen ineffective for the infecting pathogen is increased. These circumstances increase the time required to recognize the resistant pathogen and to modify the initial antibacterial regimen accordingly. Prolongation of time-to-appropriate antibacterial therapy is directly related to increased all-cause mortality.

Factors associated with an increased risk for infection by antibiotic-resistant microorganisms include prior colonization or infection by resistant bacteria (including methicillin-resistant *Staphylococcus aureus*, vancomycin-resistant *Enterococci*, extended-spectrum β-lactamase [ESBL]-producing *Enterobacteriaceae*, carbapenem-resistant *Enterobacteriaceae*, multidrug resistant afermentative Gram-negative bacilli, *Clostridium difficile*, and fungi [*Candida* spp.]), prior exposure to broad-spectrum antibacterial agents (especially third- or fourth-generation cephalosporins), serious underlying illness such as progressive or relapsed malignancy, hospital-acquired infection, prolonged or repeated hospitalization, use of indwelling urinary catheters, older age, and requirement for critical care services [46].

In a study of 726 febrile neutropenic patients having 5,840 blood cultures from 1999 to 2006 from Pakistan, 18% were positive [57]. Among the Gram-negative organisms, Enterobacteriaceae accounted for the majority (278 of 442, 62.9%) and *Pseudomonas aeruginosa* for 49 (11.1%). Between 1999 and 2006, resistance among the Enterobacteriaceae had increased from 27% to 50% for ciprofloxacin, from 24% to 56% (54% of these were ESBL-producers) for ceftriaxone, and from 0% to 11% for piperacillin/tazobactam. During this same period, resistance among *P. aeruginosa* isolates for ciprofloxacin had increased from 13% to 29%, for piperacillin/tazobactam from 0% to 11%, and for imipenem/cilastatin from 0% to 6% [57]. While these observations suggest that initial empirical antibacterial therapy with piperacillin/tazobactam- or carbapenem-based regimens would be effective in the majority of cases the observed increase in the number of resistant isolates, particularly in ESBL-producing Gram-negative bacteria, over this period is disturbing.

In a report from the National Healthcare Safety Network 2009–2012 examining the predominant isolates among cancer patients developing central venous line-associated bloodstream infections, fluoroquinolone resistance had increased 22% from 49.5% to 60.4% between 2009 and 2012 among the *E. coli* bloodstream isolates [58].

Colonization by resistant Enterobacteriaceae is a risk factor for invasive infection in patients with hematological malignancies. In a study of 497 high-risk patients from Germany, colonization by ESBL-producing Enterobacteriaceae was observed in 55 cases (11%) [59]. Of these patients, ESBL-producing Enterobacteriaceae bloodstream infections occurred in four (7.3%) compared to 1 of 442 subjects not colonized (RR 32.1, 95% CI 3.7–282.4, $p = .0006$). Colonization by carbapenem-resistant *Klebsiella pneumoniae* was observed in 31 (1%) of 2,978 autologous hematopoietic stem cell transplant recipients and in 51 (2.3%) of 2,135 allogeneic stem cell transplant recipients in an Italian study [60]. Invasive infections were due to these pathogens in 8 (25.8%) of 31 colonized autologous transplant recipients and in 20 (39.2%) of 51 allogeneic transplant recipients. Accordingly, colonization was associated with a relative risk for invasive infection of 44.7 (95% CI 20.9–95.8) and 9.4 (95% CI 6.3–13.9) for autologous and allogeneic transplant recipients, respectively [60].

In a retrospective study of 213 patients with an ESBL-producing Gram-negative bacteremia, either empirical piperacillin/tazobactam or a carbapenem was administered; pipericillin/tazobactam was associated with increased mortality (adjusted HR 1.92, 95% CI 1.07–3.45, $p = .03$) [61]. These observations argue for the wider initial empirical use of carbapenems where the risk for invasive ESBL-producing Gram-negative infection is high. However, not all studies have reached the same conclusions regarding β-lactam/β-lactamase inhibitor combinations for the treatment of ESBL bloodstream infections [62]. The wider use of carbapenems is predictably likely to enhance the risk for carbapenem resistance, as has been observed [63].

MRSA has become a significant community-acquired pathogen. MRSA has in some cancer centers replaced MSSA as the most common *S. aureus* bacteremia in febrile neutropenic patients [64]. While vancomycin remains the recommended treatment for most MRSA infections, a relationship between poor outcomes and infection with *S. aureus* strains with elevated MICs to vancomycin has been recognized [65]. Among MRSA bacteremic cancer patients, a vancomycin MIC of ≥2 mg/L has been observed to be an independent predictor of MRSA mortality [66]. The frequency of such infections in cancer patient populations is relatively low. Alternatives to vancomycin for the treatment of MRSA infections include linezolid and daptomycin.

Rates of VRE bloodstream infections early in the post-stem cell transplant period have increased and have had reported crude mortality rates as high as 85%. In one U.S. center, VRE represented the most common bloodstream isolate (53.5% of all isolates) within the first 30 days of transplant [67]. A delay in the institution of appropriate treatment for invasive VRE infections is associated with incremental 30-day all-cause mortality, from 11% on day 1 to 48% on day 4 [68]. The inclusion of linezolid or daptomycin in the initial empirical antibacterial regimen for febrile neutropenic patients known to be colonized by VRE should be considered [3,47].

References

1 Hann I, Viscoli C, Paesmans M, Gaya H, Glauser M. A comparison of outcome from febrile neutropenic episodes in children compared with adults: results from four EORTC studies. International Antimicrobial Therapy Cooperative Group (IATCG) of the European Organization for Research and Treatment of Cancer (EORTC). Br J Haematol. 1997 Dec;99(3):580–8. PubMed PMID: 9401070. Epub 1997/12/24. eng.

2 Bodey GP, Rodriguez V, Chang HY, Narboni G. Fever and infection in leukemic patients: a study of 494 consecutive patients. Cancer. 1978;41(4):1610–22.

3 Freifeld AG, Bow EJ, Sepkowitz KA, Boeckh MJ, Ito JI, Mullen CA, et al. Clinical practice guideline for the use of antimicrobial agents in neutropenic patients with cancer: 2010 update by the Infectious Diseases Society of America. Clin Infect Dis. 2011 Feb 15;52(4):e56–93. PubMed PMID: 21258094. Epub 2011/01/25. eng.

4 Mackowiak PA, Bartlett JG, Bordon BC, et al. Concepts of fever: recent advances and lingering dogma. Clin Infect Dis. 1997;35:119–38.

5 Bow EJ, Meddings JB. Intestinal mucosal dysfunction and infection during remission-induction therapy for acute myeloid leukaemia. Leukemia. 2006;20(12):2087–92.

6 Spielberger R, Stiff P, Bensinger W, Gentile T, Weisdorf D, Kewalramani T, et al. Palifermin for oral mucositis after intensive therapy for hematologic cancers. N Engl J Med. 2004;351(25):2590–8.

7 van der Velden WJ, Blijlevens NM, Feuth T, Donnelly JP. Febrile mucositis in haematopoietic SCT recipients. Bone Marrow Transplant. 2009 Jan;43(1):55–60. PubMed PMID: 18762766. Epub 2008/09/03. eng.

8 Bow EJ, Wingard JR. Overview of neutropenic fever syndromes: Wolters Kluwer; 2017 [updated December 2, 2015; cited 2017 February 9, 2017]. Available from: https://www-uptodate-com.uml.idm. oclc.org/contents/overview-of-neutropenic-fever-syndromes?source=search_result&search=febrile%20neutropenia%20low%20risk,febrile%20neutropenia%20low%20risk&selectedTitle=1~150.

9 Keng MK, Thallner EA, Elson P, Ajon C, Sekeres J, Wenzell CM, et al. Reducing time to antibiotic administration for febrile neutropenia in the emergency department. J Oncol Pract. 2015 Jul 28;10.1200/JOP.2014.002733. PubMed PMID: 26220930.

10 Bullard MJ, Unger B, Spence J, Grafstein E. Revisions to the Canadian Emergency Department Triage and Acuity Scale (CTAS) adult guidelines. CJEM. 2008 Mar;10(2):136–51. PubMed PMID: 18371252. Epub 2008/03/29. engfre.

11 Bone RC, Sibbald WJ, Sprung CL. The ACCP-SCCM consensus conference on sepsis and organ failure. Chest. 1992;101(6):1481–3.

12 Regazzoni CJ, Khoury M, Irrazabal C, Myburg C, Galvalisi NR, O'Flaherty M, et al. Neutropenia and the development of the systemic inflammatory response syndrome. Intensive Care Med. 2003;29(1):135–8.

13 Wisplinghoff H, Cornely OA, Moser S, Bethe U, Stutzer H, Salzberger B, et al. Outcomes of nosocomial bloodstream infections in adult neutropenic patients: a prospective cohort and matched case-control study. Infect Control Hosp Epidemiol. 2003;24(12):905–11.

14 Sickles EA, Greene WH, Wiernik PH. Clinical presentation of infection in granulocytopenic patients. Arch of Internal Med. 1975;135:715–9.

15 DesJardin JA, Falagas ME, Ruthazer R, Griffith J, Wawrose D, Schenkein D, et al. Clinical utility of blood cultures drawn from indwelling central venous catheters in hospitalized patients with cancer. Ann Intern Med. 1999 Nov 02;131(9):641–7. PubMed PMID: 10577325.

16 Flowers CR, Seidenfeld J, Bow EJ, Karten C, Gleason C, Hawley DK, et al. Antimicrobial prophylaxis and outpatient management of Fever and neutropenia in adults treated for malignancy: american society of clinical oncology clinical practice guideline. J Clinical Oncology. 2013 Feb 20;31(6):794–810. PubMed PMID: 23319691. Epub 2013/01/16. eng.

17 Hughes WT, Armstrong D, Bodey GP, Bow EJ, Brown AE, Calandra T, et al. 2002 guidelines for the use of antimicrobial agents in neutropenic patients with cancer. Clin Infect Dis. 2002 Mar 15;34(6):730–51. PubMed PMID: 11850858.

18 Rosa RG, Goldani LZ. Cohort study of the impact of time to antibiotic administration on mortality in patients with febrile neutropenia. Antimicrobial agents & Chemother. 2014 Jul;58(7):3799–803. PubMed PMID: 24752269.

19 Fletcher M, Hodgkiss H, Zhang S, Browning R, Hadden C, Hoffman T, et al. Prompt administration of antibiotics is associated with improved outcomes in febrile neutropenia in children with cancer. Pediatr Blood & Cancer. 2013 Aug;60(8):1299–306. PubMed PMID: 23417978.

20 Ahn S, Lee YS, Lim KS, Lee JL. Timing of antibiotic administration and outcomes in patients with chemotherapy-induced febrile neutropenia. Hematol Oncol. 2013 Dec;31(4):221–2. PubMed PMID: 23436230.

21 Ko BS, Ahn S, Lee YS, Kim WY, Lim KS, Lee JL. Impact of time to antibiotics on outcomes of chemotherapy-induced febrile neutropenia. Support Care Cancer. 2015 Sep;23(9):2799–804. PubMed PMID: 25663578.

22 Perron T, Emara M, Ahmed S. Time to antibiotics and outcomes in cancer patients with febrile neutropenia. BMC Health Services Research. 2014;14:162. PubMed PMID: 24716604. Pubmed Central PMCID: 3991909.

23 Dellinger RP, Levy MM, Rhodes A, Annane D, Gerlach H, Opal SM, et al. Surviving sepsis campaign: international guidelines for management of severe sepsis and septic shock: 2012. Crit Care Med. 2013 Feb;41(2):580–637. PubMed PMID: 23353941. Epub 2013/01/29. eng.

24 Tam CS, O'Reilly M, Andresen D, Lingaratnam S, Kelly A, Burbury K, et al. Use of empiric antimicrobial therapy in neutropenic fever. Australian Consensus Guidelines 2011 Steering Committee. Intern Med J. 2011 Jan;41(1b):90–101. PubMed PMID: 21272173. Epub 2011/01/29. eng.

25 Immunocompromised Host S. The design, analysis, and reporting of clinical trials on the empirical antibiotic managment of the neutropenic patient. J Infect Dis. 1990;161:397–401.

26 Peacock JE, Herrington DA, Wade JC, Lazarus HM, Reed MD, Sinclair JW, et al. Ciprofloxacin plus piperacillin compared with tobramycin plus piperacillin as empirical therapy in febrile neutropenic patients: a randomized, double-blind trial. Ann Intern Med. 2002;137(2):77–87.

27 Carmona-Bayonas A, Jimenez-Fonseca P, Virizuela Echaburu J, Antonio M, Font C, Biosca M, et al. Prediction of serious complications in patients with seemingly stable febrile neutropenia: validation of the Clinical Index of Stable Febrile Neutropenia in a prospective cohort of patients from the FINITE study. J Clin Oncol. 2015 Feb 10;33(5):465–71. PubMed PMID: 25559804.

28 Teh BW, Harrison SJ, Worth LJ, Spelman T, Thursky KA, Slavin MA. Risks, severity and timing of infections in patients with multiple myeloma: a longitudinal cohort study in the era of immunomodulatory drug therapy. Br J Haematol. 2015 Oct;171(1):100–8. PubMed PMID: 26105211.

29 Torres JP, De la Maza V, Kors L, Villarroel M, Piemonte P, Izquierdo G, et al. Respiratory viral infections and coinfections in children with cancer, fever and neutropenia: clinical outcome of infections caused by different respiratory viruses. Pediatr Infect Dis J. 2016 Sep;35(9):949–54. PubMed PMID: 27518750.

30 Santolaya ME, Alvarez AM, Acuna M, Aviles CL, Salgado C, Tordecilla J, et al. Efficacy and safety of withholding antimicrobial treatment in children with cancer, fever and neutropenia, with a demonstrated viral respiratory infection: a randomized clinical trial. Clin Microbiol Infect. 2017 Nov 14;23:173–8. PubMed PMID: 27856269.

31 Klastersky J, Paesmans M, Rubenstein EB, Boyer M, Elting L, Feld R, et al. The multinational association for supportive care in cancer risk index: a multinational scoring system for identifying low-risk febrile neutropenic cancer patients. J Clin Oncol. 2000;18(16):3038–51.

32 Paesmans M, Klastersky J, Maertens J, Georgala A, Muanza F, Aoun M, et al. Predicting febrile neutropenic patients at low risk using the MASCC score: does bacteremia matter? Support Care Cancer. 2011 Jul;19(7):1001–8. PubMed PMID: 20596732.

33 Bow EJ. The diagnostic approach to the febrile neutropaenic patient: clinical considerations. In: Maschmeyer G, Rolston, K.V.I., editor. Infections in Hematology. Berlin, Heidelberg: Springer-Verlag; 2015. p. 91–111.

34 Teuffel O, Ethier MC, Alibhai SM, Beyene J, Sung L. Outpatient management of cancer patients with febrile neutropenia:

a systematic review and meta-analysis. Ann of Oncol. 2011 Nov;22(11):2358–65. PubMed PMID: 21363878.

35 Paul M, Dickstein Y, Schlesinger A, Grozinsky-Glasberg S, Soares-Weiser K, Leibovici L. Beta-lactam versus beta-lactam-aminoglycoside combination therapy in cancer patients with neutropenia. Cochrane Database Syst Rev. 2013;6:CD003038. PubMed PMID: 23813455.

36 Feld R. Vancomycin as part of initial empirical antibiotic therapy for febrile neutropenia in patients with cancer: pros and cons. Clin Infect Dis. 1999;29(3):503–7.

37 Paul M, Borok S, Fraser A, Vidal L, Leibovici L. Empirical antibiotics against Gram-positive infections for febrile neutropenia: systematic review and meta-analysis of randomized controlled trials. J Antimicrob Chemother. 2005;55(4):436–44.

38 Vardakas KZ, Samonis G, Chrysanthopoulou SA, Bliziotis IA, Falagas ME. Role of glycopeptides as part of initial empirical treatment of febrile neutropenic patients: a meta-analysis of randomised controlled trials. Lancet Infect Dis. 2005;5(7):431–9.

39 Paul M, Yahav D, Fraser A, Leibovici L. Empirical antibiotic monotherapy for febrile neutropenia: systematic review and meta-analysis of randomized controlled trials. J Antimicrob Chemother. 2006 Feb;57(2):176–89. PubMed PMID: 16344285.

40 Bow EJ, Rotstein C, Noskin GA, Laverdiere M, Schwarer AP, Segal BH, et al. A randomized, open-label, multicenter comparative study of the efficacy and safety of piperacillin-tazobactam and cefepime for the empirical treatment of febrile neutropenic episodes in patients with hematologic malignancies. Clin Infectious Dis. 2006;43(4):447–59.

41 Horita N, Shibata Y, Watanabe H, Namkoong H, Kaneko T. Comparison of antipseudomonal beta-lactams for febrile neutropenia empiric therapy: systematic review and network meta-analysis. Clin Microbiol Infect. 2017 Apr 01;10.1016/j.cmi.2017.03.0242017/04/06. PubMed PMID: 28377312. Epub 2017/04/06. eng.

42 Link H, Bohme A, Cornely OA, Hoffken K, Kellner O, Kern WV, et al. Antimicrobial therapy of unexplained fever in neutropenic patients—guidelines of the Infectious Diseases Working Party (AGIHO) of the German Society of Hematology and Oncology (DGHO), Study Group Interventional Therapy of Unexplained Fever, Arbeitsgemeinschaft Supportivmassnahmen in der Onkologie (ASO) of the Deutsche Krebsgesellschaft (DKG-German Cancer Society). Ann Hematol. 2003;82 Suppl 2:S105–S17.

43 Penack O, Becker C, Buchheidt D, Christopeit M, Kiehl M, von Lilienfeld-Toal M, et al. Management of sepsis in neutropenic patients: 2014 updated guidelines from the Infectious Diseases Working Party of the German Society of Hematology and Medical Oncology (AGIHO). Ann Hematol. 2014 Jul;93(7):1083–95. PubMed PMID: 24777705. Pubmed Central PMCID: PMC4050292.

44 Kumar A, Safdar N, Kethireddy S, Chateau D. A survival benefit of combination antibiotic therapy for serious infections associated with sepsis and septic shock is contingent only on the risk of death: a meta-analytic/meta-regression study. Crit Care Med. 2010 Aug;38(8):1651–64. PubMed PMID: 20562695.

45 Legrand M, Max A, Peigne V, Mariotte E, Canet E, Debrumetz A, et al. Survival in neutropenic patients with severe sepsis or septic shock. Crit Care Med. 2012 Jan;40(1):43–9. PubMed PMID: 21926615. Epub 2011/09/20. eng.

46 Averbuch D, Orasch C, Cordonnier C, Livermore DM, Mikulska M, Viscoli C, et al. European guidelines for empirical antibacterial therapy for febrile neutropenic patients in the era of growing

resistance: summary of the 2011 4th European Conference on Infections in Leukemia. Haematologica. 2013 Dec;98(12):1826–35. PubMed PMID: 24323983. Pubmed Central PMCID: PMC3856957.

47 Averbuch D, Cordonnier C, Livermore DM, Mikulska M, Orasch C, Viscoli C, et al. Targeted therapy against multi-resistant bacteria in leukemic and hematopoietic stem cell transplant recipients: guidelines of the 4th European Conference on Infections in Leukemia (ECIL-4, 2011). Haematologica. 2013 Dec;98(12):1836–47. PubMed PMID: 24323984. Pubmed Central PMCID: 3856958. Epub 2013/12/11.

48 Bow EJ. Approach to Infection in Patients Receiving Cytotoxic Chemotherapy for Malignancy. In: Hall JB, Schmidt GA, Kress JP, editors. Principles of Critical Care4th. 4th ed. New York: McGraw-Hill; 2015. p. 600–25.

49 Bow EJ. Neutropenic fever syndromes in patients undergoing cytotoxic therapy for acute leukemia and myelodysplastic syndromes. Semin Hematol. 2009 Jul;46(3):259–68. PubMed PMID: 19549578. Epub 2009/06/25. Eng.

50 Stein RS, Kayser J, Flexner JM. Clinical value of empirical amphotericin B in patients with acute myelogenous leukemia. Cancer. 1982;50:2247–51.

51 Pizzo PA, Robichaud KJ, Gill FA, Witebsky FG. Empiric antibiotic and antifungal therapy for cancer patients with prolonged fever and granulocytopenia. Am J Med. 1982;72(1):101–11.

52 Group EIATP. Empiric antifungal therapy in febrile granulocytopenic patients. EORTC International Antimicrobial Therapy Cooperative Group. Am J Med. 1989;86(6 Pt 1):668–72.

53 Slavin MA, Szer J, Grigg AP, Roberts AW, Seymour JF, Sasadeusz J, et al. Guidelines for the use of antifungal agents in the treatment of invasive Candida and mould infections. Intern Med J. 2004;34(4):192–200.

54 Marchetti O, Cordonnier C, Calandra T. Empirical antifungal therapy in neutropaenic cancer patients with persistent fever. Eur J Cancer Suppl. 2007;5(2):32–42.

55 Akova M, Paesmans M, Calandra T, Viscoli C. A European Organization for Research and Treatment of Cancer-International Antimicrobial Therapy Group Study of secondary infections in febrile, neutropenic patients with cancer. Clin Infect Dis. 2005;40(2):239–45.

56 Sogn DD, Evans R, 3rd, Shepherd GM, Casale TB, Condemi J, Greenberger PA, et al. Results of the National Institute of Allergy and Infectious Diseases Collaborative Clinical Trial to test the predictive value of skin testing with major and minor penicillin derivatives in hospitalized adults. Arch Intern Med. 1992 May;152(5):1025–32. PubMed PMID: 1580706.

57 Irfan S, Idrees F, Mehraj V, Habib F, Adil S, Hasan R. Emergence of Carbapenem resistant Gram negative and vancomycin resistant Gram positive organisms in bacteremic isolates of febrile neutropenic patients: a descriptive study. BMC Infect Dis. 2008;8:80.

58 See I, Freifeld AG, Magill SS. Causative organisms and associated antimicrobial resistance in healthcare-associated, central line-associated bloodstream infections from oncology settings, 2009–2012. Clin Infect Dis. 2016 May 15;62(10):1203–9. PubMed PMID: 26936664. Pubmed Central PMCID: PMC4894695.

59 Vehreschild MJ, Hamprecht A, Peterson L, Schubert S, Hantschel M, Peter S, et al. A multicentre cohort study on colonization and infection with ESBL-producing Enterobacteriaceae in high-risk patients with haematological malignancies. J Antimicrob Chemother. 2014 Dec;69(12):3387–92. PubMed PMID: 25103492.

60 Girmenia C, Rossolini GM, Piciocchi A, Bertaina A, Pisapia G, Pastore D, et al. Infections by carbapenem-resistant

Klebsiella pneumoniae in SCT recipients: a nationwide retrospective survey from Italy. Bone Marrow Transplant. 2015 Feb;50(2):282–8. PubMed PMID: 25310302.

61 Tamma PD, Han JH, Rock C, Harris AD, Lautenbach E, Hsu AJ, et al. Carbapenem therapy is associated with improved survival compared with piperacillin-tazobactam for patients with extended-spectrum beta-lactamase bacteremia. Clin Infect Dis. 2015 May 1;60(9):1319–25. PubMed PMID: 25586681. Pubmed Central PMCID: 4462658.

62 Vardakas KZ, Tansarli GS, Rafailidis PI, Falagas ME. Carbapenems versus alternative antibiotics for the treatment of bacteraemia due to Enterobacteriaceae producing extended-spectrum beta-lactamases: a systematic review and meta-analysis. J Antimicrob Chemother. 2012 Dec;67(12):2793–803. PubMed PMID: 22915465.

63 Canton R, Akova M, Carmeli Y, Giske CG, Glupczynski Y, Gniadkowski M, et al. Rapid evolution and spread of carbapenemases among Enterobacteriaceae in Europe. Clin Microbiol Infect. 2012 May;18(5):413–31. PubMed PMID: 22507109.

64 Morris PG, Hassan T, McNamara M, Hassan A, Wiig R, Grogan L, et al. Emergence of MRSA in positive blood cultures from patients with febrile neutropenia—a cause for concern. Support Care Cancer. 2008 Sep;16(9):1085–8. PubMed PMID: 18274787. Epub 2008/02/16. eng.

65 Holmes NE, Johnson PD, Howden BP. Relationship between vancomycin-resistant Staphylococcus aureus, vancomycin-intermediate S. aureus, high vancomycin MIC, and outcome in serious S. aureus infections. J Clin Microbiol. 2012 Aug;50(8):2548–52. PubMed PMID: 22593595. Pubmed Central PMCID: 3421495. Epub 2012/05/18. eng.

66 Mahajan SN, Shah JN, Hachem R, Tverdek F, Adachi JA, Mulanovich V, et al. Characteristics and outcomes of methicillin-resistant staphylococcus aureus bloodstream infections in patients with cancer treated with vancomycin: 9-year experience at a comprehensive cancer center. Oncologist. 2012;17(10):1329–36. PubMed PMID: 22707509. Pubmed Central PMCID: 3481899.

67 Kamboj M, Chung D, Seo SK, Pamer EG, Sepkowitz KA, Jakubowski AA, et al. The changing epidemiology of vancomycin-resistant Enterococcus (VRE) bacteremia in allogeneic hematopoietic stem cell transplant (HSCT) recipients. Biol Blood Marrow Transplantation. 2010 Nov;16(11):1576–81. PubMed PMID: 20685257. Epub 2010/08/06.eng.

68 Zasowski EJ, Claeys KC, Lagnf AM, Davis SL, Rybak MJ. Time is of the essence: the impact of delayed antibiotic therapy on patient outcomes in hospital-onset Enterococcal bloodstream infections. Clin Infect Dis. 2016 May 15;62(10):1242–50. PubMed PMID: 26945013. Pubmed Central PMCID: PMC4845789.

Chapter 19

Infections in General Surgery

Paul A. Moroz and Christine H. Lee

19.1 Surgical Site Infections

Case Presentation 1

A 37-year-old male with underlying ulcerative colitis underwent emergency colectomy for perforated colon. Perioperatively, he received intravenous ceftriaxone and metronidazole. Within 24 hours of surgery, he developed progressively severe, generalized abdominal and right flank pain, associated with nausea, anorexia, and diaphoresis. On examination, he appeared flushed. His heart rate was 140 per minute, blood pressure 100/40, respiratory rate 26 per minute, temperature 39.4°C. Abdomen was diffusely tender. Surgical wound site revealed areas of dusky discoloration, purulent discharge, and foul odor.

19.1.1 Post-operative Site Soft-tissue Infections

It is estimated more than 46 million surgeries are performed each year in the United States [1]. Surgical site infections (SSI) are one of the most common healthcare-associated infections and occur following 16–63% of operations [2]. This, however, is likely an underestimation as the post-operative length of hospital stay has decreased significantly over the past decade, and it is estimated that 48% of SSIs occur after hospital discharge [3].

SSIs are sub-classified into *superficial incisional*, involving the skin and subcutaneous tissues; *deep incisional*, affecting the fascial and muscle layers of the incision; and *organ space*, which describes infections in any part of the organs or spaces other than the incision that was exposed during the procedure. Organ space infections include post-operative intra-abdominal abscesses, empyema, and mediastinitis.

19.1.2 Evaluation of Post-operative Patients with Suspected Infection

Fever is the most common symptom of post-operative infection occurring in approximately 30–40% of patients after a major surgery [4]. Fever during the first three days of the post-operative period is often due to a non-infectious cause: medications, atelectasis, deep vein thrombosis, transfusion reactions, or injury to tissue. In a retrospective review of patients undergoing major gynecologic surgery, Fanning et al. identified that 84% of patients, who were discharged despite experiencing fever of ⩾38.0°C, did not have an infectious etiology for the fever [4]. Presence of fever alone is not an indication for initiation of antibiotic therapy.

Evidence-Based Infectious Diseases, Third Edition. Edited by Dominik Mertz, Fiona Smaill, and Nick Daneman.
© 2018 John Wiley & Sons Ltd. Published 2018 by John Wiley & Sons Ltd.

A post-operative patient with fever requires a systematic, complete evaluation along with supportive laboratory tests, if indicated: complete blood count with differential, urinalysis, and bacteriologic cultures of blood and tissue/aspirated fluid from surgical site. Selective imaging studies, particularly computed tomography (CT) of the abdomen and pelvis, may be useful in evaluating a patient with late-onset, post-operative fever, after an abdominal surgery, without an apparent source, as it can localize occult infection or intraabdominal abscess. The common causes of non-surgical site-related, post-operative infections and fever, which include urinary, respiratory, and catheter-related infections, can be readily delineated by careful assessment of the patient. The majority of SSIs occur five or more days after surgery, but necrotizing soft tissue infections, particularly due to clostridial species or Group A streptococci, can manifest within 36 hours after an operation [5].

If the clinical assessment establishes the diagnosis of SSI, as indicated by fever, expanding inflammation, positive bacterial cultures, radiographic evidence, or presence of purulent discharge from the wound, it is accepted practice that the wound should be opened for drainage. To date, however, there are no randomized-controlled trials (RCTs) that have compared drainage to conservative management. SSIs, with the exception of uncomplicated cellulitis, may require operative intervention to open an infected wound, drain abscesses, and remove devitalized tissues. An empiric antibiotic therapy is recommended if there is extensive erythema around the wound, fever ⩾38.5°C, heart rate >110 beats/minute, or signs of systemic infection [6].

A number of factors will influence the choice of empiric antimicrobial agent(s). These include: patient-associated factors, including host immunity, presence of diabetes mellitus, and length of pre-operative hospital stay; procedure-associated factors such as the type and duration of perioperative antimicrobial prophylaxis, the duration of surgery, and class of surgical site [6]; and institution-specific factors such as the hospital's microbial antibiogram (antibiotic susceptibility profile). Many SSIs are polymicrobial, often including microbes resistant to antibiotics. Pathogens generally originate from the patient's own skin flora with *Staphylococcus aureus* being the most commonly isolated organism from SSIs, followed by Enterobacteriaceae, and Streptococci species. Based on these data, the responsible pathogens and the antibiotic susceptibility can be postulated and appropriate antibiotic(s) can be instituted until the culture results are available.

Diagnostic work-up recommendations include obtaining aerobic and anaerobic cultures from the site of infection prior to initiating antibiotic treatment to identify the bacteria involved and to institute appropriate antibiotic therapy [6]. Cultures should be transported at room temperature to the laboratory in appropriate aerobic and anaerobic transport media within two hours of specimen collection. Deep aspirates or tissue cultures are superior to swab samples in providing clinically relevant results. The results of culture and antibiotic susceptibility can help modify the antibiotic regimen, as treatment failure can occur in the presence of resistant organisms [6].

19.2 Post-operative Necrotizing Fasciitis

Case Presentation 1 (continued)

The wound was completely exposed and packed with sterile dressings. The infectious diseases service was consulted. Recommendation was made to surgically explore the wound to rule out possible necrotizing fasciitis. Surgical exploration revealed infection tracking into the transversalis fascia and internal oblique muscle. Portions of the transversalis fascia were necrotic. Infected and necrotic tissues were completely evacuated. A Jackson-Pratt drain was placed in the pelvis. Histopathology confirmed the diagnosis of necrotizing fasciitis. Culture of the tissue grew mixed facultative aerobic and anaerobic intestinal organisms.

Necrotizing fasciitis is a rare but potentially life-threatening, soft-tissue infection; it encompasses three types based on the bacteriologic entities [7]. Type 1 is a polymicrobial infection caused by both aerobic and anaerobic bacteria other than Group A streptococci. It is associated with abdominal and perineal lesions. Type 2 is caused by Group A streptococci, alone or in combination with other bacteria, most commonly *Staphylococcus aureus*. Type 3 is caused by *Vibrio vulnificus* infection and is associated with seafood ingestion or exposure to seawater. It is useful to distinguish the three types of necrotizing fasciitis as medical management among them differs, although surgical management does not. Post-operative necrotizing fasciitis, as with other necrotizing fasciitis, is usually an acute, rapidly extending inflammatory process [7]. The affected area is initially exquisitely painful and associated with rapidly progressive erythema, poorly demarcated edema, and occasionally numbness near the affected area. The course is followed by fever, hemodynamic instability, skin discoloration ranging from erythema to violaceous-gray, bullae formation, and crepitation may be present. By day 4 and 5 of onset, frank cutaneous gangrene develops. Owing to the associated morbidity and mortality with delay in diagnosis and management, it is paramount to recognize and institute immediate operative intervention when necrotizing fasciitis is clinically suspected.

During the early stage, it may be difficult to clinically distinguish necrotizing fasciitis from cellulitis as the local features of the affected area can be non-specific. Presence of severe systemic toxicity and fever while the cutaneous appearance is innocuous should alert the clinician to possible underlying necrotizing fasciitis. The diagnosis of necrotizing fasciitis is made at surgery and it is essential to extensively excise the affected skin and subcutaneous tissues beyond healthy fascia [7]. Post-debridement, a patient with necrotizing fasciitis usually requires critical care support and at times repeated surgical debridement.

Empiric antibiotic therapy and intravenous fluid must be promptly administered as soon as the diagnosis of invasive soft-tissue infection is considered. Initially, the antimicrobial therapy should consist of a regimen that reliably targets streptococci, *S. aureus*, Enterobacteriaceae, and anaerobic organisms. For type 1 necrotizing fasciitis, a broad-spectrum antibiotic regimen should be continued, as infection is due to mixed organisms. In type 2 necrotizing fasciitis, confirmed by detection of Group A streptococci, treatment should be with penicillin or a third-generation cephalosporin. Necrotizing fasciitis may be accompanied by streptococcal toxic shock syndrome (STSS), as evidenced by hypotension and signs of end-organ damage, including renal, liver, and pulmonary (adult respiratory distress syndrome) impairment in addition to rash or necrosis [7]. Intravenous immunoglobulin (IVIG) has been used successfully in some patients with STSS [7] and may be considered.

In summary, despite advances in surgical techniques and infection control practices, SSIs continue to be common healthcare-associated infections. The basic principle of SSI management is to open the infected site and allow drainage. Antibiotics have an adjunct role only when there is invasive infection. There is no guideline or study which specifically addresses the duration of antibiotic therapy for SSIs. The patient's overall clinical response to surgical and antimicrobial therapy can guide the duration and the route of antibiotic administration.

19.3 Mesh Infections After Incisional Hernia Repair

Case Presentation 2

A 59-year-old woman presents with a four-day history of purulent discharge from a previous abdominal surgical site, fever, and malaise. One month prior to this presentation, she underwent abdominal wall sarcoma resection, followed by insertion of polytetrafluoroethylene mesh and reconstruction of the abdominal wall. Abdominal examination revealed erythema and induration over the right lateral aspect of the abdomen. There were three small open areas with thick, purulent yellow secretion at the right lateral corner of the graft. The white blood cell count was 14.3×10^9/L. The skin and subcutaneous tissues are opened and the mesh was exposed. The patient was managed with surgical debridement and irrigation of the wound. The culture of the wound grew *Staphylococcus aureus*, sensitive to methicillin. Intravenous cloxacillin 2 g was started and the surgeon sought your advice for further management of this patient.

Following a midline laparotomy between 3% and 20% of patients develop incisional hernia [8]. Without prompt reduction and repair, there may be serious complications such as strangulation of the small bowel. The major risk factors for developing incisional hernia are conditions which negatively influence wound healing: obesity, diabetes, malnutrition, smoking, atherosclerosis, and wound infection [8]. After a primary repair, several studies have shown that rates of recurrent hernia can be up to 54%. Meta-analyses have found reduced relapse rates when using mesh repair compared to suture repair of the hernia, albeit slightly increased rates of SSI [9].

Mesh related infections occur in up to 8% of patients following hernia repair [10]. Although some meshes are superior to others in terms of lower infection rates, they may have reduced flexibility or strength. Infection risk is lowest in monofilament meshes with a large pore size that allow for neutrophil invasion such as polypropylene-based mesh [11]. However, bowel tissue can also invade macroporous mesh, thus increasing the risk of bowel adhesions [11]. The mesh selection process should take into consideration the surgical location, patient specific risk factors, and patient preference.

The immediate host response to mesh implantation is recruitment and infiltration of inflammatory cells. In an ideal milieu, acute inflammation is replaced by fibroblasts and multinucleated giant cells, leading to complete incorporation of deposited mesh into the neighboring tissues and induction of collagen synthesis. In a study by Amid et al. [12] the majority of complications were attributable to errors in surgical techniques, for example improper positioning of the mesh, inadequate fixation, and use of non-absorbable sutures.

Evidence to guide management of mesh infections is based on biologic principles and animal studies, as there are no cohort studies or RCTs. SSIs occurring early in the postoperative phase are usually independent of mesh utilization. These infections are primarily limited to the skin or subcutaneous layers and do not appear to interfere with proper mesh incorporation into host tissues. With administration of appropriate antibiotics, proper drainage, and debridement, it is rarely necessary to remove the mesh to eradicate the infection.

Deep mesh-related infections usually occur several weeks to months or even years after surgery and are relatively uncommon. They present with the cardinal signs of inflammation but there is a wide spectrum of severity. The factors that determine clinical presentation include: virulence of the infecting pathogen, the nature of the host tissue and its ability to support microbial growth, and the host response to the presence of these pathogens. Most patients present with a subacute to indolent course, characterized by progressive, crescendo wound pain, occasionally accompanied by cutaneous draining sinuses. Fever, soft-tissue swelling, and erythema may be absent. Rarely, some may present with acute, fulminant sepsis with high-grade fever, severe pain over the surgical site and soft tissue swelling, erythema, and exudate. The infecting organism in this acute form is typically virulent, such as *Staphylococcus aureus*, which will elicit more systemic inflammatory responses compared to other organisms. Other bacteria commonly responsible for mesh infections include Streptococci and Enterobacteriaceae species. One study found that methicillin-resistant *Staphylococcus aureus* (MRSA) was present in more than 50% of mesh infections [10].

Case Presentation 2 (continued)

After two weeks of local surgical site care and intravenous antibiotic therapy, the patient's signs and symptoms of systemic infection had resolved. The abdominal surgical site was left open, and she was discharged with intravenous antibiotic and daily surgical site care by a visiting home-care nurse. One month following the hospital discharge, the patient presented with purulent, foul-smelling greenish suppuration from the abdominal wound and the exposed mesh. She was afebrile and hemodynamically stable. The surgical site culture grew *Pseudomonas aeruginosa*. At this time, you recommend removal of the infected mesh, but the surgeon is reluctant to do so.

Based on the results from the combined European and American groups' observations, which included 12,374 cases of hernia repair using mesh, only eight patients developed mesh infection; five of the eight patients required removal of the mesh [13]. In a case report series consisting of three patients, the infections were completely eradicated in all the patients after the removal of the infected mesh [14]. Hence, based on these limited observational findings, it appears that patients who experience refractory infections despite repetitive drainage, lavage, and appropriate systemic antibiotic therapy may improve following the removal of the prosthetic material. It is improbable that an adequately powered, prospective, randomized trial of conservative therapy versus surgical

management for mesh infection will take place, given the very low rate of infectious complications.

When a patient presents with infection, the decision and the timing of the mesh removal should be individually tailored, taking into consideration the benefit and risks associated with repeat surgery. For patients who display evidence of persistent sepsis, while infected with virulent organisms, such as *S. aureus*, or aerobic enteric Gram-negative bacilli, immediate removal of the mesh is likely necessary. Some studies have found evidence to suggest that infected meshes should be replaced with absorbable or biological meshes [11].

Although mesh-related infection is rare, it is a significant complication. The risk can be minimized with strict adherence to aseptic techniques during mesh preparation and implantation, while conforming to current perioperative recommended guidelines for SSI prevention. Inflammatory symptoms that present weeks after surgery are likely mesh-related and majority of them can be managed with antibiotics and wound care.

19.4   Acute Diverticulitis

Case Presentation 3

A 62-year-old woman with a history of diverticulosis and hypertension presented with a three-day history of left lower quadrant pain, anorexia, low-grade fever, and chills. There was associated dysuria, urinary urgency, and frequency. On physical examination, blood pressure was 116/62 mmHg; heart rate 110 beats per minute; temperature 38.2°C. The jugular venous pressure was 2 cm below the sternal angle and the mucous membranes were dry. There were normal bowel sounds, moderate tenderness, and rigidity in the left lower quadrant and suprapubic area. There was no costovertebral angle tenderness. The white blood cell count was 16.7×10^9/L;

hemoglobin 104 g/L; platelets 407×10^9/L. Routine biochemical tests and urinalysis were normal. A clinical diagnosis of diverticulitis was made. You admitted the patient for intravenous hydration and for consultation with a general surgeon. You searched the literature to determine optimal evidence-based diagnosis of diverticulitis.

19.4.1 Epidemiology

Acquired colonic diverticular disease is common in industrialized countries, where it is estimated to affect approximately 5% of individuals by age 40 and nearly 65% of individuals by age 85 [15]. There is also growing evidence that the overall prevalence is increasing, particularly in younger patients, who seem to experience more severe forms of the disease compared to older patients. In younger populations, rates of diverticular disease are higher among men; in older populations, they are higher among women. Diverticulitis refers to inflammation of diverticulosis and approximately 15–20% of patients with diverticulosis will develop diverticulitis [16].

Prior to a few decades ago, diverticular disease was exceedingly rare in developing countries and Japan, attributed largely to sufficient dietary fiber consumption [15]. Recent studies indicate its increasing incidence in Africa and Japan with the introduction of a Westernized diet that is high in refined carbohydrates and low in fiber [15].

19.4.2 Pathogenesis

Colonic diverticulosis occurs due to elevated intraluminal pressure and weakening of the colonic wall. The weakening of the bowel leads to herniation of mucosa and submucosa, commonly through inherently vulnerable areas where blood vessels dive in toward the lumen. Refined carbohydrates and low dietary fiber lead to diminished stool bulk, an increase in gastrointestinal transit time, and a subsequent increase in intraluminal pressure. Diverticulitis ensues when fecal material or undigested food particles lodge in a diverticulum, causing obstruction of the diverticulum neck. This results in accumulation of mucus, bacterial overgrowth, and loss of blood supply to the already distended diverticulum. In the majority of cases, the outcome is a microscopic perforation and localized inflammatory process. Hinchey et al. created a useful method to classify inflammatory conditions associated with diverticulitis [17]. Stage I is defined as small, confined pericolonic abscesses, which can lead to larger paracolic abscesses (stage II). Stage III depicts generalized suppurative peritonitis and stage IV is fecal peritonitis. With recurrent episodes of inflammation, fibrosis and stricture of the colonic wall may emerge [18].

19.4.3 Diagnosis of Acute Diverticulitis

19.4.3.1 Clinical Features

The most common symptom of acute diverticulitis is a gradual onset of constant lower abdominal pain, particularly in the left lower quadrant, as the descending and sigmoid colons are frequently involved. Patients may report bloating, constipation, and experience pain relief following a bowel movement. Non-specific symptoms such as anorexia, nausea, and vomiting may accompany abdominal pain. When there is involvement of the bowel segment near the bladder or presence of colovesical fistula then urinary urgency, frequency, or dysuria may occur [18]. No studies were identified which specifically addressed the diagnostic accuracy of the clinical examination for diverticulitis.

Profuse rectal bleeding is unusual in acute diverticulitis, but microscopic fecal blood may be present. Often, low-grade fever, mild leukocytosis, and localized lower quadrant abdominal tenderness are found. Presence of peritonitis reflects perforation of peri-diverticular abscess or diverticulum [18,19]. Patients receiving corticosteroids may not reveal evidence of peritonitis despite extensive colonic inflammation or perforation.

Case Presentation 3 (continued)

After reviewing the literature with regard to the role of diagnostic imaging studies in the acute setting of suspected diverticulitis, you decide that your patient required a CT. The CT of the abdomen and pelvis with water-soluble contrast reveals pericolic fat inflammation, multiple diverticula, and thickening of the bowel wall. There is also a 3 cm pelvic abscess.

19.4.3.2 Imaging Studies

Since patients with acute diverticulitis may have free intraperitoneal air, it is important to include chest and abdominal radiographs in the initial management of patients presenting with a significant abdominal pain and possible underlying diverticulitis.

CT scans have been shown to be very useful in ascertaining the presence of acute diverticulitis, with a specificity of nearly 100% and a sensitivity between 93% and 97% [19]. Owing to the high risk of perforation, colonoscopy should be avoided in acute diverticulitis. Colonoscopy can be performed several weeks after the resolution of acute diverticulitis to rule out other pathology [19]. Although barium enema offers high diagnostic accuracy, it carries added risk and should be avoided unless CT scan is unavailable.

Modern CT scans, which offer rapid and high-resolution imaging, can help differentiate diverticular disease from similarly presenting diseases such as abdominal abcess, Crohn's disease, and appendicitis. CT scans can also identify cases of complicated diverticulitis. These are defined by evidence of perforation, hemorrhage, abscess, obstruction, or fistula.

Case Presentation 3 (continued)

On day 3 of the admission, the patient developed sudden onset of diffuse abdominal pain and vomiting. On examination, she was pale and diaphoretic. There was generalized abdominal guarding and rebound tenderness. A plain film of the abdomen showed increased gas in small and large intestines.

19.4.4 Treatment of Acute Diverticulitis

19.4.4.1 Medical Management

Most patients with a first episode of acute uncomplicated diverticulitis are treated with conservative management, which consists of intravenous fluid administration, bowel rest, and broad-spectrum antibiotic therapy. Meperidine can be used for pain control as it is associated with less colonic spasm than other opioids. Although patients respond to this management well, the use of antibiotics has been called into question. Recent studies have shown that antibiotics provide no additional benefit in uncomplicated diverticulitis [20]. Patients with a mild first episode of acute diverticulitis can be treated as outpatients and prescribed oral antibiotics if deemed necessary. Those with more complicated cases of diverticulitis are advised to remain in hospital for further management. These patients will benefit from treatment with broad-spectrum antibiotics [19]. Patients should be monitored for signs of disease progression such as fever, inflammation, worsening pain, and leukocytosis. Repeat CT and surgical consultation is warranted in these cases [19].

19.4.4.2 Surgical Management

Ten percent of patients with acute diverticulitis will require surgical intervention [19]. Small abscesses (<4 cm in diameter) without peritonitis usually drain spontaneously because of the development of fistulae between the colon and abscess, and they generally resolve with antibiotic treatment. Abscesses that are larger than 4 cm in diameter can be drained percutaneously under radiologic guidance [19]. With the administration of appropriate antibiotic therapy and adequate percutaneous drainage, patients in this group improve within days as indicated by a reduction in pain and normalization of leukocytosis [19]. Some of the advantages of percutaneous drainage are rapid control of sepsis, avoidance of general anesthesia for open drainage, and obviating the potential need for a second operation to restore colon contiguity.

The absolute indications for immediate colonic resection are uncontrolled sepsis, diffuse peritonitis, visceral perforation, large undrainable abcess, or failure to respond to conservative treatment [21]. Elective surgical intervention should also be considered after a patient with complicated diverticulitis has stabilized [21]. According to a recent RCT involving 109 patients, elective sigmoidectomy may offer a better quality of life than conservative management in those with recurrent or persistent abdominal complaints [22].

References

1 Defrances CJ, Lucas CA, Buie VC, Golosinskiy A. 2006 National Hospital Discharge Survey. Natl Health Stat Report. 2008;(5):1–20.

2 Lewis SS, Moehring RW, Chen LF, Sexton DJ, Anderson DJ. Assessing the relative burden of hospital-acquired infections in a network of community hospitals. Infect Control Hosp Epidemiol. 2013;34(11):1229–30.

3 Gibson A, Tevis S, Kennedy G. Readmission after delayed diagnosis of surgical site infection: a focus on prevention using the American College of Surgeons National Surgical Quality Improvement Program. Am J Surg. 2014;207(6):832–9.

4 Fanning J, Brewer J. Delay of hospital discharge secondary to postoperative fever—is it necessary? J Am Osteopath Assoc. 2002;102(12):660–1.

5 Barie PS. Surgical infections and antibiotic use. In: Townsend CM, Beauchamp DR, Evers MB, et al. ed. Sabiston Textbook of Surgery, 20th ed. Philadelphia, PA: Elsevier Saunders, 2017:241–80.

6 Stevens DL, Bisno AL, Chambers HF, et al. Practice guidelines for the diagnosis and management of skin and soft tissue infections: 2014 update by the Infectious Diseases Society of America. Clin Infect Dis. 2014;59(2):e10–52.

7 Salcido RS. Necrotizing fasciitis: reviewing the causes and treatment strategies. Adv Skin Wound Care. 2007;20(5):288–93.

8 Sanders DL, Kingsnorth AN. The modern management of incisional hernias. BMJ. 2012;344:e2843.

9 Nguyen MT, Berger RL, Hicks SC, et al. Comparison of outcomes of synthetic mesh vs suture repair of elective primary ventral herniorrhaphy: a systematic review and meta-analysis. JAMA Surg. 2014;149(5):415–21.

10 Falagas ME, Kasiakou SK. Mesh-related infections after hernia repair surgery. Clin Microbiol Infect. 2005;11(1):3–8.

11 Brown CN, Finch JG. Which mesh for hernia repair? Ann R Coll Surg Engl. 2010;92(4):272–8.

12 Amid PK. Classification of biomaterials and their related complications in abdominal wall hernia surgery. Hernia. 1997;1:15–21.

13 Phillips EH, Arregui M, Carroll BJ, et al. Incidence of complications following laparoscopic hernioplasty. Surg Endosc. 1995;9(1):16–21.

14 Avtan L, Avci C, Bulut T, Fourtanier G. Mesh infections after laparoscopic inguinal hernia repair. Surg Laparosc Endosc. 1997;7(30):192–5.

15 Weizman AV, Nguyen GC. Diverticular disease: epidemiology and management. Can J Gastroenterol. 2011;25(7):385–9.

16 Stollman NH, Rakin JB. Diverticular disease of the colon. J Clin Gastroenterol. 1999;29:241–52.

17 Hinchey EJ, Schaal PH, Richards GK. Treatment of perforated diverticular disease of the colon. Adv Surg. 1978;12:85–109.

18 Boulos PB. Complicated diverticulosis. Best Prac Resear Clin Gastroenterol. 2002;16:649–62.

19 Jacobs DO. Clinical practice. Diverticulitis. N Engl J Med. 2007;357(20):2057–66.

20 Daniels L, Ünlü Ç, De korte N, et al. Randomized clinical trial of observational versus antibiotic treatment for a first episode of CT-proven uncomplicated acute diverticulitis. Br J Surg. 2017;104(1):52–61.

21 Feingold D, Steele SR, Lee S, et al. Practice parameters for the treatment of sigmoid diverticulitis. Dis Colon Rectum. 2014;57(3):284–94.

22 van de Wall BJ, Stam MA, Draaisma WA, et al. Surgery versus conservative management for recurrent and ongoing left-sided diverticulitis (DIRECT trial): an open-label, multicentre, randomised controlled trial. Lancet Gastroenterol Hepatol. 2016;0(0).

Chapter 20

Infections in Healthcare Workers

Gregory W. Rose

20.1 A Note on Evidence Sources

Healthcare workers (HCWs) represent a unique epidemiologic stratum—healthy adults who are frequently exposed to virulent, contagious, or difficult-to-treat infections. Despite this, there is no well-developed population-specific literature. Many of the practices in this field are drawn from secondary sources: analogy to patient groups, retrospective analyses of outbreaks, and expert opinion informed by the dual (and sometimes conflicting) principles of precaution and duty-of-care.

20.2 General Measures

The HCW's primary defense is a bundle of activities termed routine practices and additional, syndrome-specific, precautions [1]. Routine practices assume that any patient encounter could transmit known or unknown pathogens to the healthcare worker. Routine practices include environmental controls, administrative controls, personal protective equipment (PPE) to prevent contact with blood or body fluids, on-going risk assessment during patient care, and adequate hand hygiene.

Infection control programs often stress the patient safety aspect of hand hygiene, but there is evidence among non-HCW populations that hand hygiene is self-protective. A Cochrane systematic review concluded that hand hygiene reduces incidence of diarrheal illness by 30% in a wide range of socioeconomic strata [2]. Hand hygiene alone, however, may be insufficient to prevent acute respiratory infection (ARI), specifically influenza, without additional precautions [3].

> **Case Presentation 1**
>
> An emergency department nurse asks you about a patient she treated during her last shift. The patient is an elderly woman presenting with fever, cough, and shortness of breath. The nurse tended to this patient in an open stretcher bay for some time prior to the initial physician assessment, and afterward was dismayed to learn that the patient had presumed influenza. The nurse declined influenza vaccine this year, citing concern regarding possible adverse reactions. She is now worried about becoming ill. She wants to know what steps can be taken to ameliorate her risk now and for future exposures.

20.3 Influenza

Influenza is one of the most important causes of acute respiratory infection. Transmission of influenza in healthcare settings results in

Evidence-Based Infectious Diseases, Third Edition. Edited by Dominik Mertz, Fiona Smaill, and Nick Daneman.
© 2018 John Wiley & Sons Ltd. Published 2018 by John Wiley & Sons Ltd.

closure of clinical units, generating additional healthcare costs and impacting patient care [4]. Infected HCWs become part of the chain of influenza transmission to patients.

Vaccination is the principal prevention mechanism specific to influenza [5]. A Cochrane review of influenza vaccine in healthy adults demonstrated a 53% reduction in laboratory confirmed cases of influenza (95% confidence interval [CI] 38–65) for the live aerosolized vaccine and a 60% reduction (95% CI 53–66) for the inactivated parenteral vaccine [6]. Vaccination was also associated with a modest reduction in work absenteeism. Live aerosolized vaccine was associated with local upper respiratory tract symptoms, for example, cough, sore throat (Relative Risk [RR] 1.56, 95% CI 1.22–2.27 vs. placebo), while inactivated parenteral vaccine significantly increased injection site adverse effects (RR 2.44, 95% CI 1.82–3.28) and minor systemic symptoms such as myalgia (RR 1.77, 95% CI 1.4–2.24).

The institutional infection control benefit to vaccinating HCWs is less clear. A Cochrane review of influenza vaccination for HCWs working in long-term care institutions could only demonstrate a reduction in the incidence of lower respiratory tract infection among institutional residents (Risk Difference -0.02, 95% CI -0.04–0.01) [7]. Among institutional residents, there was no reduction in laboratory-confirmed influenza or hospital admission due to respiratory illness. The clearest benefit at the institutional level is a reduction in HCW absenteeism: economic evaluation using U.K. data suggests that HCW vaccination saves approximately £12 in healthcare costs per vaccinee [8].

The uptake of influenza vaccine among HCWs varies widely between studies, from as low as 2% (8) to as high as 82% [9]. The major barriers to vaccination were: (a) HCWs' misperception of the need for vaccination, (b) perceived lack of conveniently available vaccine, (c) misperception of vaccine effectiveness, (d) fear of adverse effects, (e) fear that vaccine causes influenza, and (f) fear of needles [8,9]. A systematic review of promotional campaigns for HCW influenza vaccination yielded variable results, limited by bias, confounding, incomplete reporting, and lack of long-term follow-up [8]. These studies reported baseline vaccination rates of 5–17%, increasing to 5–45% in response to vaccination campaigns. Uncertainty remains around whether behavioral interventions can improve HCW influenza vaccination coverage in a sustained manner.

A Cochrane meta-analysis reviewed studies of neuraminidase inhibitor prophylaxis in children and adults, including one trial in HCWs [10]. This analysis demonstrated a reduction in symptomatic influenza in healthy adults for both oseltamivir (RR 0.45, 95% CI 0.3–0.67) and zanamivir (RR 0.39, 95% CI 0.22–0.70). This was countered by an increased risk of psychiatric symptoms (RR 1.8, 95% CI 1.05–3.08), headache (RR 1.18, 95% CI 1.05–1.33), and nausea (RR 1.96, 95% CI 1.2–3.2).

20.3.1 Summary

Influenza vaccination should be offered to HCWs, with the intention of reducing HCW illness and absenteeism. Expert opinion supports presenting vaccination as a measure for patient protection, but the evidence is lacking. In the absence of influenza vaccination, neuraminidase inhibitors may be offered as influenza prophylaxis.

Case Presentation 2

A phlebotomist presents to you with a needle stick injury from a patient known to have advanced HIV and hepatitis C infections. She used the needle to draw blood and injected a small amount of blood into her finger accidentally while re-sheathing the needle before disposal. She is fully vaccinated against hepatitis B and had her antibody levels checked within the last six months. You counsel her about the risk of transmission of HIV and hepatitis C.

20.4   Blood and Body Fluid Exposures

Blood and body fluid exposures, by percutaneous sharps injury or mucous membrane contact, are common among HCWs. Data from the 2014 US EPINet Research Group demonstrate annual incidences of 24.7 sharps injuries and 8.9 non-sharp body fluid exposures per 100 occupied hospital beds [11]. The World Health Organization (WHO) estimates that blood-borne pathogen exposures among HCWs are responsible for 66,000 cases of hepatitis B, 16,000 cases of hepatitis C, and 200–5,000 cases of human immunodeficiency virus (HIV) annually as well as a smaller number of other infections such as tuberculosis or malaria [12].

20.4.1   HIV: Infection and Risk Assessment

A summary of 25 case control studies found that the risk of HIV transmission after percutaneous exposure was 0.32% (95% CI 0.18–0.45) and the risk after mucocutaneous exposure was 0.03% (95% CI 0.006–0.19) [13].

A Cochrane review [14] identified only one study on the effect of post-exposure prophylaxis (PEP) on HIV transmission following occupational exposure. It was a case-control study of cases of HCWs who acquired HIV infection after percutaneous exposure and controls of HCWs who remained HIV seronegative [15]. Multivariate analysis demonstrated that HIV infection was 81% less likely in HCWs who received post-exposure zidovudine compared with those who did not (95% CI 43–94). The Cochrane review in 2007 identified no studies evaluating the efficacy of other PEP regimens following occupational exposure [14], nor have there been any such studies since. A recent systematic review of PEP regimens (for occupational and non-occupational exposures) demonstrated that tenofovir-based regimens were more tolerable than traditional zidovudine-based regimens and were more frequently completed [16]. In particular, a regimen of tenofovir, emtricitabine, and raltegravir was least likely to be discontinued due to adverse drug reaction (1.9%, 95% CI 0–3.8). This has subsequently become the standard regimen recommended by a number of national and international guideline bodies.

20.4.2   Hepatitis B Virus (HBV) Infection

Unvaccinated HCWs are at risk of occupational exposure to HBV. Depending on the e antigen status of the surface antigen positive "source" patient, exposed HCWs have a 23%–62% risk of seroconversion and a 1%–31% risk of developing clinical hepatitis [17].

Effective vaccines prevent occupational acquisition of HBV. A Cochrane review supports occupational health guidelines that all HCWs should be offered HBV vaccination [18]. Evaluating clinical outcomes, older plasma-derived HBV vaccines were effective for preventing HBV infection in HCWs (RR 0.51, 95% CI 0.35–0.73). Newer recombinant DNA HBV vaccines were evaluated for adequacy of antibody titre, as a proxy marker for prevention of hepatitis B infection. They appear to be as safe and immunogenic as plasma derived vaccines.

Approximately 10% of HCWs fail to respond to HBV immunization. Persons who do not respond to an initial three-dose vaccine series have a 30%–50% chance of responding to a second three-dose series [19], otherwise are termed non-responders.

When a non-immune HCW is exposed to HBV, post-exposure measures include vaccination and hepatitis B immune globulin (HBIG) [19]. The effectiveness of combined vaccination and HBIG following exposure has not been evaluated in the occupational setting; however, efficacy of this combination in preventing perinatal transmission provides indirect evidence [20]. Unvaccinated (or incompletely vaccinated) HCWs should receive a single HBIG dose plus HBV vaccine following a significant exposure, while vaccine "non-responders" should receive two doses of HBIG [19].

20.4.3 Hepatitis C Virus (HCV) Infection

HCV is not efficiently transmitted by occupational exposure. One study of 11,000 exposed HCWs from six countries demonstrated an incidence of 0.5% (95% CI 0.39–0.65) [21]. Transmission occurs through percutaneous or mucosal exposure; no occupational transmission has been documented from intact or non-intact skin exposures [19].

There are currently no recommended post-exposure regimens to prevent HCV transmission. Animal studies and retrospective human studies have demonstrated no benefit to immune globulin, and there have been no clinical trials evaluating the efficacy of antiviral prophylaxis [19]. Until recently, HCV antiviral regimens—ribavirin and pegylated interferons—had substantial adverse effects and viral genotype-dependent heterogeneity of efficacy. It is possible we may see HCV PEP evaluated using newer regimens with better efficacy and tolerability in future. To date, the only such registered clinical trial was withdrawn in 2014 prior to enrolling any subjects [22].

At present, antiviral therapy is recommend only for chronic HCV [19], but there is low-level evidence for early therapy of acute infection. Arguments for early therapy include shorter duration of therapy and higher likelihood of sustained virologic response (cure), but is balanced against treatment cost, adverse effects, and the possibility that acute infection will spontaneously clear [23]. Unfortunately, studies have lacked homogeneity in terms of initiation, duration, and composition of therapy, making it difficult to interpret the value of early therapy.

One early open-label study followed 44 patients given a 24-week course of single-agent interferon-α2b, preventing chronic HCV infection in 98% of patients [24]. More recently, another small open-label study did not demonstrate any benefit to early administration of a six-week course of sofosbuvir and ribavirin [25].

Current guidelines do not establish an optimal approach for treating HCWs occupationally exposed to HCV, but we suggest surveillance at one, three, and six months for seroconversion, confirmation with quantitative HCV PCR and genotyping, observation over 8 to 12 weeks for spontaneous viral clearance, then consideration of antiviral therapy.

20.4.4 Prevention of Blood and Body Fluid Exposures

Risk factors for blood-borne pathogen exposure include less-experienced or less-educated HCWs, HCWs in higher-workload centres, and extended duration of work-shifts [26]. These are largely non-modifiable, but there are numerous studies evaluating training programs and safety-engineered sharps systems to reduce risk. One systematic review of 17 studies demonstrated benefit to risk reduction training (RR 0.66, 95% CI 0.5–0.89), safety-engineered devices (RR 0.51, 95% CI 0.4–0.64), and a combination of both (RR 0.38, 95% CI 0.28–0.50) [27].

20.4.5 Summary

Harm prevention strategies should incorporate training about safer work practices, particularly for more inexperienced health care workers, and incorporate safety-engineered devices. Should a blood-borne pathogen exposure occur, HCW require prompt evaluation and management. For high-risk exposures, combination antiretroviral therapy should be initiated promptly and rapid testing performed on the source patient. There is good evidence to support universal HBV vaccination of HCWs, but weak evidence for post-exposure use of HBIG and vaccination. Occupational exposures to HCV should be managed by surveillance for, and consideration of, early treatment of acute disease.

Case Presentation 3

At the end of his 24-hour on-call shift, a resident asks his attending staff to look at his rash. It is chickenpox. You are promptly called for advice regarding management of the resident and his contacts. The resident believed he had chickenpox as a child, but had not been tested further. As a result of exposure to this resident, 15 healthcare workers spent 14 days of paid leave off work, and 8 exposed patients were kept in respiratory isolation during the period they were potentially infectious. You must review the prevention and screening protocols for varicella among healthcare workers.

20.5 Varicella Zoster Virus (VZV) Infections

Nosocomial transmission of VZV is well-recognized, and control measures in healthcare facilities are strongly recommended [5,28]. VZV is transmitted from person to person via contact with infected lesions or airborne spread from respiratory tract secretions. Patients with localized zoster are less contagious than those with primary chickenpox or disseminated zoster.

Pre-placement immunity is the bedrock of HCW protection from VZV. A childhood history of chickenpox predicts serologic immunity in HCWs with a high positive predictive value (PPV) (95%), but a negative predictive value of 11% [29]. Overall, less than 5% of HCWs in the western world lack serologic immunity to VZV [29]; however, HCWs from Africa, the Middle East, and East Asia may be at higher risk (12 to 19% lack seroprotection [30]).

Vaccination for VZV is highly effective. A qualitative review of the literature demonstrates vaccination decreases any disease due to varicella from 70–90%, and severe disease by 95–100% [31]. Several studies demonstrated that a two-dose regimen offers greater protection from varicella disease than a single dose [31]. For this reason, current guidelines recommend that all susceptible HCWs be immunized with two doses of standard-dose live attenuated VZV vaccine [5,28].

Properly applied pre-placement procedures should prevent the situation of a susceptible HCW being exposed to VZV, but yet this scenario still arises. Possible post-exposure strategies include vaccination, varicella-zoster immune globulin (VZIG), and antivirals. A Cochrane review of three RCTs of post-exposure vaccination demonstrated substantial reduction in incidence of post-exposure disease (from 78% to 22%), but deemed the studies too heterogeneous for meta-analysis [32]. Furthermore, the population of these studies was children, therefore benefit to adult HCWs is inferred, rather than demonstrated.

There is no evidence to support the routine use of VZIG in healthy HCWs exposed to chickenpox. A systematic review of the literature for VZIG in pregnancy reported that among 640 pregnant women in the 3 prospective cohort studies included, VZIG reduced the risk of congenital varicella syndrome from 2.81% to 0% [33]. As such, VZIG is recommended post-exposure for immunocompromised or pregnant HCWs who are susceptible [5,28].

There are almost no studies evaluating the use of acyclovir as post-exposure prophylaxis in adults. In a single report, two varicella-susceptible resident physicians were deliberately exposed to VZV and then given a seven-day course of acyclovir beginning 9 to 11 days post-exposure. Both residents developed limited disease [34]. Based on current evidence, the prophylactic use of acyclovir is not recommended; post-exposure vaccination remains the approach of choice for otherwise healthy susceptible individuals, and VZIG is recommended for immunocompromised individuals [5,28].

20.5.1 Summary

Healthcare facilities should ensure HCWs are immune to VZV prior to employment, either by serologically demonstrated immunity or documented evidence of receipt of two doses of varicella vaccine. Susceptible HCW exposed to VZV should receive post-exposure vaccination within three days of exposure as a secondary prevention measure. The indications for prophylactic VZIG are very limited, and prophylactic acyclovir is not recommended.

References

1 Ontario Agency for Health Protection and Promotion, Provincial Infectious Diseases Advisory Committee. Routine Practices and Additional Precautions in All Health Care Settings. 3rd edition. Toronto, ON: Queen's Printer for Ontario; November 2012.

2 Ejemot-Nwadiaro RI, Ehiri JE, Arikpo D, Meremikwu MM, Critchley JA. Hand washing promotion for preventing diarrhoea. Cochrane Database Syst Rev. 2015 Sep 03(9):CD004265. PubMed PMID: 26346329. Pubmed Central PMCID: 4563982.

3 Wong VW, Cowling BJ, Aiello AE. Hand hygiene and risk of influenza virus infections in the community: a systematic review and meta-analysis. Epidemiol Infect. 2014 May;142(5):922–32. PubMed PMID: 24572643. Pubmed Central PMCID: 4891197.

4 Hansen S, Stamm-Balderjahn S, Zuschneid I, Behnke M, Ruden H, Vonberg RP, et al. Closure of medical departments during nosocomial outbreaks: data from a systematic analysis of the literature. J Hosp Infec. 2007 Apr;65(4):348–53. PubMed PMID: 17350731.

5 Health Canada. Prevention and control of occupational infection in health care. An infection control guideline. CCDR. 2002;28S1:1–264.

6 Demicheli V, Jefferson T, Al-Ansary LA, Ferroni E, Rivetti A, Di Pietrantonj C. Vaccines for preventing influenza in healthy adults. Cochrane Database Syst Rev. 2014 Mar 13(3):CD001269. PubMed PMID: 24623315.

7 Thomas RE, Jefferson T, Lasserson TJ. Influenza vaccination for healthcare workers who care for people aged 60 or older living in long-term care institutions. Cochrane Database Syst Rev. 2016 Jun 02(6):CD005187. PubMed PMID: 27251461.

8 Burls A, Jordan R, Barton P, Olowokure B, Wake B, Albon E, et al. Vaccinating healthcare workers against influenza to protect the vulnerable—is it a good use of healthcare resources? A systematic review of the evidence and an economic evaluation. Vaccine. 2006 May 08;24(19):4212–21. PubMed PMID: 16546308.

9 Hofmann F, Ferracin C, Marsh G, Dumas R. Influenza vaccination of healthcare workers: a literature review of attitudes and beliefs. Infect. 2006 Jun;34(3):142–7. PubMed PMID: 16804657.

10 Jefferson T, Jones MA, Doshi P, Del Mar CB, Hama R, Thompson MJ, et al. Neuraminidase inhibitors for preventing and treating influenza in healthy adults and children. Cochrane Database Syst Rev. 2014 Apr 10(4):CD008965. PubMed PMID: 24718923.

11 International Safety Center. U.S. EPINet Sharps Injury and Blood and Body Fluid Exposure Surveillance Research Group. Sharps injury data report for 2014; Blood and body fluid exposure report for 2014 [Online] 2014. Accessed Nov 19, 2016. Available from: internationalsafetycenter.org.

12 Pruss-Ustun ARE, Hutin Y. Sharps injuries: Global burden of disease from sharps injuries to health-care workers. Environmental burden of disease series No 3. Geneva, Switzerland: World Health Organization; 2003.

13 Public Health Laboratory Service. Occupational transmission of HIV. Summary of published reports. London, UK: Public Health Laboratory Service; 1997.

14 Young TN, Arens FJ, Kennedy GE, Laurie JW, Rutherford G. Antiretroviral post-exposure prophylaxis (PEP) for occupational HIV exposure. Cochrane Database Syst Rev. 2007 Jan

24(1):CD002835. PubMed PMID: 17253483. Epub 2007/01/27. eng.

15 Cardo DM, Culver DH, Ciesielski CA, Srivastava PU, Marcus R, Abiteboul D, et al. A case-control study of HIV seroconversion in health care workers after percutaneous exposure. Centers for Disease Control and Prevention Needlestick Surveillance Group. N Engl J Med. 1997 Nov 20;337(21):1485–90. PubMed PMID: 9366579.

16 Ford N, Shubber Z, Calmy A, Irvine C, Rapparini C, Ajose O, et al. Choice of antiretroviral drugs for postexposure prophylaxis for adults and adolescents: a systematic review. Clin Infect Dis. 2015 Jun 01;60 Suppl 3:S170–6. PubMed PMID: 25972499. Epub 2015/05/15. eng.

17 Werner BG, Grady GF. Accidental hepatitis-B-surface-antigen-positive inoculations. Use of e antigen to estimate infectivity. Ann Internal Med. 1982 Sep;97(3):367–9. PubMed PMID: 7114632.

18 Chen W, Gluud C. Vaccines for preventing hepatitis B in health-care workers. Cochrane Database Syst Rev. 2005 Oct 19(4):CD000100. PubMed PMID: 16235273.

19 Centers for Disease Control and Prevention. Updated U.S. Public Health Service Guidelines on the management of occupational exposures to HBV, HCV, and HIV and recommendations for postexposure prophylaxis. MMWR. 2001;50(RR11):1–42.

20 Beasley RP, Hwang LY, Stevens CE, Lin CC, Hsieh FJ, Wang KY, et al. Efficacy of hepatitis B immune globulin for prevention of perinatal transmission of the hepatitis B virus carrier state: final report of a randomized double-blind, placebo-controlled trial. Hepatol. 1983 Mar-Apr;3(2): 135–41. PubMed PMID: 6339349.

21 Jagger J, Puro V, De Carli G. Occupational transmission of hepatitis C virus. JAMA. 2002 Sep 25;288(12):1469; author reply -71. PubMed PMID: 12243628.

22 U.S. National Institutes of Health. Search for "hepatitis C" and "exposure." [En ligne]

Accessed 19 Nov 2016. Available from: clinicaltrials.gov.

23 Blackard JT, Shata MT, Shire NJ, Sherman KE. Acute hepatitis C virus infection: a chronic problem. Hepatol. 2008 Jan;47(1):321–31. PubMed PMID: 18161707. Pubmed Central PMCID: 2277496.

24 Jaeckel E, Cornberg M, Wedemeyer H, Santantonio T, Mayer J, Zankel M, et al. Treatment of acute hepatitis C with interferon alfa-2b. N Engl J Med. 2001 Nov 15;345(20):1452–7. PubMed PMID: 11794193.

25 Martinello M, Gane E, Hellard M, Sasadeusz J, Shaw D, Petoumenos K, et al. Sofosbuvir and ribavirin for 6 weeks is not effective among people with recent hepatitis C virus infection: The DARE-C II study. Hepatol. 2016 Dec;64(6):1911–21. PubMed PMID: 27639183.

26 Clarke SP. Hospital work environments, nurse characteristics, and sharps injuries. Am J Infect Control. 2007 Jun;35(5):302–9. PubMed PMID: 17577476.

27 Tuma S, Sepkowitz KA. Efficacy of safety-engineered device implementation in the prevention of percutaneous injuries: a review of published studies. Clin Infectious Dis. 2006 Apr 15;42(8):1159–70. PubMed PMID: 16575737. Epub 2006/04/01. eng.

28 Marin M, Guris D. Prevention of varicella: recommendations of the Advisory Committee on Immunization Practices (ACIP). MMWR. 2007;56:1–40.

29 Gallagher J, Quaid B, Cryan B. Susceptibility to varicella zoster virus infection in health care workers. Occup Med. 1996 Aug;46(4):289–92. PubMed PMID: 8854707.

30 Almuneef MA, Memish ZA, Balkhy HH, Otaibi B, Helmi M. Seroprevalence survey of varicella, measles, rubella, and hepatitis A and B viruses in a multinational healthcare workforce in Saudi Arabia. Infect Control Hosp Epidemiol. 2006 Nov;27(11):1178–83. PubMed PMID: 17080374.

31 Javed S, Javed SA, Tyring SK. Varicella vaccines. Current Opinion Infect Dis. 2012 Apr;25(2):135–40. PubMed PMID: 22123665.

32 Macartney K, Heywood A, McIntyre P. Vaccines for post-exposure prophylaxis against varicella (chickenpox) in children and adults. Cochrane Database Syst Rev. 2014 Jun 23(6):CD001833. PubMed PMID: 24954057.

33 Cohen A, Moschopoulos P, Stiehm RE, Koren G. Congenital varicella syndrome: the evidence for secondary prevention with varicella-zoster immune globulin. CMAJ. 2011 Feb 08;183(2):204–8. PubMed PMID: 21262937. Pubmed Central PMCID: 3033924.

34 White CB, Hawley WZ, Harford DJ. The pediatric resident susceptible to varicella: providing immunity through postexposure prophylaxis with oral acyclovir. Pediatr Infect Dis J. 1994 Aug;13(8):743–5. PubMed PMID: 7970978.

Index

Page numbers in *italic* refer to figures.
Page numbers in **bold** refer to tables.

Evidence-Based Infectious Diseases, Third Edition. Edited by Dominik Mertz, Fiona Smaill, and Nick Daneman.
© 2018 John Wiley & Sons Ltd. Published 2018 by John Wiley & Sons Ltd.

Printed and bound by CPI Group (UK) Ltd, Croydon, CR0 4YY